PATIENT SAFETY INFORMATICS

Studies in Health Technology and Informatics

This book series was started in 1990 to promote research conducted under the auspices of the EC programmes' Advanced Informatics in Medicine (AIM) and Biomedical and Health Research (BHR) bioengineering branch. A driving aspect of international health informatics is that telecommunication technology, rehabilitative technology, intelligent home technology and many other components are moving together and form one integrated world of information and communication media. The complete series has been accepted in Medline. Volumes from 2005 onwards are available online.

Volume 166

Recently published in this series

Vol. 165. L. Stoicu-Tivadar, B. Blobel, T. Marčun and A. Orel (Eds.), e-Health Across Borders Without Boundaries – E-salus trans confinia sine finibus – Proceedings of the EFMI Special Topic Conference, 14–15 April 2011, Laško, Slovenia

Vol. 164. E.M. Borycki, J.A. Bartle-Clar, M.S. Househ, C.E. Kuziemsky and E.G. Schraa (Eds.), International Perspectives in Health Informatics

Vol. 163. J.D. Westwood, S.W. Westwood, L. Felländer-Tsai, R.S. Haluck, H.M. Hoffman, R.A. Robb, S. Senger and K.G. Vosburgh (Eds.), Medicine Meets Virtual Reality 18 – NextMed

Vol. 162. E. Wingender (Ed.), Biological Petri Nets

Vol. 161. A.C. Smith and A.J. Maeder (Eds.), Global Telehealth – Selected Papers from Global Telehealth 2010 (GT2010) – 15th International Conference of the International Society for Telemedicine and eHealth and 1st National Conference of the Australasian Telehealth Society

Vol. 160. C. Safran, S. Reti and H.F. Marin (Eds.), MEDINFO 2010 – Proceedings of the 13th World Congress on Medical Informatics

Vol. 159. T. Solomonides, I. Blanquer, V. Breton, T. Glatard and Y. Legré (Eds.), Healthgrid Applications and Core Technologies – Proceedings of HealthGrid 2010

Vol. 158. C.-E. Aubin, I.A.F. Stokes, H. Labelle and A. Moreau (Eds.), Research into Spinal Deformities 7

Vol. 157. C. Nøhr and J. Aarts (Eds.), Information Technology in Health Care: Socio-Technical Approaches 2010 – From Safe Systems to Patient Safety

ISSN 0926-9630 (print)
ISSN 1879-8365 (online)

Patient Safety Informatics

Adverse Drug Events, Human Factors and IT Tools for Patient Medication Safety

Edited by

Vassilis Koutkias

Aristotle University of Thessaloniki, Thessaloniki, Greece

Julie Niès

MEDASYS, Gif-sur-Yvette Cedex, France

Sanne Jensen

Capital Region of Copenhagen, Copenhagen, Denmark

Nicos Maglaveras

Aristotle University of Thessaloniki, Thessaloniki, Greece

and

Régis Beuscart

CHRU de Lille, Lille Cedex, France

IOS Press

Amsterdam • Berlin • Tokyo • Washington, DC

ISBN 978-1-60750-739-0 (print)
ISBN 978-1-60750-740-6 (online)
Library of Congress Control Number: 2011926828

Publisher
IOS Press BV
Nieuwe Hemweg 6B
1013 BG Amsterdam
Netherlands
fax: +31 20 687 0019
e-mail: order@iospress.nl

Distributor in the USA and Canada
IOS Press, Inc.
4502 Rachael Manor Drive
Fairfax, VA 22032
USA
fax: +1 703 323 3668
e-mail: iosbooks@iospress.com

PRINTED IN THE NETHERLANDS

Patient Safety Informatics
V. Koutkias et al. (Eds.)
IOS Press, 2011

Preface

Patient safety has become an important theme of the research agenda in the course of the last decade, both throughout Europe and worldwide. Improving patient safety and the quality of healthcare poses many challenges, and information technology (IT) has always been seen as having the potential to support the measures necessary to address these. But the risk of adverse events is unfortunately rising alongside the increasing sophistication and maturity of the health IT systems incorporated into the hospital environment. One major source of such errors is related to medication, i.e. adverse drug events (ADEs), which can incur considerable extra healthcare costs, as well as posing a risk to the safety of patients.

From a research perspective, different approaches have been introduced to eliminate ADEs, such as reporting systems, records and chart reviews, detection methods (with varying degrees of automation), etc. The major concerns raised by all of these approaches and methods are related to reliability and quality of results, reproducibility or generalisation of the conclusions drawn, appropriate identification of the contributing factors and interpretation of the outcomes, and knowledge management.

From a practical perspective, the transferability and use of such tools in clinical practice is a major challenge. Aspects related explicitly to the healthcare environment have to be taken carefully into account, such as organisational and procedural parameters, contextualisation issues, human factors and usability features, to name but a few. The adoption of these tools into real clinical settings is only possible by means of a holistic, validated and qualitative approach.

Following the success of the first workshop, organised in the context of the EU-funded Patient Safety through Intelligent Procedures in medication (PSIP) project and held in Belgirate, Italy, in September 2009, this second workshop presents current, novel methods and applications that have achieved concrete results and that are relevant to the domain of patient safety as a whole. Reading the papers of this book, which review the state-of-the-art, it is evident that significant progress has been made in the field, but that even greater challenges must still be faced if a successful transfer of research ideas and outcomes into clinical practice is to be accomplished. It is the diversity of these challenges and the complexity of the domain which indicate and justify the necessity to introduce a new direction in healthcare IT devoted to patient safety per se. Hence the title of this book: "*Patient Safety Informatics*".

To this end, the contributions in this book include: (a) *designing IT systems for patient safety*, coping in particular with information contextualisation, human factor engineering, the design aspects of clinical decision support systems, and e-prescription frameworks; (b) *methods and technologies for developing patient safety systems*, devoted to medical information extraction via semantic mining techniques, multi-terminology systems linked with semantic interoperability, knowledge representation techniques and standardisation aspects, etc.; (c) *novel applications of patient safety informatics*, such as an ADE retrospective analysis framework, the exploitation of decision support services for ADE prevention via a variety of systems (i.e. a commercial electronic health record, a commercial computerised physician order entry system, and an autonomous web-based platform), a standardised patient summary framework, a terminology mapping framework applicable in several domains, etc., and (d) *validation and impact assessment studies for patient safety informatics outcomes*, analysing in particular patient empowerment solutions, clinical decision support systems and knowledge bases targeting ADE prevention, an ADE retrospective analysis system, medical information extraction from discharge letters, etc.

In addition, this workshop is an opportunity for experts active in the field, including the contributors to this book, to meet and confront ideas and experiences arising from many different perspectives, i.e. research, clinical practice and healthcare IT industry oriented, as well as from several EU projects funded to contribute to patient safety as a whole.

We would like to express our gratitude to Prof. David Bates, Prof. Jos Aarts and Dr. Beth Lilja for their participation and their keynote speeches; to Mr. Michele Carenini, Prof. Peter Elkin, Dr. Zoi Kolitsi, Prof. Andre Kushniruk and Prof. Gianluca Trifirò for accepting the invitation to participate in the Workshop; to all the participants and the authors of the Workshop; to the Scientific Committee and the reviewers who helped in the preparation of qualitative contributions in the Workshop and, last but not least, to the European Commission which, by funding European projects in the domain of patient safety, have made the organisation of this workshop possible, as well as the editing and publication of this book.

The book cover is inspired by the paper entitled "Implementation of a Taxonomy Aiming to Support the Design of a Contextualised Clinical Decision Support System" by Stéphanie Bernonville, Romaric Marcilly, Radja Messai, Nicolas Leroy, Emma Przewozny, Nathalie Souf and Marie-Catherine Beuscart-Zéphir which is published in this book (pp. 74–83). The picture denotes the design approach proposed by the authors for developing contextualised clinical decision support systems (CDSS) for medication safety.

Vassilis Koutkias, Julie Niès, Sanne Jensen, Nicos Maglaveras and Régis Beuscart (editors)

May 2011

Contents

Part A

Keynote Papers on Patient Safety Informatics

Patient Safety Informatics
V. Koutkias et al. (Eds.)
IOS Press, 2011

doi:10.3233/978-1-60750-740-6-3

PSIP: An Overview of the Results and Clinical Implications

Régis BEUSCART [1]
CHU Lille, UDSL EA2694, Univ Lille Nord de France, F-59000 Lille, France

Abstract. Adverse Drug Events (ADEs) are injuries due to medication management rather than the underlying condition of the patient. They endanger the patients and most of them could be avoided and prevented. The detection of ADEs usually relies on spontaneous reporting or medical chart reviews. The first objective of the PSIP Project is to automatically detect cases of ADEs by means of Data Mining, and to provide these cases to healthcare professionals. The second objective is to prevent ADEs by means of contextualised Clinical Decision Support Systems (Cx-CDSS) connected with Computerised Physician Order Entry (CPOE) or Electronic Health Record (EHR) systems. The detection of ADEs has been made possible through a set of rules able to identify relevant cases is a set of 92,000 medical cases. The results of this detection are provided through "ADE Scorecards". Contextualized Decision Support Systems have been developed by using the same set of rules and implemented in different software environments. The initial objectives of the PSIP project have been reached. The evaluation of the clinical impact has to be completed.

Keywords. Adverse drug event (ADE), prevention, ADE occurrence, reporting system, clinical decision support system (CDSS), context

Introduction

Adverse Drug Events (ADEs), caused by product safety problems, and medication errors due to Human Factors (HF), are a major Public Health issue [1]. They endanger the patients' safety and instigate considerable extra hospital costs.

Normally, they should be systematically declared by physicians when they are observed in medical units. But, in practice, this declaration is not systematic and, in most of the countries, this declaration rarely exceeds 5% [2].

It is also difficult to identify ADEs through the retrospective analysis of medical records. This necessitates chart reviews and records review. These reviews can be realized by trained Healthcare Professionals (physicians and nurses) through a time consuming, if effective, process. In most of the hospitals, such reviews are never organized and the prevalence of ADEs is only based upon estimations.

Most often, these reviews are performed on the paper records, summarized under the form of charts [1, 2]. Yet today there are Electronic Health Records in most of the hospitals of developed countries. For example, the Lille University Hospital gathers 1.5 millions of Electronic Health Records. It seems natural to exploit and analyse these Electronic Health Records to detect the occurrences of ADEs.

[1] Corresponding Author: regis.beuscart@univ-lille2.fr

The first objective of the PSIP (Patient Safety through Intelligent Procedures in medication) project will contribute to identify, by state-of-the-art Data and Semantic Mining techniques, healthcare situations where patient safety is at risk. Data Mining will permit to acquire new and more profound knowledge on the occurrence of ADEs and of their characteristics.

By applying semi-automatically data and semantic mining techniques on existing healthcare data repositories of large Medical Data Bases (Electronic Health Records), statistical analyses based upon this knowledge will allow the calculation of the prevalence of ADEs and of their characteristics, per hospital, per region, per country.

The second objective of the PSIP project is to improve the decision support tool related to medication cycle and deliver contextualised alerts, just-in-time and at the point of care, or relevant information to healthcare professionals and patients. These alerts are triggered by decision rules derived from the results of the previous phase. The alerts have to be contextualized according to the frequency and prevalence of ADEs in different countries, different hospitals, and different medical units.

The last objective of the project is, through a rigorous evaluation of the project in the medical field, to demonstrate a significant reduction of patient risk in a sub-set of diseases and practices in the hospital setting.

After 3 years of work, some results have been achieved and milestones attained, in the different stages of the project. They will be detailed in some chapters of this book. In this introductory paper, we will give an overview of the main goals attained. In the discussion, we will present the most important problems we have been confronted with, and present some recommendations to improve the quality of the results of the project.

1. Automatic Detection of Adverse Drug Events in Electronic Health Records

1.1. Result 1: Exploitable Data Structures

The first result addresses the definition of a "Common Data Model" [3] to make possible the extraction of data from the Electronic Medical Records, including Demographic data, Medical data, Lab results, Procedures results, and Drugs from Computerised Physician Order Entry (CPOE), free text letters and reports.

This model has been developed to conduct data extraction from the various data repositories and has been designed in order to be compatible with a large set of hospital databases and to gather the necessary information to detect and identify ADEs.

Figure 1 shows a simplified representation of the data scheme. In this illustration, fields are replaced using groups of fields.

By this mean, more than 90,000 complete Electronic Health Records have been extracted from hospitals of different countries: France (3 hospitals), Denmark (2 hospitals), Bulgaria (1 hospital). Data have been anonymised and exported under a coded format in a global Data Repository so that the following steps should be realized.

1.2. Result 2: Data Mining for Knowledge Discovery

Data Mining has been performed routinely through the medical cases collected in the data warehouse of the project. By using multivariate analyses (decision trees, association rules), it has been possible to provide a large set of rules that has been filtered and validated by experts (physicians, pharmacologists, pharmacists) [4].

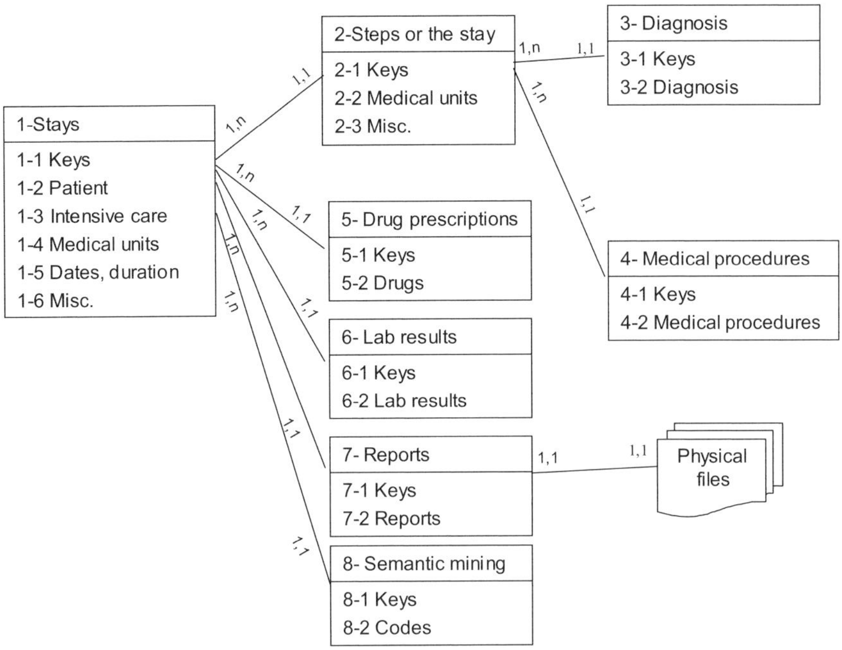

Figure 1. Simplified representation of the PSIP data scheme.

A corpus of 236 rules (an example of rule is presented in Figure 2) has been validated, organised, to be used by the two main applications developed in PSIP:

- the ADE Scorecards application, in order to identify ADEs by mining Electronic Medical Records, and
- the contextualized Clinical Decision Support Systems (Cx-CDSS) for the prevention of ADEs through a tight connection with CPOEs, Electronic Health Record (EHR) systems, or even Web applications.

Obviously, this corpus of rules represents the central result of the PSIP project.

Their validation by pharmacists, pharmacologists, and physicians is central for their future usage in the ADE Scorecards and the Cx-CDSS modules.

For each rule, various statistical features are computed such as confidence, support, prevalence, risk ratio, etc. These features help to have a better knowledge on the occurrence, prevalence, and severity of the detected ADEs.

These rules are currently being tested in different environments: simulation tests in Capital Region of Denmark, real ground tests in Denain hospitals, acceptability tests in the University Hospital of Lille.

Improvement, maintenance, update, parameterization of this corpus of rules will be one of the main challenges in the next phases of the project.

Rule: renal failure **&** low weight heparin **&** age $\geq 70 \rightarrow$ hyperkalemia (K+>5.3)

Comments on the Rule:

- *LMWH can induce hyperkaliemia, specially with renal insufficiency.*
- *Somes aldosteronism or metabolic acidosis cases have been described with heparins. The risk is increased in case of a kidney insufficiency [5].*
- *In case of a low molecular weight heparin treatment, the dosage has to be adapted and the clinical and biological monitoring has to be increased.*

Figure 2. Example of an ADE detection rule.

Information on rules and statistics issued from PSIP is available in the deliverable D2.3 “Results of data and semantic mining”. This document is available for registered users on the PSIP Website.

This corpus of rules, its conceptualization, its organization, represent one of the major results of the PSIP project. They can be compared to the corpus of 150 rules used by Partners in the Boston Hospitals for alerting healthcare professionals on the risks linked with the prescription of drugs.

1.3. Result 3: The ADE Scorecards

Statistical analysis, based on the rules previously mined and validated, can be performed each month on the medical cases collected in the different hospitals of the consortium, to provide epidemiological reports on the occurrence of ADEs in hospitals, per medical department.

These statistics are supposed to be used by the physicians, the pharmacists and other related healthcare professionals to support the quality and safety patient policies at the hospital level. With larger databases, they could also be used at the regional or the national level.

The “ADE Scorecards” is the application designed to describe the statistical results and to improve the awareness of the healthcare professionals on the ADEs occurring in their medical unit or in their hospital (Figure 3).

Fields of the upper part of Figure 3 provide the information on the hospital, the medical unit, the involved healthcare professionals, the period of the data extraction, and the periodicity of the report (here monthly reports). The ADEs and the corresponding rules are described in the “blue” table. The frequencies, percentages (cases, rules) are computed on a given period.

Diagrams describe the total number of ADEs per month (left) and the delay between the prescription and the outcome (right) in days.

On the lower part of Figure 3, the characteristics of the patients are described: number of cases, age, gender, clinical contexts.

ADE Scorecards can be used as statistical reports to obtain a simple view of the prevalence of ADEs occurring in a medical unit or a medical department. They can also be used as indicators for Quality of Care, particularly in the field of Patient Safety.

In our experience, ADEs Scorecards per se cannot be considered as sufficient to determine any change in the way of treating patients. They have to be used through a Quality of Care procedure that will use the ADE Scorecards to increase the awareness of the physicians, nurses and pharmacists in the possibility of occurrence of ADEs. By demonstrating that ADEs really occur in the medical units; by showing the frequency of occurrence of the various ADEs; by displaying the decision rules that allowed to identify the ADEs; by giving access to the medical records of the patients who suffered from an ADE, the ADEs scorecards can be the support for discussions and improvements in the way of treating patients. The follow-up and surveillance of the number of ADEs occurring per month can demonstrate the decrease of identified ADEs through significant changes in the treatment procedures.

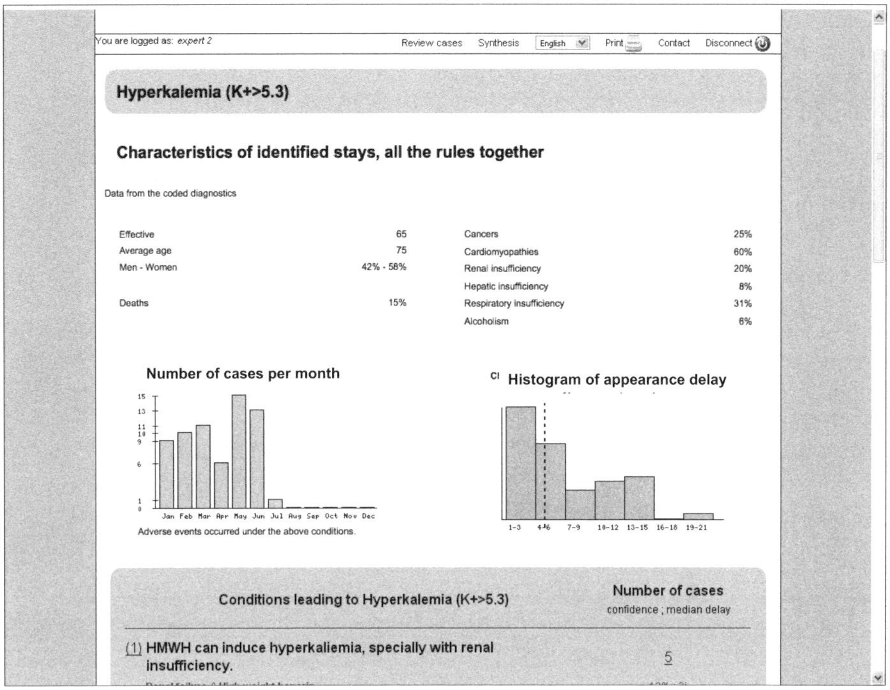

Figure 3. ADE scorecards screenshot.

2. Prevention of Adverse Drug Events: The PSIP Global Knowledge Platform

To provide healthcare professionals with relevant information helping them to prevent ADEs [6, 7], the PSIP project developed innovative knowledge-based applications, conceptualised within a Global Knowledge Platform (GKP).

The PSIP GKP enables the communication of any medical application with a Knowledge Base (KB) system for ADE prevention thanks to a Connectivity Platform (CP). Thus CPOE system, Electronic Healthcare Record (EHR) system or other medical application can access to the PSIP knowledge to get complementary information that can be used by the requiring system under various forms (alerts, complementary information, triggering a Web system, etc.).

The PSIP GKP consists of three principal components (Figure 4): (1) The PSIP KB providing the representation and management services of Decision Rules; (2) A CP providing transformation and routing services between medical applications and the PSIP KB System; (3) User interface module allowing the display of PSIP knowledge within medical applications.

2.1. Result 1: The PSIP Knowledge Base System

The PSIP KB system has been designed to constitute the basis for the construction of contextualized Clinical Decision Support System (CDSS) for ADE prevention. More precisely, it enables to systematically represent and manage an ADE detection rule base developed by the consortium (236 rules constitute the PSIP rule base) [8]. The PSIP

KB uses the GASTON framework that provides guidelines for the design, the development, the validation and the implementation of CDSS.

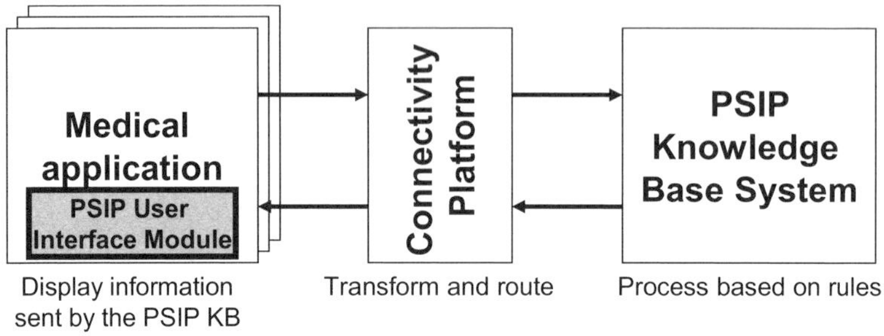

Figure 4. Major components of the PSIP GKP architecture.

2.2. Result 2: The Connectivity Platform

The objective of the CP is to provide an interoperability platform to centralize and support the communication of two kinds of entities, medical applications and the PSIP KB, therefore providing the medical applications with knowledge on ADEs.

The development of the CP is based on Oracle© products. It enables to minimize the effort needed to increase system integration regardless of system structure, language and platform. The CP currently offers a specific service to enable the medical applications communication and a specific service to enable the PSIP KB communication.

2.3. Result 3: User Interface Module

To allow the display of the PSIP knowledge in any medical application, user interface modules have to be developed according to the requirements of the systems that want to host the PSIP CDSS. Those modules will depend on the structure of the medical applications and consequently will allow displaying ADE information in different ways.

To test the portability of the PSIP GKP, three PSIP user interface modules have been designed to show the use of the same PSIP KB in three different medical applications for ADE prevention.

The first PSIP user interface module (the PSIP IBM prototype) integrates the PSIP KB in a Danish CPOE system developed by the Danish IBM© Company. This prototype allows visualising patient data and providing potential ADE information during the prescription by the physician.

The second PSIP user interface module (the PSIP Medasys prototype) integrates the PSIP KB in a French EHR system, DxCare© edited by the Medasys Company. This prototype takes into account the medication use process and allows displaying potential ADE information on different places of the system and makes easier the sharing of information about risks of potential ADEs between the healthcare professionals.

The third PSIP user interface module (the PSIP Web prototype) integrates the PSIP KB in an independent Web application. This prototype allows providing ADE information independently of any CPOE system via Web access. It gives the possibility of displaying patient data, simulating patient prescriptions and displaying risks of potential ADEs for a patient. A screen shot of this prototype is presented in Figure 5.

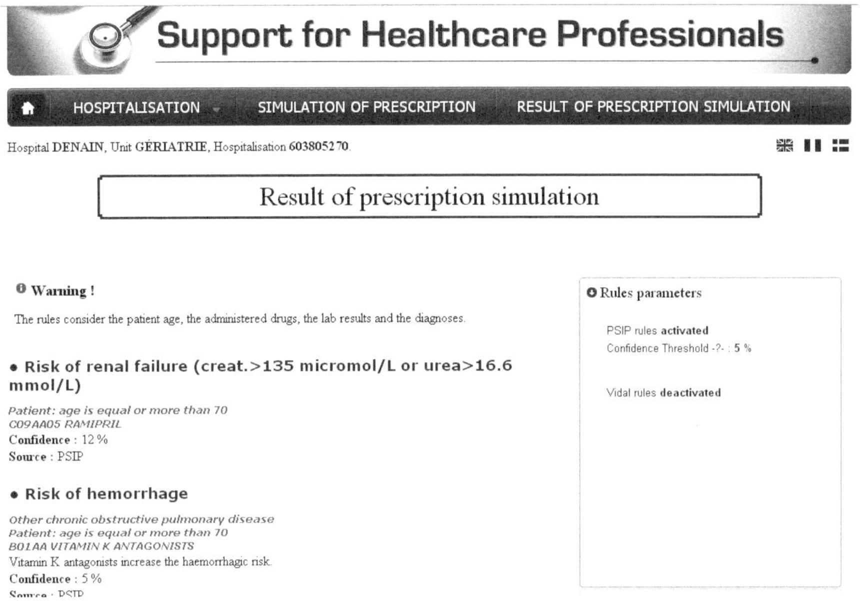

Figure 5. Example of a user interface module developed in the PSIP project: the Web prototype.

2.4. Result 4: Contextualization

2.4.1. Definition of "Context" in the PSIP Project

One of the objectives of the PSIP project is to focus on the context handling to provide contextualized PSIP alerts to the medical staff. Thus, it was mandatory to define the dimensions of "context" that are applicable in the application domain and to elaborate on a strategy to take into account them in the CDSS design and development. After a literature review [9, 10], we proposed a definition of context that takes into account:

- the USER (knowledge of habits, emotional state, biophysiological conditions…);
- the ENVIRONMENT (co-location of others, social interaction, group dynamics, location…);
- the TASKS (activity, engaged tasks, general goals…), and
- the TIME or TEMPORAL ASPECTS, which must be considered to preserve the integrity of information.

2.4.2. Contextualisation in Scorecards

The Scorecards application is constructed to take into account the "ENVIRONMENT" aspects (hospital, department, medical unit) and the "TIME" dimension. Data Mining can be performed at each level to identify special rules of knowledge, while statistics on ADEs are computed per hospital, medical unit and for different periods.

As an example, in Table 1 the comparative results of six hospitals are displayed. For each hospital, the different lines show the various statistics when computed in every medical department at the same time. Then, when available, the statistics are computed per department.

Table 1. Example of confidence statistics computed for a rule in six hospitals.

Department		Confidence (PPV)
Hospital 1, All departments		8/106=**7.5%**
	Medicine A	1/6=**16.7%**
	Medicine B	3/48=**6.3%**
	Pneumology	5/40=**12.5%**
Hospital 2, All departments		5/146=**3.4%**
	Cardio endocrino	3/62=**4.8%**
	Geriatrics	1/4=**25%**
	ICU	1/15=6.7%
	Obstetrics	0/0
	Urology	1/21=**4.8%**
Hospital 3		1/8=**12.5%**
Hospital 4		1/46=**2.2%**
Hospital 5		0/0
Hospital 6		2/11=**18.2%**

2.4.3. Contextualisation in the CDSS

To take into account the "ENVIRONMENT" and the "TIME" dimensions in the PSIP KB system, statistics on ADEs are computed per hospital and medical unit, as well as for different periods. Thus, PSIP alerts can be displayed adaptively, according to different hospital and medical unit.

In the obstetrical unit of Hospital 1 (Table 1): only few ADEs are detected. 90% of them are in relation with NSAID (Non-steroidal anti-inflammatory drugs). From this result, and after validation by the physicians, it is proposed that in the Cx-CDSS all the rules will be weighed by low confidence coefficients, except the rules involving NSAID. In this context, alerts will not be frequent, and appropriate for a limited number of patients.

In the geriatrics unit of Hospital 1: a greater number of ADEs are identified, particularly in people who are more than 70, and who suffer from renal insufficiency. All the rules involving "Patients older than 70 with renal insufficiency", will have high confidence coefficients and high severity coefficients. In this context, alerts will be frequent, but oriented to patients at risk.

3. The Evaluation

The challenge is to evaluate the potential impact of the prototype solutions that are not yet available in routine care. We solve this challenge by choosing and combining the following state-of-the-art evaluation methodologies for the prediction and evaluation of impact.

We evaluate PSIP solutions from the point of view of different stakeholders, including test users, potential future users, and CPOE experts. Different stakeholders will have different views on the potential impact of Cx-CDSS and how to best design them; thus, by combining and confronting these general views, we will be able to generate new insights.

For this stakeholder evaluation, we use validated survey instruments as far as possible. We also apply the method of Delphi studies which is a way to come to a consensus among experts.

4. Discussion

PSIP is a complex project, including a wide range of partners, including hospitals, companies involved in the development of medical information systems, companies involved in information processing, managing large repositories, and academic teams from universities or from academic hospitals. PSIP involves also academic teams specialized in Human Factors Engineering.

The first objective of the project considered the possibility to improve the knowledge on ADEs occurring in European hospitals. For this purpose, it was necessary to develop a set of decision rules allowing to the automatic detection of ADEs in computerized medical records. This set of decision rules was elaborated by mining medical records to associate significant outcomes with demographic, clinical and biological items. These rules have been validated by experts (pharmacologists, pharmacists, physicians, healthcare professionals) and improved by addition of decision rules already existing in databanks (such as the one provided by the partner VIDAL). Most of these rules are already known, but some associations have been suspected and ADEs discovered by means of this first phase of data mining.

This set of rules is now used in routine to detect automatically ADEs in EHRs. This allows providing statistics on the ADEs occurring per hospital or per medical department for a determined period of time. In particular, it is expected that the "ADE Scorecards" will improve the knowledge on ADEs really occurring in hospitals, and increase the awareness of the healthcare professionals on ADEs.

The validity of the detection achieved via the Scorecards has to be carefully established. It is essential that the healthcare professionals, particularly the physicians and the pharmacists, will be confident in the results provided by such applications. It seems obvious that the quality of these statistics is highly dependent on the quality of the data existing in the EHRs. Demographic data are reliable. Lab results are more often reliable but there are some errors (abnormalities in the measurement of Potassium levels or INR, for example) that have to be detected to avoid over-alerting. Diagnoses are most often reliable but, due to their potential economical usage through the DRGs, some bias can be observed. In the PSIP experience there are also some errors and imprecision in the drug information (dosage, prescription vs. administration, ATC codes). So, the data quality management is an essential aspect of this type of project.

The validation of the ADEs potentially identified by PSIP is currently realised in routine with the medical partners of the project working in the clinical units. This helps to refine the decision rules used in the PSIP applications, to fine-tune the confidence coefficients associated with the rules, and to improve the CDSS according to the last international recommendations [11].

The PSIP project has to gain in generalization. That is why the PSIP applications have to be integrated in different environments. The PSIP+ project is dedicated to implement the PSIP applications in new hospitals by integrating them in the hospital information systems of two Bulgarian hospitals. The first results show that this integration is feasible in a short period of time (less than 3 weeks).

5. Conclusion

The PSIP project has been built on the hypothesis that it would be possible to automatically detect ADEs by means of automatic analysis of EHR data, and that it would be possible, from the computed statistics to deliver relevant information to healthcare professionals by means of statistical scorecards and by means of a contextualized Clinical Decision Support System. The first hypothesis has been verified. The second one has to be carefully checked to verify that over-alerting is avoided but also to prove that no dangerous situation has been neglected.

This work has allowed a close collaboration between European teams involved in computer science and Human Factors Engineering, in a difficult domain where it is difficult to provide the right information in the right place.

Acknowledgements

The research leading to these results has received funding from the European Community's Seventh Framework Programme (FP7/2007-2013) under grant agreement n° 216130 – the PSIP project.

References

[1] D.W. Bates, R.S. Evans, H. Murff, P.D. Stetson, L. Pizziferri, G. Hripcsak, Detecting adverse events using information technology, *JAMIA* **10** (2003), 115–28.
[2] A.K. Jha, J. Laguette, A. Seger, D.W. Bates, Can surveillance systems identify and avert adverse drug events? A prospective evaluation of a commercial application, *JAMIA* **15** (2008), 647–53.
[3] E. Chazard, B. Merlin, G. Ficheur, J.C Sarfati, PSIP Consortium, R. Beuscart, Detection of adverse drug events: proposal of a data model, *Stud Health Technol Inform* **148** (2009), 63–74.
[4] E. Chazard, G. Ficheur, B. Merlin, E. Serrot, PSIP Consortium, R. Beuscart, Adverse drug events prevention rules: multi-site evaluation of rules from various sources, *Stud Health Technol Inform* **148** (2009), 102–11.
[5] Martindale, *The complete drug reference- 34ème edition*, The Pharmaceutical Press, London, 2005, 927–31.
[6] P.M. Kilbridge, U.C. Campbell, H.B. Cozart, M.G. Mojarrad, Automated surveillance for adverse drug events at a community hospital and an academic medical center, *JAMIA* **13** (2006), 372–7.
[7] G.J. Kuperman, et al., Detecting alerts, notifying the physician, and offering action items: a comprehensive alerting system, *Proc AMIA Annual Fall Symposium* (1996), 704–8.
[8] V. Koutkias et al., A Knowledge Engineering Framework towards Clinical Support for Adverse Drug Event Prevention: The PSIP Approach, *Stud Health Technol Inform* **148** (2009), 134–44.
[9] A.K. Dey, Understanding and using Context, *Personal Ubiquitous Computing* **5** (2001), 4–7.
[10] A. Schmidt, M. Beigl, H.W. Gellersen, There is more to context than location, *Computers and Graphics Journal* **23** (1999), 893–902.
[11] D.F. Sittig et al., Grand challenges in clinical decision support, *J Biomed Inform* **41** (2008), 387–92.

Patient Safety Informatics
V. Koutkias et al. (Eds.)
IOS Press, 2011

doi:10.3233/978-1-60750-740-6-13

The Future of Electronic Prescribing

Jos AARTS [1]
Institute of Health Policy and Management, Erasmus University Rotterdam, The Netherlands

Abstract. Implementing electronic prescribing in health care has been a slow process. Health authorities are now requiring mandatory electronic prescribing because of patient safety concerns. Electronic prescribing is not yet a mature technology, and may therefore pose a risk if especially organizational conditions are not taken into account. The paper offers some thoughts on the future of electronic prescribing in practice. It is especially important to extend electronic prescribing to the continuum of care in order avoid that medication safety falls in the cracks of fragmented health care organizations.

Keywords. Electronic health record systems, electronic prescribing systems, CPOE systems

Introduction

In September 2010 the Director-General of the Dutch Health Inspectorate announced that electronic prescribing of medications would be mandatory for all Dutch physicians beginning January 1, 2012. This is a bold statement, since it presumes that the technology and organizational infrastructure is ready, but it also reflects the urgency of health authorities to reduce medication errors, which still count as the most important threat to patient safety [1].

A doctor on an American discussion list addresses his concern about the impending introduction of electronic prescribing: “As I am getting closer and closer to e-prescribing in my office, I am starting to have a problem with it. As it is now, I can write “Fluoxetine 20 mg” and the pharmacist can fill with either capsules or tablets depending on what he has in stock and what the patient prefers. As part of E-Rx I have to specify, and I don’t want to. With Diltiazem—a calcium channel blocker for treatment of heart problems—sustained release there are at least 4 different dosage forms for each strength and I don’t know the difference between them. I am concerned that, if I chose the wrong one from the table, I will get a call from the pharmacist and it’ll be a big pain for both of us. Does anyone have any experience with this? Is there a liaison between the medical and pharmacy professions that can help? Is there a course that we all need to take to learn about these differences or does there need to be legislation to permit greater substitution so we don’t all get bogged down in minutia?”

In this paper I will address the apparent gap between expectations and reality of electronic prescribing in medical practice and offer some thoughts on its future.

[1] Corresponding Author: aarts@bmg.eur.nl

1. Uptake of Electronic Prescribing

The first computerized physician order entry (CPOE) system, or electronic prescribing system, was implemented in the early 1970s, initially intended for cost savings limiting choices for approved formularies. It quickly became evident that, the system offered other advantages in the form of clear presentations of dosage options and reminders, if physicians deviated from approved standards. When the safety problems of medicine became more apparent, CPOE was seen as the technology to reduce errors [2]. However, a study by Aarts and Koppel in 2009 showed that implementation in hospitals in Western countries is still rare [3]. Even in countries with the largest penetration, the United States and the Netherlands, the figure does not exceed 20%. The study that other factors, such as lack of technology integration, poorly functioning decision support systems, unsatisfactory user interfaces, insufficient funding, professional attitudes and organization of health, may be more consequential.

Most electronic prescribing systems have a stand-alone background. They were developed with the specific purpose of prescribing medications. They are therefore not well integrated with electronic patient record systems, let alone with systems across organizational boundaries. For the same reason the fit with professional workflow is often poor and users often devise a whole set of workarounds to make prescribing doable [4]. A decision support system is an integral component of electronic prescribing. In combination with a drug information database it has the facility to generate reminders and alerts. Its quality leaves much to be desired. A study of the functionality of drug safety alerting of CPOE systems available in the Netherlands showed huge differences in sensitivity and specificity and lacked integration with laboratory patient data [5]. User interfaces have been noted as problematic as well. The main issue is about presenting information in such a way that its meaning is unambiguous and prompts for the right action. Despite the fact that in some countries governments invest huge sums in health IT adoption, funding remains a problem, especially when interests have to be balanced: does extra money need to be spent on direct patient care and personnel at the bedside or in technology, of which the benefits are not direct clear. A sensitive issue is the professional attitudes. Physicians are very protective of their professional autonomy; they may conceive electronic prescribing—especially when their prescribing behavior is logged electronically—as an infringement of their discretionary decision space and the doctor-patient relationship. It may help explain why in some countries virtually no CPOE system has been implemented. In the Netherlands the fact that pharmacists are legally co-responsible for patient care has proved to be an important incentive to adopt electronic prescribing. And finally, it is still next to impossible to implement electronic prescribing across organizational boundaries. Electronic prescribing may be well implemented within a hospital, but breaks down as soon as the patient is transferred to primary or long-term care.

2. Challenges of Electronic Prescribing

The decision of the Dutch director-general shows that there is great sense of urgency to reduce the number of medication related errors. It means that the pressure is put up to implement electronic prescribing system across the board. The time of gratuitousness is clearly over. Yet, the decision may be flawed. First, an electronic prescribing must be integrated with decision support. Many systems, especially in primary care, do not have this functionality. There is little added value in replacing a written prescription by a computer print that the patient still has to bring to the pharmacy. Different systems have to be integrated. In many countries primary care, long-term care and hospital health information systems are not connected. In the previous paragraph I have outlined how integration is still in its infancy because of technological, professional and organizational reasons. Since January 1st, 2011 it is mandatory in the Netherlands to provide a medication summary when referring, transferring or discharging a patient. It may provide a sound basis for the next step of using this information for electronic prescribing. Countries are working towards infrastructures to exchange information electronically. Currently, different approaches are being adopted. The United Kingdom focuses on a centralized backbone to store and exchange patient data. In the United States the responsibility for exchanging data sits with regional health information networks. The Netherlands has chosen for an infrastructure that allows providers to Google for patient information in local systems. Mindful to protect patient privacy strictly Germany has chosen for credit card size patient card to store essential medical data. Whatever solution is being chosen, interoperability is key.

The quote above from a doctor's message in a discussion list shows that professional issues play an important role as well. There is uncertainty about what dosage works and uneasiness what strength from a medication list would work and to get in bogged-down discussions with the pharmacist. Also it shows how discretionary space that he favors might be taken away by the system. Implementation requires close examination of prescription practices, establishment of new rules and modes of collaboration between professionals, especially between nurses and doctors. And not the least, implementation requires appropriate and well-timed education and training for prospective users.

3. The Future of e-Prescribing

Electronic prescribing can reach its full potential, if a number of conditions in the short and long term can be met. In the short term efforts should be directed to mandatory interoperability using open standards. The health IT market is fragmented and there are hundreds of vendors, thus encouraging many differing and proprietary systems, few of which communicate with each other. Interoperability will enhance effective communication about medicines taken by patients. Use of national standards for a medication choice list with dosing ranges and routes of administration and decision-support reminders and alerts are expected to speed adoption. In the Netherlands there is one national standard for drug-drug interaction alerts that is adopted by all IT vendors [6]. These measures do not require large investments in developing new technology, but their emphasis is on creating the organizational conditions, which may prove already difficult enough.

I have already noted that CPOE technology is still far from mature. Van der Sijs and Aarts have found that customizing reminders is hard to achieve [7]. CPOE systems generate many alerts and too many can lead to alert fatigue among physicians, carrying the risk that important ones can be overlooked as well [8]. Koppel et al. found that CPOE systems may even induce errors [9]. Customization that takes into account the context of a specific patient and medical expertise is therefore crucial for a successful system. At the crude level of medical specialties distinctions can already be made between surgery and general internal medicine. Surgeons usually have a limited choice of medications that they use; it does not make sense to present alerts for medications that they hardly use and then only in very specific circumstances. It becomes more difficult to take into account differences between subspecialties in internal medicine. An even more complicating factor is the level of expertise within a specialty. Junior doctors will rely much more on factual knowledge that they gradually incorporate to become experts. Prescribing systems that are able to incorporate medical expertise require complex knowledge acquisition and machine learning technology that for the foreseeable future will not be available in practice.

The other approach is linking electronic prescribing with electronic patient records and clinical guidelines. The project "Patient Safety through Intelligent Procedures in medication" is an example of developing technologies to detect adverse drug events and incorporating them in electronic prescribing systems. Alerting can be customized by extending the rules of decision support technology incorporating patient data such as lab results. Patient data is often sitting in diverse, heterogeneous databases, but modern data mining techniques have proven to be effective. I foresee as the next step the extension of electronic prescribing to the continuum of care in the form of linking with personal health records that make use of even more diverse and heterogeneous databases in different organizations.

4. Conclusion

A number of steps have been outlined to implement electronic prescribing systems successfully, both in the short and long term. It must be emphasized that despite my plea for interoperability, heterogeneity of systems will still be the norm. Implementing electronic prescribing is a thoroughly sociotechnical process that not only changes technology, but foremost prescribing practices of physicians. Prescribing medication is prone to errors, and therefore much effort has been devoted to develop advanced prescribing systems, but it affects the whole medication process. Shifting from oral orders to nurses to computerized order entry of medications has changed the process of notifying of nurses to administer medications. The changes of workflow are fundamental, and may even not improve patient safety. Being able to support the continuum of care in a fragmented health care system is the challenge for future electronic prescribing systems.

References

[1] A.J. Leendertse et al., Frequency of and risk factors for preventable medication-related hospital admissions in the Netherlands, *Arch Intern Med* **168** (2008), 1890–6.

[2] D.W. Bates et al., The impact of computerized physician order entry on medication error prevention, *J Am Med Inform Assoc* **6** (1999), 313–21.

[3] J. Aarts and R. Koppel, Implementation of computerized physician order entry in seven countries, *Health Aff (Millwood)* **28** (2009), 404–14.

[4] Z. Niazkhani et al., The impact of computerized provider order entry systems on inpatient clinical workflow: a literature review, *J Am Med Inform Assoc* **16** (2009), 539–49.

[5] H. van der Sijs et al., Functionality test for drug safety alerting in computerized physician order entry systems, *Int J Med Inform* **79** (2010), 243–51.

[6] E.N. van Roon et al., Clinical relevance of drug-drug interactions: a structured assessment procedure, *Drug Saf* **28** (2005), 1131–9.

[7] H. van der Sijs et al., Turning off frequently overridden drug alerts: limited opportunities for doing it safely, *J Am Med Inform Assoc* **15** (2008), 439–48.
[8] H. van der Sijs et al., Overriding of drug safety alerts in computerized physician order entry, *J Am Med Inform Assoc* 13 (2006), 138–47.
[9] R. Koppel et al., Role of computerized physician order entry systems in facilitating medication errors, *JAMA* **293** (2005), 1197–203.

Patient Safety Informatics
V. Koutkias et al. (Eds.)
IOS Press, 2011

doi:10.3233/978-1-60750-740-6-18

Accelerating Patient Safety through the Innovative Use of Information Technology

Beth LILJA [a,b] and Jonas EGEBART [a,1]
[a] *Unit for Patient Safety, Capital Region of Denmark*
[b] *Danish Society for Patient Safety*

Abstract. Numerous studies have confirmed that the patient safety challenge remains tangible. Innovative use of healthcare IT (Information Technology) could play a part in the solution, if the costs of development and implementation are weighed against the major potential savings by improving quality and safety. It is suggested through the "Safe Seven"-checklist, that the design of supporting eHealth solutions lends principles from the patient safety and physical design domains.

Keywords. Patient safety, eHealth, healthcare IT, Safe Seven, checklist

Introduction

Patient Safety was solidly put on the healthcare agenda in 1999 with the Institute of Medicine report "To err is human" [1]. Now, more than 10 years later our knowledge of the domain is broader, but our efficacy remains debated [2].

In the Capital Region of Denmark (pop. 2010: 1.68 mill.) a reporting system was put in place in 2001 for all healthcare professionals to report patient safety incidents. Reporting has since 2004 been mandatory and non-punitive by law [3]. Each year more reports are submitted, totaling more than 17,000 in 2010 [4]. 23% of these are medication errors and in 31 % of these are the regions Computerized physician order entry's (CPOE) mentioned. In an internal study all reports from January 1st 2007 to September 30th 2008 concerning the CPOE were reviewed. Whereas it was not possible to attribute cause-and-effect relations between the reported medication incidents and the CPOE, the reporting healthcare professional did in 59% indicate the user interface as possible cause of the error.

Many countries have implemented patient satisfaction surveys, including Denmark. The patients are among other questions asked, whether they experienced a patient safety incident during their hospital stay. In the 2009 survey 23% answered "yes" to that question. In a recent Eurobarometer [5], 25% of respondents claim that they, themselves, or a member of their family, experienced a patient safety incident. Half of the responders felt that they could be harmed by the healthcare system.

Numerous studies have tried to estimate the prevalence of patient safety incidents through chart review. A Danish study from 2001 [6] found preventable incidents in 9% of the charts reviewed, which is of similar range to the studies conducted in other European countries for instance Sweden [7], England [8] and France [9].

[1] Corresponding Author: jonas@regionh.dk

The patient safety challenge therefore remains tangible.

This paper outlines a keynote talk at the "Adverse Drug Events, Human Factors & IT Tools for Patient Medication Safety"-conference, addressing current challenges in patient safety, how we seek to overcome them, and how IT can play a part in the effort.

1. Challenges in a Time of Demographic Change

An increasingly older population and a decreasing number of persons in the workforce in the near future signify an enormous pressure on the healthcare sector in order to increase the productivity. All over the world the sector is struggling to reduce the raise in expenditures. Large investments in improvement projects, and IT to support them, might not be top of the agenda everywhere.

We know that patient safety events are costly. At the Veterans Health Administration (VA) it has been documented that an admission *without* an adverse event on average costs $14,500 whereas an admission *with* one of nine defined adverse events costs an extra $9,500 to $42,000, resulting in 2.42% of the total budget [10].

In some countries and organizations the strategy in order to solve the financial and demographic challenge is to strengthen quality and safety [11]. The simple explanation is, that it will be less costly, if we do things right the first time:

- Instead of treating a pressure ulcer, it should be prevented in the first place;
- instead of treating a ventilator-associated pneumonia (VAP), it should be prevented;
- instead of treating a septic patient, he could have had his central venous line removed before the bacteria entered the bloodstream in the first place;
- instead of transferring a patient suffering from a medication error to the intensive care unit, the right drug and dosage should be given every time.

Some institutions have successfully reduced or eliminated several of these events, which for years have been perceived as an inseparable part of being sick.

2. What We'll Do

In order to successfully follow this quality and safety-driven strategy numerous actions are to be taken.

2.1. Support Clinical and Management Decision

All kinds of decision support are needed, ranging from simple checklists to advanced computerized decision support programs, and operating on all organizational levels.

It has been shown that the use of a simple checklist, the Safe Surgery Checklist, introduced by the WHO and developed by Atul Gawande [12], has proved to reduce mortality by 30% and has shown a substantial reduction in morbidity was seen as well.

The Danish Naestved Hospital confirmed a 35 % reduction of postoperative surgery following the implementation of the WHO Safe Surgery Checklist [13].

The checklist method, as shown by Gawande [14], bears an immense potential to act as an integrated part of how healthcare processes are supported by IT.

2.2. Massive Scaling of Best Practice Solution with Demonstrated Effect

The quality and safety practices, where effect has been demonstrated, must be disseminated to large scale in order to reach a broader population.

The Danish Society for Patient Safety began in 2010 the Danish Safer Hospital Programme [15] with expert assistance from the Institute for Healthcare Improvement (IHI). The Safer Hospital Programme is inspired by other initiatives in Europe: for instance the Scottish Patient Safety Programme and the Welsh "1000 Lives Plus"-initiative and correspond with recognized and accepted best practices, promoting only agreed upon knowledge in quality improvement. The aims are to achieve 15% reduction in mortality and 30% reduction in harm, by i.e. reducing the number of cardiac arrests, eliminating hospital infections, reducing pressure ulcers, and preventing medication errors. The results will be shared and disseminated to be an inspiration for the country's other hospitals. The key to success with the program is to use reliability research which relies heavily on different ways of using decision support tools.

2.3. Use Patient and Relatives as a Source for Knowledge Improvement

Patients and their families both have the desire and the legitimate wish to be an active part of the healthcare team. They want to be seen and listened to as individuals. Illness and medical treatment often make patients feel vulnerable and powerless. In order to build a system where patients is in the center of the care and, where no decisions are made without their participation, organizations are providing different Shared decision-making tools.

Shared decision-making is an approach where:

- clinicians and patients communicate together using the best available evidence,
- patients are supported to inquire about the possible attributes and consequences of options, to arrive at informed preferences in making a determination about the best action in respect for their autonomy,
- the involvement of patients and relatives is desired, ethical and legal.

To some extent these tools are in fact decision support tools. The more active and engaged the patient is in deciding his own care, the more likely it is, that he will be able to function as a "barrier" to adverse events and medical errors.

2.4. Design for Safety

The Danish government and the hospital owners have decided to replace 50% of all hospital building in Denmark during a period of more than 20 years. This poses a great opportunity not only for innovative physical design, but also to rethink the content of these new buildings.

Unsurprisingly the design principles for building safe hospitals also apply to design of IT and human-computer interfaces:

- Set fundamental principles against which all aspects of design are checked;
- conduct risk assessment at every stage in the design process;
- use full-size mock-ups for testing;
- develop specific design for the vulnerable patient or high-risk situation (e.g. patients in anti-coagulative treatment), and
- consider human factors at every stage.

3. The "Safe Seven" – A Checklist for Supporting Safety in Healthcare IT

The "Safe Seven" checklist is suggested as a synthesis of patient safety best practice, lessons learned from the Patient Safety through Intelligent Procedures in Medication and experience from incident reports, analysis and management. The checklist is meant to be used when developing new eHealth solutions, in specification and contracts and when testing new solutions or changes to current systems.

Table 1. The "Safe Seven" checklist for supporting safer eHealth solutions.

#	Item	Notes
1	Communicate maintenance, errors and notices to healthcare professionals at the point-of-use.	Experience from several large disruptions of service all had in common, that it was difficult or impossible to communicate directly with the affected user base.
2	Ensure a safe user-interface.	Is all the needed information present without the need to scroll or shift to different tabs/screens? Is it clear which patient is in context?
3	Use existing data for decision support.	Leverage the potential from using already-present data to support the clinical decisions.
4	Integrate to known data-sources and eliminate redundant data.	
5	Support the safe practice. Make the right path the easy path.	Alert fatigue is common, thus guiding the user with alerts might not ensure a continuous safe practice.
6	Implement emergency system to handle down-time. Test in full-scale.	Healthcare relies heavily on its IT supporting systems. Downtime not only threatens productivity but safe care of patients.
7	Avoid courses and class-room training. Design systems that are intuitive to use without education.	Staff turnover and lack of retaining knowledge make courses and class-room training at best expensive, at worst ineffective.

References

[1] L.T. Kohn, J.M. Corrigan, M.S. Donaldson (Eds.), *To err is human: building a safer health system*, Committee in Quality of Health Care in America, Institute of Medicine, National Academy Press, Washington DC, 1999.
[2] C.P. Landrigan et al., Temporal trends in rates of patient harm resulting from medical care, *N Engl J Med* **363(22)** (2010 Nov 25), 2124-34, Erratum in *N Engl J Med* **363(26)** (2010 Dec 23), 2573.
[3] Sundhedsloven, kap. 61, § 198-§202 Patientsikkerhed, LBK nr. 913 af 13/07/2010. Indenrigs- og Sundhedsministeriet 2010.
[4] Årsrapport DPSD 2009, Sundhedsstyrelsen 2010.
[5] SPECIAL EUROBAROMETER 327. Patient safety and quality of healthcare. Conducted by TNS Opinion & Social at the request of Directorate-General for Health and Consumers.
[6] T. Schøler et al., Forekomsten af utilsigtede hændelser på sygehus. En retrospektiv gennemgang af journaler, *Ugeskriftet Læger* **163(39)** (2001), 5331.
[7] M. Soop, U. Fryksmark, M. Kšster, B. Haglund, The incidence of adverse events in Swedish hospitals: a retrospective medical record review study, *Int J Qual Health Care* **21(4)** (2009), 285–91.

[8] C. Vincent, G. Neale, M. Woloshunowych, Adverse events in British hospitals: preliminary retrospective record review, *BMJ* **322(7285)** (2001), 517–9.
[9] P. Michel, J.L. Quenon, A. Djihoud, S. Tricaud-Vialle, A.M. de Sarasqueta, Error management. French national survey of inpatient advers events prospectively assessed with ward staff, *BMJ Qual Saf Health Care* **16** (2007), 369–77.
[10] K. Carey, T. Stefos, Measuring the cost of hospital adverse patient safety events, *Health Econ* (2010 Oct 20) [Epub ahead of print].
[11] J. Easton, Leading for Quality in Tough Times, ISQUA Paris, Oct. 2010 and National Health Forum, Orlando, Dec. 2010.
[12] A.B. Haynes et al., A Surgical Safety Checklist to Reduce Morbidity and Mortality in a Global Population, *N Engl J Med* **360** (2009), 491–9.
[13] http://internationalforum.bmj.com/doc/2010/posters/WHO_Halberg_Implementation_of_Safe_Surgery_Checklist.pdf, last access on March 2011.
[14] A. Gawande, *The Checklist Manifesto: How to Get Things Right*, Profile Books, London, 2010.
[15] http://www.sikkerpatient.dk/about-sikker-patient, last access on March 2011.

Part B

Invited Papers on Patient Safety Informatics

Patient Safety Informatics
V. Koutkias et al. (Eds.)
IOS Press, 2011

doi:10.3233/978-1-60750-740-6-25

EU-ADR Healthcare Database Network *vs.* Spontaneous Reporting System Database: Preliminary Comparison of Signal Detection

Gianluca TRIFIRÒ [a, 1], Vaishali PATADIA [a,b], Martijn J. SCHUEMIE [a], Preciosa M. COLOMA [a], Rosa GINI [c], Ron HERINGS [d], Julia HIPPISLEY-COX [e], Giampiero MAZZAGLIA [f], Carlo GIAQUINTO [g], Lorenza SCOTTI [h], Lars PEDERSEN [i], Paul AVILLACH [j,k], Miriam C.J.M. STURKENBOOM [a] and Johan VAN DER LEI [a], on behalf of the EU-ADR group

[a] *Department of Medical Informatics, Erasmus University Medical Center, Rotterdam, The Netherlands*
[b] *Astellas Pharmaceuticals*
[c] *Agenzia Regionale di Sanità della Toscana, Florence, Italy*
[d] *PHARMO Institute, Utrecht, The Netherlands*
[e] *University of Nottingham, UK*
[f] *Società Italiana di Medicina Generale, Florence, Italy*
[g] *Pedianet-Società Servizi Telematici SRL, Padova, Italy*
[h] *Department of Statistics, Università di Milano-Bicocca, Milan, Italy*
[i] *Department of Clinical Epidemiology, Aarhus University Hospital, Aarhus, Denmark*
[j] *Université Victor Segalen Bordeaux, France*
[k] *LERTIM, Faculté de Médecine, Université de la Méditerranée, Marseille, France*

Abstract. The EU-ADR project aims to exploit different European electronic healthcare records (EHR) databases for drug safety signal detection. In this paper we report the preliminary results concerning the comparison of signal detection between EU-ADR network and two spontaneous reporting databases, the Food and Drug Administration and World Health Organization databases. EU-ADR data sources consist of eight databases in four countries (Denmark, Italy, Netherlands, and United Kingdom) that are virtually linked through distributed data network. A custom-built software (Jerboa©) elaborates harmonized input data that are produced locally and generates aggregated data which are then stored in a central repository. Those data are subsequently analyzed through different statistics (i.e. Longitudinal Gamma Poisson Shrinker). As potential signals, all the drugs that are associated to six events of interest (bullous eruptions - BE, acute renal failure - ARF, acute myocardial infarction - AMI, anaphylactic shock - AS, rhabdomyolysis - RHABD, and upper gastrointestinal bleeding - UGIB) have been detected via different data mining techniques in the two systems. Subsequently a comparison concerning the number of drugs that could be investigated and the potential signals detected for each event in the spontaneous reporting systems (SRSs) and EU-ADR network was made. SRSs could explore, as potential signals, a larger number of drugs for the six events, in comparison to EU-ADR (range: 630-3,393 vs. 87-856), particularly for those events commonly thought to be

[1] Corresponding Author: g.trifiro@erasmusmc.nl

potentially drug-induced (i.e. BE: 3,393 vs. 228). The highest proportion of signals detected in SRSs was found for BE, ARF and AS, while for ARF, and UGIB in EU-ADR. In conclusion, it seems that EU-ADR longitudinal database network may complement traditional spontaneous reporting system for signal detection, especially for those adverse events that are frequent in general population and are not commonly thought to be drug-induced. The methodology for signal detection in EU-ADR is still under development and testing phase.

Keywords. Pharmacovigilance, electronic health records, drug safety, signal detection, spontaneous reporting database

Introduction

World Health Organization defines a drug safety signal as information on a possible causal relationship between an adverse event and a drug, which is unknown or incompletely documented [1]. Historically, spontaneous reporting systems (SRSs) for adverse drug reactions (ADRs) have been the cornerstone of signal detection in pharmacovigilance for the last four decades [2]. Cerivastatin and more recently rofecoxib stories highlighted the limitations of spontaneous reporting system with respect to the early detection of ADRs. The increasing availability of electronic healthcare records (EHRs) offers opportunities to investigate a wide spectrum of adverse drug effects and to detect signals closer to real time [3]. EHR databases present the additional advantage of large populations and long follow-up periods. A number of data mining techniques have been specifically developed for automatic detection of drug safety signals [2]. Currently, a number of ongoing international initiatives (SENTINEL [4], EU-ADR [5], PROTECT [6], and OMOP [7]) are aimed at testing the potential of signal detection using longitudinal electronic health record databases.

The EU-ADR (Exploring and Understanding Adverse Drug Reactions by integrative mining of clinical records and biomedical knowledge) project was funded by the European Commission and started in February 2008. The overall objective of the project was to design, develop, and validate a computerized integrative system that exploits data from EHRs and biomedical databases for the early detection of ADRs. Beyond the current state-of-the-art, EU-ADR led to the federation of different databases of EHRs, creating a resource of unprecedented size for drug safety monitoring in Europe (over 30 million patients from eight different databases). The initial stage of signal generation is followed by signal substantiation through causal reasoning, semantic mining of literature, and computational analysis of pharmacological and biological information, all with the aim of finding possible pathways that explain the drug-event associations.

As regard signal generation, in the EU-ADR project an event-based approach was adopted. A set of events warranting priority for monitoring in pharmacovigilance have been selected and inspected for their association with all possible drugs [8].

In this paper we describe the preliminary results of the comparison between EU-ADR healthcare network and two spontaneous reporting systems databases (Food and Drug Administration - Adverse Event Reporting System (FDA-AERS) and World Health Organization (WHO) Vigibase). As potential signal in the two systems, for the preliminary analyses we considered all the drugs being associated with the following six events that are deemed to be important in pharmacovigilance: Upper Gastrointestinal Bleeding (UGIB), Anaphylactic Shock (AS), Acute Myocardial

Infarction (AMI), Rhabdomyolysis (RHABD), Acute Renal Failure (ARF) and Bullous Eruption (BE).

1. Methods

1.1. Signal Detection in EU-ADR

The EU-ADR database network currently comprises of anonymised healthcare data from eight established European databases located in four countries: Health-Search (HSD, Italy). Integrated Primary Care Information (IPCI, Netherlands), Pedianet (Italy) and QResearch (United Kingdom) are general practice (GP) databases, while Aarhus University Hospital Database (Denmark), PHARMO (Netherlands), and the regional Italian databases of Lombardy and Tuscany are all comprehensive record-linkage systems in which drug dispensing data of a well-defined population is linked to a registry of hospital discharge diagnoses and other medical registries.

Due to the difference in coding schemes across various databases, the Unified Medical Language System (UMLS) was initially used as the terminology to define the events of interest [9]. Subsequently projection of the selected UMLS concept into different terminologies (i.e. READ, ICD9-CM, ICD10, and ICPC) was carried out.

In the EU-ADR project we adopted a distributed network approach that requires standardization of input files from the different databases. These input files (patient, drug, and event files) have been created locally by each database owner and have been subsequently elaborated through the purpose-built software called Jerboa© [10]. The software queries patient-level data in the different databases, which is later aggregated, and sent in encrypted format to a central repository for further analyses. For the analysis described in this paper, data from 1996 till 2010 has been contributed from six databases (QResearch and UNIMIB databases could not contribute data for this analysis). Several statistics were generated to detect all the associations between all the covered drugs and the six events of interest. Currently, the Longitudinal Gamma Poisson Shrinker (LGPS) posterior expectation of the incidence rate ratio higher than 2 and $p\text{-value}<0.05$ are the criteria that have been considered to distinguish between potential signals and non-signals [11]. The LGPS is a modification of the GPS method used in some spontaneous reporting system databases. These statistical approaches apply shrinkage to the frequentist estimates to reduce the chance of a false positive result. For the incidence rate ratios exposed time was compared with all non-exposed time including time exposed to other drugs. Based on empirically determined background incidence rates, for each event the minimum required amount of exposure was determined and the drugs not reaching this threshold were not tested as potential signals.

1.2. Signal Detection in FDA-AERS and WHO

Food and Drug Administration (FDA) - Adverse Event Reporting System (AERS) and World Health Organization (WHO) spontaneous reporting databases have been used as comparators. The FDA-AERS database is a computerized spontaneous reporting database that was established in 1969 to support the FDA's post-marketing safety surveillance program and currently contains over 4 million reports of suspected adverse drug reactions (ADRs). FDA-AERS collects most of its reports from the USA.

The WHO spontaneous report database (Vigibase) was established in 1968 and is maintained by the Uppsala Monitoring Centre (UMC) [12]. VigiBase contains at the moment more than 4 million reports of suspected ADRs that are sent from the national centers of 95 countries participating in the WHO Programme for International Drug Monitoring.

Both databases collect reports from marketing authorization holders, healthcare professionals and consumers. Overlapping of the collected report in the two databases is present. The suspected adverse drug reactions are coded using the Medical Dictionary for Regulatory Activities (MedDRA). All the Preferred Terms (PTs) of MedDRA corresponding to the six events have been used.

As regard the drug coding, an internal mapping between the generic name and the ATC code has been created. A disproportionality analysis was performed using the above mentioned PTs and the drug-ATC mapping in FDA-AERS and WHO database from the beginning (1968-9) through the 3Q2010 data. Empirical Bayes Geometric Mean (EBGM) was used to detect signals. A threshold of EB05>2 (with number of reports>0) was applied, with EB05 being the lower band of 95% Confidence Interval of EBGM [13].

As preliminary comparison for signal detection in SRSs and EU-ADR, for each of the six events we calculated the number of drugs that could be investigated and we identified the potential signals. The number of drugs that can be investigated depends on the presence of at least one report of suspected ADR in spontaneous reporting databases and on the presence of at least one exposed case patient (i.e. patients exposed to the drug when the event occurred) in the EU-ADR database network.

Table 1. Overview of signal detection in FDA-AERS and EU-ADR for the six events under consideration.

	Spontaneous reporting databases				EU-ADR		
	FDA-AERS		WHO VigiBase				
Event	**N. of drugs that could be studied**	**Potential signals N (%)**	**N. of drugs that could be studied**	**Potential signals N (%)**	**N. of drugs that could be studied**	**Potential signals N (%)**	**Potential signals in both systems, N**
Acute myocardial infarction	791	38 (4.8)	630	37 (5.9)	856	143 (16.7)	6
Acute renal failure	2,626	354 (13.5)	3,002	302 (10.1)	461	171 (37.1)	40
Anaphylactic shock	1,443	144 (10.0)	2,679	269 (10.0)	265	47 (17.7)	13
Bullous eruption	2,053	289 (14.1)	3,393	225 (6.6)	228	42 (18.4)	13
Rhabdomyolysis	1,302	94 (7.2)	1,164	51 (4.4)	87	30 (34.5)	3
Upper GI bleeding	1,937	115 (5.9)	2,419	175 (7.2)	695	218 (31.4)	31

Legend: *N. of drugs that could be studied*=number of drugs that could be investigated as potential signals, which depends on the presence of at least one report of suspected adverse drug reactions in FDA-AERS and on at least one exposed case patient in EU-ADR. *Potential signal:* statistically significant association between drug and event, based on specific analyses as described in paragraphs 1.1 and 1.2.

2. Results

Table 1 shows for each event the number of drugs that could be tested as potential signals and the number of signals being detected in the two spontaneous reporting databases and the EU-ADR system. The unit of analysis for signals is represented by single drug-event association. Overall, spontaneous reporting systems could explore, as potential signals, a larger number of drugs in association with the six events under study, in comparison to EU-ADR (range: 630-3,393 vs. 87-856). This difference was even higher for the events that are thought to be potentially drug-induced (i.e. BE: 2,053 in FDA and 3,393 in WHO vs. 228 in EU-ADR; ARF: 2,626 in FDA and 3,002 in WHO vs. 461 in EU-ADR). On the contrary, concerning the analysis for AMI a larger number of drugs could be investigated in EU-ADR (856) than SRSs (791 in FDA and 630 in WHO).

Overall, higher proportion of potential signals is detected in EU-ADR as compared to SRSs (17-37% vs. 5-14%). For the signal generation new methodologies are currently under development in EU-ADR.

The potential for signal detection in both EU-ADR and spontaneous reporting systems varies across events. The highest proportion of signals detected in SRSs was reported for BE, ARF and AS, while for ARF, UGIB and RHABD (for this event however a very low number of drugs could be tested) in EU-ADR.

3. Conclusion

The potential of EU-ADR database network for drug safety signal detection is promising particularly for those adverse events that have high frequency (i.e. acute myocardial infarction) in general population. Data mining of longitudinal electronic medical records may particularly complement traditional analyses on spontaneous reporting systems in the signal detection, especially for those frequent adverse events that are not traditionally thought to be drug induced. The implementation of additional analyses in the EU-ADR system is still ongoing. In the final EU-ADR system, a panel of statistical analyses will allow a greater precision of signal detection. In addition, automatic search in the scientific literature and summary of product characteristics will filter out the already known signals among those being initially identified in EU-ADR. On the other hand, signals will be substantiated by a computer-assisted exploration of biological plausibility in the context of current biomedical knowledge to reduce the false positive signals.

Acknowledgments

This research has been funded by the European Commission Seventh Framework Programme (FP7/2007-2013) under grant no. 215847 – The EU-ADR Project.

The authors also wish to thank the NLM for making UMLS available free of charge.

References

[1] M. Stahl et al., Assessing the impact of drug safety signals from the WHO database presented in "SIGNAL": results from a questionnaire of National Pharmacovigilance Centres, *Drug Saf* **26** (2003), 721–7.

[2] E.M. Rodriguez, J.A. Staffa, D.J. Graham, The role of databases in drug postmarketing surveillance, *Pharmacoepidemiol Drug Saf* **10** (2001), 407–10.

[3] S. Schneeweiss, J. Avorn, A review of uses of health care utilization databases for epidemiologic research on therapeutics, *J Clin Epidemiology* **58** (2005), 323–37.

[4] http://www.fda.gov/Safety/FDAsSentinelInitiative/ucm2007250.htm, last access on March 2011.

[5] G. Trifirò et al., The EU-ADR project: preliminary results and perspective, *Stud Health Technol Inform* **148** (2009), 43–9.

[6] Pharmacoepidemiological Research on Outcomes of Therapeutics by a European Consortium – PROTECT project. Available at: http://www.imi-protect.eu/, last access on March 2011.

[7] P.E. Stang et al., Advancing the science for active surveillance: rationale and design for the Observational Medical Outcomes Partnership, *Ann Intern Med* **153** (2010), 600–6.

[8] G. Trifirò et al., Data mining on electronic health record databases for signal detection in pharmacovigilance: which events to monitor?, *Pharmacoepidemiol Drug Saf* **18** (2009), 1176–84.

[9] P. Avillach et al., Design and evaluation of a semantic approach for the homogeneous identification of events in eight patient databases: a contribution to the European EU-ADR project. *Stud Health Technol Inform* **160** (2010), 1085–9.

[10] P.M. Coloma et al., Combining electronic healthcare databases in Europe to allow for large-scale drug safety monitoring: the EU-ADR Project, *Pharmacoepidemiol Drug Saf* **20** (2011), 1–11.

[11] M.J. Schuemie, Methods for drug safety signal detection in longitudinal observational databases: LGPS and LEOPARD, *Pharmacoepidemiol Drug Saf* 2010 Oct 13 [Epub ahead of print].

[12] M. Lindquist, The WHO Adverse Reaction Database: Basic Facts. In: http://www.who-umc.org/graphics/4789.pdf. Uppsala: Uppsala Monitoring Centre; 2004, last access on March 2011.

[13] A. Szarfman, S.G. Machado, R.T. O'Neill, Use of screening algorithms and computer systems to efficiently signal higher-than-expected associations of drugs and events in the US FDA's spontaneous reports database, *Drug Safety* **25** (2002), 381–92.

Patient Safety Informatics
V. Koutkias et al. (Eds.)
IOS Press, 2011

doi:10.3233/978-1-60750-740-6-31

3,520 Medication Errors Evaluated to Assess the Potential for IT-based Decision Support

Kristine BINZER and Annemarie HELLEBEK [1]
Unit for Patient Safety, Capital Region of Denmark

Abstract. We have previously studied system failures involved in medication errors using a limited number of root cause analyses as source. The aim of this study was to describe a larger number of medication errors with respect to harm, involved medicines and involved system problems – thus providing information for the development of IT-based decision support. We evaluated 3,520 medication error reports derived from 12 months of consecutive reporting from 13 hospitals in the Capital Region of Denmark. We found 0.65% errors with serious harm and 16% with moderate harm. A small number of medicines were involved in the majority of the errors. The problems in the medication error process were heterogeneous. Some were related to specific medicines and others were related to the computerized order entry system. Accordingly decision support targeted at specific medicines and improved IT systems are part of the continuing work to reduce the frequency of medication errors.

Keywords. Medication error, decision support, reporting system

Introduction

Medication errors (ME) are errors in the medication process resulting in the patient not receiving the right medicinal product in the right dose, in the right dispensing form, at the right time using the right route. Medication errors may be harmful or not harmful to the patient [1]. Adverse drug events are harmful events happening to the patient during treatment with medicines, these maybe caused by ME [2].

Medication errors constitute a global problem and numerous attempts have been made to reduce them [1]. Probably the largest attempt to reduce ME has been the implementation of computerized physician order entry systems (CPOE). Some authors have shown that these systems reduce ME; others are more reluctant [3].

We have previously shown that root cause analyses are an important source of knowledge about system failures related to serious ME [4].

Root cause analyses are, however, few and time consuming to conduct. The aim of the present study is to evaluate a larger source of ME using data from the patient safety incident reporting system, with focus on medicines and system failures thereby shaping the direction for the development of decision support.

[1] Corresponding Author: annemarie.hellebek@regionh.dk

1. Methods

All incident reports on ME from October 1st 2009 to September 31st 2010 were extracted from the regional patient safety reporting system into a spreadsheet. Categories (at which step in medication process did the incident occur and what was the level of harm to the patient) derived from the initial evaluation at hospitals were kept. Reports were additionally categorized by a junior doctor and a research assistant with respect to incident or near miss, and involved medicinal products. The initial categorizing from hospitals on level of harm was reevaluated and eventually corrected to obtain minimal inter observer difference. In addition reports causing moderate or serious harm were evaluated for specific system failures.

The scale used for harm evaluation was the Severity Assessment Code (SAC) score developed by the Veterans Administration. This scale has been used in the Capital Region of Denmark since 2002.

2. Results

3,520 reports about ME were reviewed. In 2,914 reports it was possible to identify the involved medicinal product at an Anatomical Therapeutic Classification (ATC) level of two or more.

The medicine most frequently reported as ME was antibiotics totalling 19% of all reports (Table 1). Antibiotics, analgetics, antithrombotics and insulins together were involved in 42% of the errors.

Table 1. Medicines most frequently involved in errors.

Medicine	Frequency
Antibiotics (J01)	18.6%
Analgesics (N02)	11.5%
Antithrombotics (B01A)	6.6%
Insulin (A10)	5.1%

Among the 483 reported ME with moderate or severe harm to the patient, it was possible to identify the medicinal product at generic drug level (ATC code 5) in 324 ME (56%). 101 of these reports were caused by 13 medicinal products (Table 2).

The medicinal products involved most frequently in ME, where harm reached the patient were: human soluble insulin, warfarin, cefuroxim, vaccine for measles, methotrexate and quetiapin (Table 2).

Opioides, insulin, potassium, quetiapin and antibiotics were all involved in more than one ME with severe harm (Table 3). The step of the medication process involved in the error could be described in 18 of the 23 ME where severe harm occurred (Table 3). Failures in dose calculation (5), medicine reconciliation (2) and delay in administration of medicinal product (2) were identified more than once.

Table 2. Medication errors involved in at least 2% of 324 ME with moderate or severe harm.

Medicinal product	**Percent of ME with moderate or severe harm**
Human insulin soluble	4
Warfarin	4
Cefuroxim	3
Vaccine against measles, rubella and parotitis	3
Methotrexat	3
Quetiapin	3
Ciprofloxacin	2
Tinzaparin	2
Digoxin	2
Phentanyl	2
Morphine	2
Haloperidol	2
Methadone	2

Table 3. Severe ME described with medicinal product, error, problem in medication process and harm.

Medicinal product	**Error**	**Problem in medication process**	**Harm**
Potassium oral solution	Administration in Central Venous Catheter	Wrong route of administration	Cardiac Arrest wit resuscitation
Potassium and insulin	Patient with diabetes, hyperkalemia and decreased renal function receives a wrong mixture of potassium, insulin and glucose due to error in instruction	Complicated instruction	Hypoglycemia
Solution for hydration	Overdose of hydration in patient with rhabdomyolysis during forced diuresis	Unknown	Referral to intensive care
Insulin	Insulin in diabetic patient omitted due to lack of medicine reconciliation in patient with diabetes	Medicine reconciliation	Patient gets Keto acidosis
Insulin	Insulin in diabetic patient omitted despite several measurements of increased plasma glucose	No use of relevant parameter in medication order	Patient gets ketoacidosis
Warfarin	Overdose of warfarin	Unknown	Gastro intestinal bleeding with need of acute life saving treatment
Digoxin	Error in dose calculation when patient changed from oral to intravenous treatment	Dose calculation	Transfer to intensive care due to arrhythmia

Atropine	Ordered and administered by mistake to child with astma. Should have been Atrovent	Mix up of names	Harm not described in report
Ephedrine	Ordering or administration of an over dose to woman in labor	Dose calculation	Child shows signs on asphyxia and acute Cesarian section is instituted
Nifedipine	Dispensing of overdose for administration in naso gastric tube	Dose calculation	Hypotension
Antibiotics	Iv antibiotics delayed more than 12 hours to patient with pneumonia	Delay	Patient dies
Antibiotics	Antibiotics delayed 2 hours in patient with sepsis	Delay	Referral to intensive care
Morphine	Error in dose calculation when patient changed from intravenous to oral treatment	Dose calculation	Referral to Intensive care due to morphine over dose
Morphine	Error in dose calculation for child	Dose calculation	Referral to intensive care and ventilator assistance
Morphine and Diazepam	Overdose in patient with Parkinson's disease	Unknown	Severe respiratory failure
Metadone	Over dose due to administration of medicine from previous medication list with medication reconciliation	Medicine reconciliation	Referral to intensive care
Diazepam	Overdose during treatment of alcohol abstinence	Unknown	Referral to intensive care
Quetiapin	Administration to wrong patient	Wrong patient	Patient admitted to department of cardiology for observation
Quetiapin	Double administration (patient and staff) resulting in over dose	Double administration	Patient admitted to department of cardiology for observation
Thiopental	Mix up of syringes with thiopental and cefuroxim	Mix up of syringes	Immediate life saving treatment by manual ventilation
Fospheyntoin	Administration of fosphenytoin is omitted in patient with severe epilepsy	Unknown	

Steps in the medication process for the medicinal products most frequently involved in errors (Table 1) were extremely heterogeneous. Errors were related not only to lack of decision support, but also to usability problems with the computer systems. Some problems were described for more products (i.e. ordering despite allergy), whereas others were closely related to the exact product (Table 4).

Table 4. Problems in the medication process for medicines most frequently involved in ME.

Medicines	Problem in medication process
Antibiotics	Ordering despite known allergy
	Ordering despite decreased renal function
	Double ordering or dispensing due to double documentation
	Ordering or dispensing wrong dose when calculating dose from patient weight and when changing route from intravenous to oral route
	Dispensing wrong dose due to wrong interpretation of medicine weight and dispensable units
	Dispensing omitted for prophylaxis before surgery
	Dispensing delayed due to differences in medication lists between computer order system and paper chart with notes
	Dispensing delayed due to difficulties for staff in interpretation of computer screens
	Administration using wrong route
Analgesics	Ordering or dispensing wrong dose due to mix up of strengths
	Ordering wrong drug due to mix up of names
	Ordering and dispensing despite known allergy
	Double ordering or dispensing due to double documentation
	Dispensing using out dated medication lists
	Continuous dispensing of stopped medicine due to difficulties for staff in interpretation of computer screens
	Administration delayed when patients are referred between wards
	Administration of wrong drug or wrong dose due to up between patches
	Administration of wrong dose using adhesives due to no removal of old patch or administration of two patches
	Administration devices (pumps) defect
Antithrombotics	Omitted reordering after treatment pause
	Omitted antithrombotic medicine for patients with coronary syndrome
	Omitted administration due to missing documentation
	Routinely ordering wrong dose in computer system due to no possibility of marking medicines for which dose is ordered on paper
	Ordering wrong dose due to mix up between medicine weight and dispensable units
	Wrong ordering at discharge due to double documentation
	Delayed dispensing due to unclear placement of responsibility between departments
	Administration at wrong time due to improper default administration time in computer system
	Administration using wrong route
	No stopping of low molecular weight heparins at discharge

Insulin	Administration of double dose due to missing documentation of first administration
	Ordering of insulin in paper system omitted due to double documentation system
	Monitoring of insulin drip missing
	Dispensing insulin drip without label or without insulin
	Ordering of insulin drip unclear due to instruction difficult to interpret
	Administration of insulin to patient with hypoglycemia
	Administration of insulin because patient gives wrong information and information is not checked in computer system
	Dispensing wrong dose due to calculation error when dispensing from bottle instead of pen
	Administration of wrong dose due mix up of patients

3. Discussion

The present study confirms that insulin, analgesics, antibiotics and antithrombotic are the medicines most frequently involved in ME in hospitals – constituting almost 42% of the errors in 2009-2010 at the hospitals of the Capital Region of Denmark. The exact step in the medication process related to ME are heterogeneous and related not only to lack of decision support, but also to general problems with the CPOE system.

A previous study based on root cause analyses from the same hospitals in the years 2002-2008 [4] found similar problems as those identified in the present study – despite the fact that a CPOE system was implemented in 2006-2007.

In a literature review paper we have claimed that CPOE and decision support is helpful – and the more sophisticated the better [3]. The present study confirms that CPOE providing allergy warnings, dose calculations and inclusion of lab data for ordering should be able to reduce error frequencies. Evaluating new CPOE systems is difficult and a successful evaluation tool for the ability of the systems to reduce serious errors remains to be developed [5]. The CPOE system implemented in the hospitals of the Capital Region of Denmark does, at the current version, not provide sophisticated decision support, indicating an explanation of the persistence of specific errors. A new version of the CPOE system is under implementation in 2010-2011 and current research activities aim at improving the decision support (http://www.psip-project.eu/).

Interestingly - medicinal products used less frequently (vaccine against measles, methotrexate and quetiapin) are included in the list of errors resulting in moderate or severe harm. They were each involved in 3% of harmful ME. The errors caused by quetiapin resulted in referral to cardiac monitoring. Quetiapin is not previously specifically mentioned as a high alert drug. We suggest that quetiapin is added to lists of high alert medicinal products.

Another problem detected in the study is lack of usability of the CPOE system. This was confirmed by errors related with misinterpretation of dose caused by small size letters on the screen and omission of dispensing caused by difficulties in understanding the presentation of medicinal products for dispensing on the screen.

While waiting for computer documentation systems with sophisticated decision support, we propose to considerate the use of warnings in the medication information systems for specific error types with the potential of causing severe harm. This kind of warnings has been in effect in Denmark since 2009. A similar approach has been used in the US with an increased adherence to specific clinical protocols [6]. We also propose that hand-over in clinical work includes specific attention to patients treated with medicinal products known to cause specific errors and not usually used in the department. A possible method for this could be the use of structural information "score cards". Such cards are under development in the PSIP project although currently only based on historical data [7].

In the present study we reported the errors without a denominator related to the consumption of medicines or hospital days. To target decision support and warnings to only the most dangerous medicinal products "high alert medications", we propose further research in denominators for ME. Such research could include the use of ME data from audit of medical records (e.g. using Global Trigger Tools [8]) using bed days as denominator and on a combination of data on errors and data on drug consumption.

References

[1] M. Cohen (Ed.), *Medication Errors*, American Pharmacists Association, Washington DC, 2007.

[2] J.R. Nebeker, P. Barach, M.H. Samore et al., Clarifying adverse drug events: A clinician's guide to terminology, documentation and reporting, *Ann Intern Med* **140** (2004), 795–801.

[3] L.I. Rabøl, J. Anhoj, A. Pedersen, B.L. Pedersen, A. Hellebek, Clinical decision support: Is the number of medication errors reduced, *Ugeskr Laeger* **168** (2006), 4179–84.

[4] A. Hellebek, P. Skjoet, Aggregated review of route cause analyses related to medication, *Stud Health Technol Inform* **157** (2010), 15–7.

[5] J. Metzger, E. Welebob, D. Bates, S. Lipsitz, D.C. Classen, Mixed results in the safety performance of computerized physician order entry, *Health Aff (Millwood)* **29** (2010), 655–63.

[6] D.T. Yu, D.L. Seger, K.E. Lasser et al., Impact of implementing alerts about medication black-box warnings in electronic health records, *Pharmacoepidemiol Drug Saf* **20** (2011), 192–202.

[7] R. Marcilly, E. Chazard, M.C. Beuscart-Zéphir et al., Design of adverse drug events-scorecards *Stud Health Technol Inform* **164** (2011), 377–81.

[8] M. Carter, Measuring harm levels with the Global Trigger Tool, *Clin Risk* **16** (2010), 122–6.

Patient Safety Informatics
V. Koutkias et al. (Eds.)
IOS Press, 2011

doi:10.3233/978-1-60750-740-6-38

Drug Knowledge Expressed as Computable Semantic Triples

Peter L. ELKIN [a,1], John S. CARTER [b], Manasi NABAR [b], Mark TUTTLE [b], Michael LINCOLN [c] and Steven H. BROWN [c]
[a] *Mount Sinai School of Medicine*
[b] *Apelon Corporation*
[c] *Veterans Health Administration*

Abstract. The majority of questions that arise in the practice of medicine relate to drug information. Additionally, adverse reactions account for as many as 98,00o deaths per year in the United States. Adverse drug reactions account for a significant portion of those errors. Many authors believe that clinical decision support associated with computerized physician order entry has the potential to decrease this adverse drug event rate. This decision support requires knowledge to drive the process. One important and rich source of drug knowledge is the DailyMed product labels. In this project we used computationally extracted SNOMED CT™ codified data associated with each section of each product label as input to a rules engine that created computable assertional knowledge in the form of semantic triples. These are expressed in the form of "Drug" HasIndication "SNOMED CT™ code". The information density of drug labels is deep, broad and quite substantial. By providing a computable form of this information content from drug labels we make these important axioms (facts) more accessible to computer programs designed to support improved care.

Keywords. Medical information, ontologies, knowledge representation, clinical decision support

Introduction

The US National Library of Medicine's (NLM) DailyMed Web site contains freely downloadable XML formatted US Food and Drug Administration (FDA) drug labels (package inserts) for legally prescribable drugs in the United States [1]. Each label is produced by the drug's manufacturer according to specifications regulated by the U.S. Food and Drug Administration (FDA) (See 21 CFR part 207) [2]. Manufactures submit labels in electronic format for "marketing applications for human drug and biologic products, including new drug applications (NDAs), abbreviated new drug applications (ANDAs), and biological license applications (BLAs) for biological products that meet the definition of drug in the Federal Food, Drug, and Cosmetic Act" [3].

These package inserts were only printed on paper until the recent development of the Structured Product Label (SPL) standard from Health Level 7 (HL7) [4]. The SPL standard is an XML markup designed to hold the content associated with each package

[1] Corresponding Author: ontolimatics@gmail.com

insert in a computable format, displayable on the web. The extraction of the SNOMED CT™ content from the labels has been previously reported [5]. This project takes the output of the parsed labels and uses a set of computable rules to generate the Semantic Triples [6]. The volume of knowledge derived is reported in this manuscript.

Drug labels contain information regarding:

- Description – A description of the drug including its chemical characteristics
- Clinical Pharmacology – The drugs methods of absorption, metabolism and excretion.
- Indications and Usage – The indications for the drug for both treatment and prevention.
- Contraindications – Any conditions or other medication use that would indicate that this medication was not an appropriate choice for this patient.
- Warnings – Important conditions, laboratory abnormalities, other medication usage and patient states that would be concerning or require monitoring if the patient were to be treated with this medication
- Precautions – Conditions that would indicate a need for monitoring or a higher risk of adverse reactions in certain patient populations. Also this area of the label discusses the need for required monitoring, often by laboratory examination, in patients on this medication.
- Adverse Reactions – Potential undesirable outcomes known to be associated with taking this medication. These can be qualified by the frequency of their occurrence and the populations at risk for certain complications.
- Overdosage – This area of the label provides advice regarding what to do in the case of an overdose of the medication.
- Dosage and Administration – This area of the label provides prescribing information including any dose adjustments in children or the elderly or people with renal impairment or hepatic dysfunction.
- How Supplied – Provides data often with images of the product and its markings along with lot sizes.
- Patient Counseling Information – Provides suggestions for topics and knowledge that should be shared with patients or their families who are taking this medication.
- Boxed Warnings – These are the most serious potential complications associated with taking this medication. This information is not to be missed by anyone prescribing or taking this medication. Often these outcomes can be life threatening. As such these are highlighted at the beginning of the label and standout with a box printed around the text of this section.
- Medication Guide – Is a patient oriented view of the information in an easy to read and understand set of instructions and advice for patients taking this medication or for their family members who help care for these patients.

The U.S. Department of Veterans Affairs was interested in evaluating clinically relevant codified semantic triples as one potential underpinning of future clinical decision support systems. Medication labels in the SPL standard were selected as an exemplar because of the importance of their content and computer accessibility of their structure.

On September 30th, 2010 there were 16,691 drug labels in the DailyMed. We downloaded these labels and extracted information from the text of the label using the intelligent natural language processor (iNLP) and codified the information where possible with SNOMED CT™ [7]. We used the July 2010 release of SNOMED CT™ which contains 292,073 concepts and 760,903 terms, our terminology server creation process adds an additional 1,395,332 terms plus word normalization variants to make the terminology more compatible with the needs of natural language processing. Previous research has shown that for disorders and findings the iNLP processor has sensitivity (recall) of 99.7% and a positive predictive value (precision) of 99.8%. The sections we included in this effort were the Black Box Warnings, the Warnings, the Precautions, the Indications and Usage, the Adverse Reactions, the Overdose and the Contraindications sections. For each label parsed an XML document was written which extended the markup of the original SPL label to include the concept based data derived in this process. We followed the HL7 SPL standard in adding the additional XML markup. For compositional expressions we included a Tip variable within the Phrase tag to hold a displayable form of the compositional expression. The same data was simultaneously stored in a relational database for easy access and evaluation.

The semantic triples are based on a semantic model of drug knowledge and have been designed to support at least the following use cases:

- A patient has a drug ordered for which the patient has a known contraindication to the medication in their prior medical record. The system alerts the clinician that the drug is contraindicated and the order does not move forward. The clinician orders a drug that is not contraindicated in this patient population.
- A patient presents to their clinician with the new onset of a sign or symptom. The system alerts the clinician that one or more of the patient's medications could be causing the patients complaint. This speeds time to diagnosis and saves inappropriate testing.
- The patient presents with a common illness but with multiple allergies to the most common treatments for that condition. The clinician pushes one button and the system informs the clinician of which other drugs have that condition as one of its indications.

The relational database of the content associated with the drug labels was the input used to generate the set of Semantic Triples. We report the information density of the assertional knowledge found in the labels by section of the record and we provide a useful resource for clinical decision support.

1. Methods

The iNLP solution has been installed and used at the VA for the last four years [8]. It has the capability to codify clinical free text data using any standardized Ontology or terminology. The accuracy of this method has been previously reported. We used a version of SNOMED CT™ released by IHTSDO in July of 2010.

In a previous study a drug XML parser was written that knew the format of the structured product label. For each of these 16,691 labels, the sections identified were read and the free text sections marked with the text tags were parsed using the iNLP processor. The output data was written to a set of relational tables. These tables were the input to an expert rules engine that determined to which semantic each eligible piece of data was to be written. The semantic tree used to represent the knowledge is shown in Figure 1. Figure 2 shows the overall workflow for the generation of the semantic roles and Figure 3 shows the specific technical implementation of the rules that generated the semantic triples from the parsed drug labels.

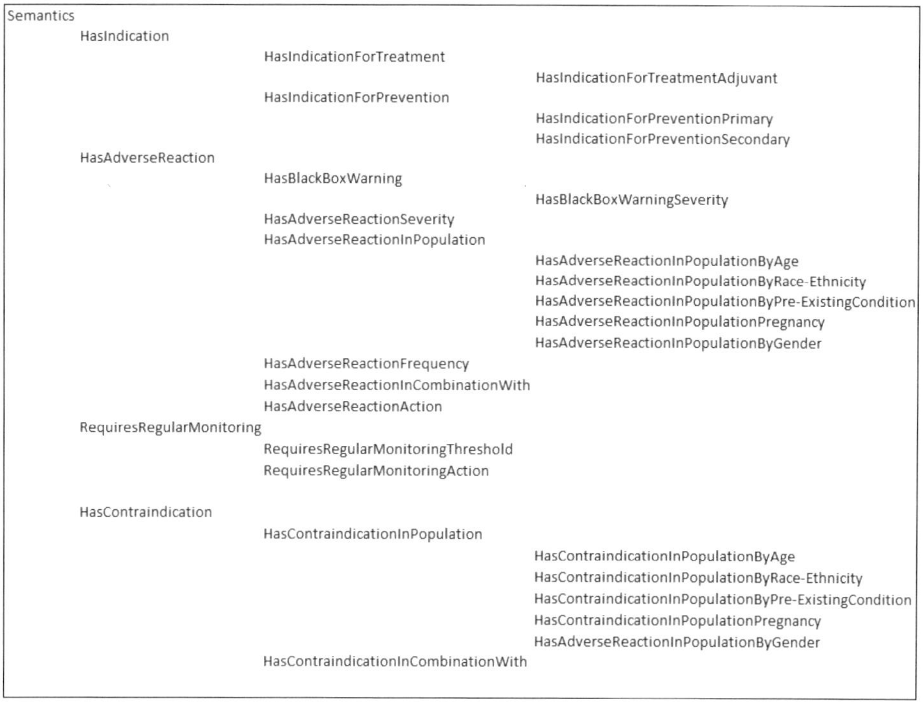
Semantics
HasIndication
HasIndicationForTreatment
HasIndicationForTreatmentAdjuvant
HasIndicationForPrevention
HasIndicationForPreventionPrimary
HasIndicationForPreventionSecondary
HasAdverseReaction
HasBlackBoxWarning
HasBlackBoxWarningSeverity
HasAdverseReactionSeverity
HasAdverseReactionInPopulation
HasAdverseReactionInPopulationByAge
HasAdverseReactionInPopulationByRace-Ethnicity
HasAdverseReactionInPopulationByPre-ExistingCondition
HasAdverseReactionInPopulationPregnancy
HasAdverseReactionInPopulationByGender
HasAdverseReactionFrequency
HasAdverseReactionInCombinationWith
HasAdverseReactionAction
RequiresRegularMonitoring
RequiresRegularMonitoringThreshold
RequiresRegularMonitoringAction
HasContraindication
HasContraindicationInPopulation
HasContraindicationInPopulationByAge
HasContraindicationInPopulationByRace-Ethnicity
HasContraindicationInPopulationByPre-ExistingCondition
HasContraindicationInPopulationPregnancy
HasAdverseReactionInPopulationByGender
HasContraindicationInCombinationWith

Figure 1. Semantic hierarchy of Drug Roles.

Examples of the rules by Section of the label in which they were found used for the assignment of knowledge to a specific semantic triple are shown below and the semantic triple output relational table is shown in Table 1.

2) HasBlackBoxWarning Detail

1. All Disorders, Findings and Morphological Abnormalities from the "Black Box Warning" section.

    1. Default
    2. HasBlackBoxWarningSeverity
        1. All codes in this section = Death (event) [419620001]
        2. (Exp) or Severity of illness (qualifier value) [43749003]
        3. Note this if possible needs to be linked to the concept code from the section as in 2.1.1.1 in the same sentence as the concept from 2.1.1.2.1

A more complex set of semantic rules is depicted in the rules for the Adverse Reactions in Population section. Exploded codes are shown using the "(Exp)" label and denote concepts where all of their subtypes in SNOMED CT™ are to be included in the logic:

5. HasAdverseReactionInPopulation
    1. HasAdverseReactionInPopulationByAge

1. 3.1.1.1 plus Person categorized by age (person) [410598002] (Exp) or Child (Subject Relationship Context) [67822003]
2. or Age (observable entity) [397659008]
3. or Age (qualifier value) [397669002]
4. or Aging (finding) [248280005]

2. HasAdverseReactionInPopulationByRace-Ethnicity
   1. Ethnic group finding (finding) [397731000] (Exp) or Racial group (racial group) [415229000] (Exp)

3.HasAdverseReactionInPopulationByPreExisting Condition
   1. History of (contextual qualifier) (qualifier value) [392521001]
   2. or Diathesis, function (observable entity) [76522002]
   3. or Susceptibility (property) (qualifier value) [118588007]
   4. in the sentence within the Adverse Reaction Section

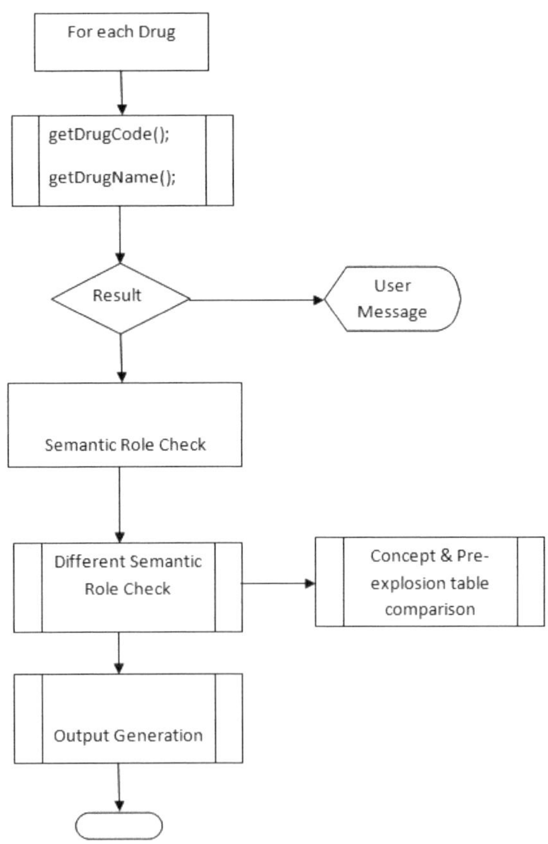

Figure 2. Workflow for the semantic role generation.

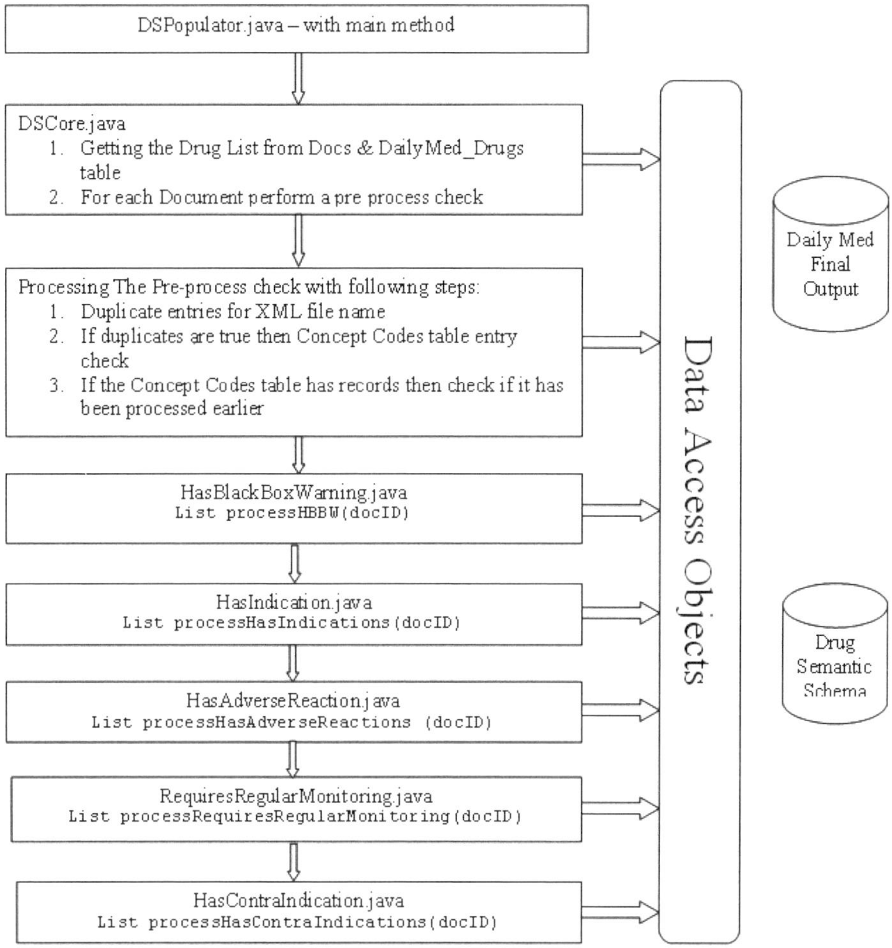

Figure 3. Program Flow of the Semantic Triples Rules Engine.

2. Results

7,571,417 SNOMED CT™ concept codes were generated from the 16,691 labels organized by Section, Sentence, Phrase and where available, Compositional Expression (post-coordination). There were 12,408 Unique Drugs (NDC Codes) identified in the labels. There were 16,259 Unique SNOMED CT™ codes instantiated. Each parsed section (Are represented in the HL7 SPL standard as LOINC codes) had considerable codified content (See Table 2). From this content 1,511,917 semantic triples were generated using 7,836 unique SNOMED CT™ concepts. The distribution of these triples is shown in Table 3 below.

Table1. Semantic Triple Output Table.

Column	Data Type	Description
DOC_ID	Numeric	Document ID from the docs table
SEC_ID	Numeric	Section ID for the parsed and processed section
SEC_NAME	Var char	Section Name
DRUG_CODE	Var char	Drug Code from the XML – dailymed_drugs table
ROLE_ID	Numeric	Role ID from the Semantic_roles table
CONCEPT_CODE	Numeric	Concept code from concept table
DRUG_NAME	Var char	Drug Name from the XML – dailymed_drugs table
ROLE_NAME	Var char	Role Name from the Semantic_role table
CONCEPT_NAME	Var char	Concept Name from concept table
SENTENCE_ID	Numeric	Sentence ID from CE_CODES table
PHRASE_ID	Numeric	Phrase ID from CE_CODES table
CE_ID	Numeric	CE ID from CE_CODES table
SEQUENCE_ID	Numeric	Sequence Id generated within the Section
DISTINCTION	Var char	Distinction from the Concept table
AGGREGATION_CONCEPT_ID	Numeric	Aggregation concept code from concept table
AGGREGATION_CONCEPT_NAME	Var char	Aggregation concept name from concept table

Table 2. Number of SNOMED CT concepts identified stratified by section of the drug label [6].

Section	LOINC Section ID	Total # SNOMED CT Concepts	Distinct SNOMED CT Concepts
Boxed Warning	34066-1	153,374	2,686
Adverse Reactions	34084-4	1,686,671	9,231
Indications and Usage	34067-9	528,417	7,970
Contraindications	34070-3	174,097	4,263
Warnings	34071-1	1,503,154	7,416
Overdosage	34088-5	530,986	4,538
Precautions	42232-9	3,000,152	10,088
Total		**7,576,851**	**16,259**

Table 3. Distribution of semantic content of the labels stratified by ROLE. The PARENT_ID provides the hierarchical relationships between the various roles.

ROLE_ID	ROLE_NAME	PARENT_ID	Number of triples identified
1	HasIndications	-1	0
2	HasIndicationsForTreatment	1	65
3	HasIndicationsForTreatmentAdjuvant	2	0
4	HasIndicationsForPrevention	1	86,267
5	HasIndicationsForPreventionPrimary	4	0
6	HasIndicationsForPreventionSecondary	4	0
7	HasAdverseReaction	-1	551,158
8	HasBlackBoxWarning	7	20,790
9	HasBlackBoxWarningSeverity	8	2,017
10	HasAdverseReactionSeverity	7	2,331
11	HasAdverseReactionInPopulation	7	0
12	HasAdverseReactionInPopulationByAge	11	7,1124
13	HasAdverseReactionInPopulationByRace-Ethnicity	11	291
14	HasAdverseReactionInPopulationByPre-ExistingCondition	11	415
15	HasAdverseReactionInPopulationPregnancy	11	254
16	HasAdverseReactionInPopulationByGender	11	2,180
17	HasAdverseReactionFrequency	7	28,636
18	HasAdverseReactionInCombinationWith	7	105,305
19	HasAdverseReactionAction	7	55,885
20	RequiresRegularMonitoring	-1	5,517
21	RequiresRegularMonitoringThreshold	20	14,821
22	RequiresRegularMonitoringAction	20	565,925
23	HasContraindication	-1	25,747
24	HasContraindicationInPopulation	23	0
25	HasContraindicationInPopulationByAge	24	726
26	HasContraindicationInPopulationByRace-Ethnicity	24	0
27	HasContraindicationInPopulationByPre-ExistingCondition	24	1,838
28	HasContraindicationInPopulationPregnancy	24	2,128
29	HasContraindicationInPopulationByGender	24	397
30	HasContraindicationInCombinationWith	23	31,264

Some of the semantics such as "HasAdverseReactionInPopulation" are only used for aggregation purposes and not for storage of primary data and some leaf nodes by their rules generated no instantiation of triples, such as "HasIndicationsForPreventionPrimary" (See Table 3).

Figure 4 presents examples of semantic triples identified for Ticlid (ticlopidine) a ADP-induced platelet-fibrinogen binding inhibitor.

DOC_ID	SEC_ID	SEC_NAME	DRUG_CODE	ROLE_ID	CONCEPT_CODE	DRUG_NAME	ROLE_NAME	CONCEPT_NAME
198100000	1	BLACKBOXWARNING	0004-0018	8	281647001	TICLID	HasBlackBoxWarning	Adverse reaction
198100000	1	BLACKBOXWARNING	0004-0018	8	17182001	TICLID	HasBlackBoxWarning	Agranulocytosis
198100000	1	BLACKBOXWARNING	0004-0018	8	165517008	TICLID	HasBlackBoxWarning	Neutropenia
198100000	1	BLACKBOXWARNING	0004-0018	8	78129009	TICLID	HasBlackBoxWarning	Thrombotic thrombocytopenic purpura
198100000	1	BLACKBOXWARNING	0004-0018	8	306058006	TICLID	HasBlackBoxWarning	Aplastic anemia
198100000	1	BLACKBOXWARNING	0004-0018	8	230690007	TICLID	HasBlackBoxWarning	Cerebrovascular accident
198100000	1	BLACKBOXWARNING	0004-0018	8	165517008	TICLID	HasBlackBoxWarning	Neutropenia
198100000	1	BLACKBOXWARNING	0004-0018	8	230690007	TICLID	HasBlackBoxWarning	Cerebrovascular accident
198100000	1	BLACKBOXWARNING	0004-0018	8	126729006	TICLID	HasBlackBoxWarning	Thrombotic microangiopathy
198100000	1	BLACKBOXWARNING	0004-0018	8	71677004	TICLID	HasBlackBoxWarning	Injury due to exposure to external cause
198100000	1	BLACKBOXWARNING	0004-0018	8	126729006	TICLID	HasBlackBoxWarning	Thrombotic microangiopathy
198100000	1	BLACKBOXWARNING	0004-0018	8	306058006	TICLID	HasBlackBoxWarning	Aplastic anemia
198100000	1	BLACKBOXWARNING	0004-0018	8	230690007	TICLID	HasBlackBoxWarning	Cerebrovascular accident
198100000	1	BLACKBOXWARNING	0004-0018	8	71677004	TICLID	HasBlackBoxWarning	Injury due to exposure to external cause
198100000	1	BLACKBOXWARNING	0004-0018	8	306058006	TICLID	HasBlackBoxWarning	Aplastic anemia
198100000	1	BLACKBOXWARNING	0004-0018	8	281647001	TICLID	HasBlackBoxWarning	Adverse reaction
198100000	1	BLACKBOXWARNING	0004-0018	8	126729006	TICLID	HasBlackBoxWarning	Thrombotic microangiopathy
198100000	1	BLACKBOXWARNING	0004-0018	8	165517008	TICLID	HasBlackBoxWarning	Neutropenia
198100000	1	BLACKBOXWARNING	0004-0018	8	306058006	TICLID	HasBlackBoxWarning	Aplastic anemia
198100000	1	BLACKBOXWARNING	0004-0018	8	281647001	TICLID	HasBlackBoxWarning	Adverse reaction
198100000	1	BLACKBOXWARNING	0004-0018	8	165517008	TICLID	HasBlackBoxWarning	Neutropenia
198100000	1	BLACKBOXWARNING	0004-0018	8	126729006	TICLID	HasBlackBoxWarning	Thrombotic microangiopathy
198100000	1	BLACKBOXWARNING	0004-0018	8	306058006	TICLID	HasBlackBoxWarning	Aplastic anemia
198100000	1	BLACKBOXWARNING	0004-0018	8	281647001	TICLID	HasBlackBoxWarning	Adverse reaction
198100000	1	BLACKBOXWARNING	0004-0018	8	165517008	TICLID	HasBlackBoxWarning	Neutropenia
198100000	1	BLACKBOXWARNING	0004-0018	8	126729006	TICLID	HasBlackBoxWarning	Thrombotic microangiopathy
198100000	1	BLACKBOXWARNING	0004-0018	8	281647001	TICLID	HasBlackBoxWarning	Adverse reaction
198100000	3	INDICATIONSANDUSAGE	0004-0018	2	371040005	TICLID	HasIndicationsForTreatment	Thrombotic stroke
198100000	3	INDICATIONSANDUSAGE	0004-0018	2	230690007	TICLID	HasIndicationsForTreatment	Cerebrovascular accident
198100000	3	INDICATIONSANDUSAGE	0004-0018	2	371040005	TICLID	HasIndicationsForTreatment	Thrombotic stroke
198100000	3	INDICATIONSANDUSAGE	0004-0018	2	78129009	TICLID	HasIndicationsForTreatment	Thrombotic thrombocytopenic purpura
198100000	3	INDICATIONSANDUSAGE	0004-0018	2	17182001	TICLID	HasIndicationsForTreatment	Agranulocytosis
198100000	3	INDICATIONSANDUSAGE	0004-0018	2	165517008	TICLID	HasIndicationsForTreatment	Neutropenia
198100000	3	INDICATIONSANDUSAGE	0004-0018	2	306058006	TICLID	HasIndicationsForTreatment	Aplastic anemia
198100000	3	INDICATIONSANDUSAGE	0004-0018	2	293660003	TICLID	HasIndicationsForTreatment	5-aminosalicylic acid allergy
198100000	3	INDICATIONSANDUSAGE	0004-0018	2	439127006	TICLID	HasIndicationsForTreatment	Thrombosis

Figure 4. Examples of semantic triples identified for Ticlid (ticlopidine) a ADP-induced platelet-fibrinogen binding inhibitor.

3. Discussion

Drug related information accounts for most of the questions that arise on hospital teaching rounds [9]. The IOM report "To Err is Human" reported that adverse reactions account for as many as 98,000 deaths per year in the United States [10]. Adverse drug reactions account for a significant portion of these errors. Authors have reported that clinical decision support associated with computerized physician order entry has the potential to decrease this adverse drug event rate [11-12]. Decision support begins with knowledge that are integrated into a rule based or algorithm driven system. The DailyMed product labels are one important and rich source of drug knowledge. The information density of drug labels provides a rich source of knowledge that can be used to link clinical notes with expert rules aimed at decreasing drug related medical error. Codifying the content of the drug labels makes the knowledge more accessible to computer programs that would operate on this knowledge to try to improve the practice of medicine.

This project identified over 1.5 million semantic triples that can be used to provide the knowledge necessary for important decision support use cases to help prevent adverse drug reactions and in doing so improve patient safety. SNOMED CT™ has a rich set of content which proved quite useful in our efforts to represent drug related knowledge. In the course of this project we made several important observations. First is that the facts in the drug labels often appear to be order dependent with the most important information usually coming earlier in the relevant section of the label. Second is that the majority of drug indications are for prevention or prevention and treatment rather than treatment alone. Third is that it is important for Adverse reactions and Contraindications to know what is the population in which these reactions or contraindications occur and what is their frequency and severity.

Much medical knowledge exists in free text sources such as journal articles, textbooks and clinical guidelines. Natural language processing has the ability to unlock this knowledge and provide rich substrate for clinical decision support systems that seek to deliver that knowledge to clinicians at the point of care.

Future work should seek to further validate the semantic triples in a clinical setting and to integrate this knowledge, represented as semantic triple axioms, into clinical decision support modules of electronic health records.

References

[1] http://dailymed.nlm.nih.gov/dailymed/about.cfm, last access on March 2011.
[2] http://ecfr.gpoaccess.gov/cgi/t/text/text-idx?c=ecfr&tpl=/ecfrbrowse/Title21/21cfr207_main_02.tpl, last access on March 2011.
[3] http://www.fda.gov/downloads/Drugs/GuidanceComplianceRegulatoryInformation/Guidances/UCM072331.pdf, last access on March 2011.
[4] http://www.hl7.org/implement/standards/spl.cfm, last access on March 2011.
[5] P.L. Elkin et al., An evaluation of the content coverage of SNOMED-CT for clinical problem lists, *Mayo Clin Proc* **81** (2006), 741–8.
[6] P.L. Elkin, J.S. Carter, S.H. Brown, Drug Labels Knowledge Representation, submitted to MIE 2011.
[7] http://www.ihtsdo.org/, last access on March 2011.
[8] S.H. Brown et al., eQuality: Automatic assessment from narrative clinical reports, *Mayo Clin Proc* **81** (2006), 1472–81.
[9] J.A. Osheroff et al., Physicians' information needs: analysis of questions posed during clinical teaching, *Ann Intern Med* **114** (1991), 576–81.
[10] http://www.iom.edu/Reports/1999/To-Err-is-Human-Building-A-Safer-Health-System.aspx
[11] B.L. Hug et al., Adverse drug event rates in six community hospitals and the potential impact of computerized physician order entry for prevention, *J Gen Intern Med* **25** (2010), 31–8.
[12] D.W. Bates, Using information technology to reduce rates of medication errors in hospitals, *BMJ* **320** (2000), 788–91.

Patient Safety Informatics
V. Koutkias et al. (Eds.)
IOS Press, 2011

doi:10.3233/978-1-60750-740-6-48

Exploring the Relationship between Usability and Technology-Induced Error: Unraveling a Complex Interaction

Andre KUSHNIRUK[1] and Elizabeth BORYCKI
School of Health Information Science, University of Victoria, Victoria, British Columbia, Canada

Abstract. The effective evaluation of the usability of health information systems is currently a major challenge. It is essential that the applications we develop are not only usable, but that they are also shown to be safe and do not inadvertently introduce errors. Furthermore, to provide appropriate feedback to designers of systems new methods for evaluation are needed as applications become more complex and distributed. To ensure system usability and safety a variety of methods have emerged from the area of usability engineering that have been adapted to healthcare. The authors have applied and adapted methods of usability engineering, working with hospitals and other healthcare organizations for designing and evaluating a range of health information systems over a number of years. We describe a methodological framework for considering some of these advances and show how a range of usability evaluations can be used to evaluate both the usability and safety of healthcare information systems both in artificial mocked up and real clinical settings using in-situ testing approaches. We conclude with a discussion of recent trends in the area of usability engineering in healthcare that have potential for improving the safety of healthcare information systems.

Keywords. Usability engineering, system safety, technology-induced error, usability testing, system evaluation, clinical simulations, in-situ system testing, patient safety

Introduction

Although innovations in health informatics have the potential to dramatically improve and streamline health care, there are a number of critical problems and issues related to their successful implementation and acceptance by end users. One of the main areas of concern involves the following question: how can we ensure that health informatics applications that we develop are usable, meet user information and workflow needs and are safe to use? The design of applications that are intuitive to use and that support human information processing is essential. This has become increasingly recognized as critical as more and more complex software and hardware applications appear in healthcare. Usability is a measure of how effective, efficient and enjoyable a system is to use, and additionally safety is becoming recognized as a component of usability [1]. Closely related to issues of usability are issues of software safety and workflow, with the need to ensure that new devices and software increase patient safety and that workflow can be carried out in an effective, efficient and safe manner. In addition,

[1] Corresponding Author: andrek@uvic.ca

applications targeted to health consumers (e.g. patients and lay people) must also be developed so that they are usable and that the information and advice they provide is both understandable and safe. This is yet another area where evaluation of health information applications is essential.

There are a wide range of approaches to the evaluation of health information systems from the end users' perspective including traditional approaches to evaluation such as surveys, interviews and focus group methods. Additionally, evaluations such as observational studies have been employed to assess system safety after a system has already been deployed for use – i.e. after it has been implemented for use in patient care. Although such approaches are useful for conducting summative evaluations, they may provide limited feedback into specific system redesign and improvement [2]. Furthermore, approaches applied after system deployment do not prevent errors from occurring in the first place that may jeopardize patient safety (i.e. they typically involve observation or interview after a system is already being used for patient care). Questionnaires, focus groups and interviews with users of such applications may provide us with useful information about users' overall perceptions and impressions. However, they are limited in providing detailed information to designers of such systems about how to specifically improve user interfaces and prevent specific problems and errors in complex real world settings. Furthermore, results from such studies may be limited by recall bias and do not give us detailed information about the cognitive processes involved in the often complex interaction between health professionals and information systems [2]. Over the past two decades approaches from the field of usability engineering [3] and cognitive science [2] have appeared in healthcare in an attempt to overcome some of these limitations and provide a complementary set of techniques for the analysis of the impact of systems. This paper describes our work in the development of a framework for considering such approaches to assessing the usability and safety of healthcare information systems based on experience in applying human factors engineering methods in healthcare.

1. Technology-Induced Error in Healthcare Information Technology

Health information technology has the potential to facilitate and improve healthcare processes as well as to increase patient safety. However, over the past several years, it has become clear that poorly designed healthcare systems (and in particular problematic user interfaces to these systems) may be associated with the occurrence of a new class of errors. These errors are termed "technology-facilitated" errors by Koppel and colleagues [4] and in parallel work, they have been termed "technology-induced" errors by Kushniruk, Borycki and colleagues [5]. These types of error may be considered a subclass of unintended consequences of the implementation of information technology in healthcare [6]. In the remainder of this paper we describe our work in identifying and preventing such error through application of approaches emerging from usability engineering and in particular the usability testing prior to widespread system release. This work spans two decades with an initial focus on improving the user experience with healthcare information technology. However, from our earliest work in this area, it was clear that usability problems were inextricably linked to health professional problems in using systems that could result in error [2].

2. Methodological Approach from Usability Testing

The authors have been involved in adapting methods that have been used in the general software industry for improving healthcare systems that can be categorized under the term "usability engineering". The main approach to usability engineering is known as usability testing [3], which is a practical yet scientific approach towards evaluating how usable systems are and can also provide feedback to designers about ways of improving their usability, safety and their integration with workflow. In healthcare, the basic approach involves observing representative end users (i.e. 5-10 participants) of a system (e.g. doctors, nurses or patients) as they carry out representative tasks using health information applications (e.g. entering patient information into a patient record system). Observing users interacting with a system under study typically involves video-recording all the user's interactions with the system (including video recording their physical behavior and also recording all the computer screens). In running such tests the users of such systems may be asked to "think aloud" or verbalize their thoughts as they use the system, while they are video and audio recorded [7].

In healthcare, a number of researchers have applied varied methods adapted from usability engineering to the design and evaluation of healthcare information systems. In the early 1990's a number of groups and laboratories emerged. Their work involved testing and designing healthcare applications. For example, Elkin and colleagues were among the early usability researchers who engaged in testing in a laboratory setting for purpose of designing healthcare applications [8]. Kushniruk, Patel, Cimino and Barrows [9] also described application of usability methods by employing a portable approach to data collection within clinical settings during this period. Over the past two decades a variety of usability laboratories and centers have appeared world-wide [10, 11]. The findings from studies conducted at these labs have been applied not only to provide input into improving user interfaces [9] but have also been used to assess the complex impact of systems on human reasoning [12,13] and more recently workflow and technology-induced error [14,15]. It is interesting to note that the application of usability engineering methods in healthcare has led to the development of new approaches and differing foci as compared to other domains (e.g. aviation and business), with a strong emphasis in healthcare IT around the cognitive aspects and impact of system usability [7]. This may be due to a number of factors, including the complexity of healthcare, a strong cognitive component in many healthcare activities, complex workflows that are very different from many other domains (such as business) and the life critical nature of healthcare applications.

3. Towards a Framework for Considering Usability Studies in Healthcare

As the field of usability engineering in healthcare has progressed and has been demonstrated to differ from other domains, there has been a need for the development of frameworks for considering usability evaluation in healthcare in order to place previous work in context and provide guidance for design of future studies. Figure 1 illustrates a range of possible and future usability studies in healthcare. Along the horizontal axis of the figure a continuum is depicted that ranges from artificial laboratory-based analyses (see left-hand side of Figure 1) to analysis of usability of systems in naturalistic settings in-situ (see right-hand side of Figure 1). In the top portion of the figure is a second continuum related to the level at which usability impacts healthcare (forming a second dimension for considering study design and results). This continuum ranges from impact on individuals using a technology in isolation to the study of the impact of systems at the organizational and health systems levels. In the remainder of this paper this framework will be used to describe current and future work in the area of usability engineering in healthcare, with a particular focus on identifying usability problems that may lead to technology-induced error.

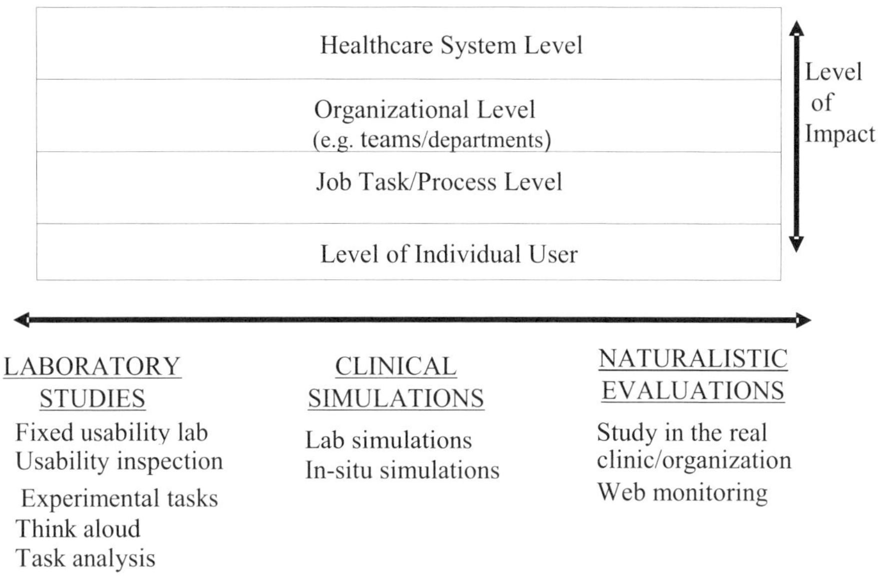

Figure 1. Framework for applying usability engineering to study system safety.

3.1. Laboratory-based Usability Studies Related to Technology-Induced Error

Studies at the laboratory end of the continuum in Figure 1 are typically conducted under artificial conditions. Such studies may attempt to control factors and vary independent variables in the evaluation. Under this category of evaluation we have also included usability inspection methods [16] where a usability analyst evaluates a system in terms of design principles (as no users are involved in such analyses we have classified them at this end of the continuum). Laboratory studies can be conducted for a number of reasons, including the identification of specific usability problems and the impact of specific features of a system (which can be manipulated and evaluated in terms of their impact on cognition or performance) [2]. In the context of healthcare usability studies, laboratory approaches have typically involved testing of subjects interacting with computer systems with one or more variables (e.g. display format) manipulated during testing, with the test being conducted under controlled artificial conditions. Early work by Kushniruk and colleagues [12] and Patel and colleagues [13] is illustrative of these types of studies and examined the impact of computerized patient record systems on an individual user's cognition. In one study, subjects were asked to think aloud while entering patient data into a computerized patient record system while arriving at a diagnosis. In this study case complexity was manipulated as subjects were given cases of varying difficulty, while controlling variables such as the environment and technology used. This type of study could be characterized as being a laboratory-based study (as illustrated in Figure 1) assessing the level of impact of the system at the individual interacting with the system in isolation under artificial conditions. It should be noted that these studies identified not only surface level usability problems, but for the context of analysis of safety, the studies also identified that systems could induce sub-optimal diagnostic reasoning that was associated with medical error.

More recent work using a laboratory style approach examined the potential impact of health information systems in inducing medical error if not designed properly – i.e. technology-induced error. Along these lines we have employed an experimental approach whereby subjects (e.g. physicians) are given tasks (e.g. to enter medications into a handheld prescription writing applications. Our studies using this approach have been run on a range of platforms from palm pilot to more recent work studying the impact of form factor (e.g. iPhones and iPads) on potential for medication error. In many of these studies we have instructed subjects to "think aloud" [5]. The data has then been collected and coded for the occurrence of both usability problems and errors in entering medications [5]. In one study along these lines, the task, study environment and technology were controlled so that the effects of the interface layout on medical error could be isolated. It was found that the occurrence of usability problems in the coded transcripts could be used to predict the likelihood of technology-induced error occurring in medication entry [5]. Specifically, the occurrence of particular usability problems (including problems with the visibility of medication dosages in menus and listing of inappropriate default dosages) was found to be highly related to the occurrence of medication errors. For example, a large percentage of the time inappropriate default appeared in a menu (e.g. for dosage), there was occurrence of one or more deviations from the desired medication administration (i.e. medication errors). The implication of this work is that ineffective user interface designs that might have a negative impact by facilitating medical error could be detected in laboratory settings prior to system release (in order to rectify potentially dangerous usability problems before they have a chance to be widely distributed). In addition, we have extended this laboratory work by using base error rates obtained in these studies as inputs to computer-based simulations and models of error rates once a system would be deployed on a large scale [17].

3.2. In-Situ Clinical Simulation Studies

From Figure 1 it can be seen that we situate simulations halfway along the continuum ranging from artificial laboratory studies to naturalistic evaluations. Such studies typically involve simulations of both the interactions of subjects with computer systems as well as their physical activities in carrying out health related work tasks (e.g. simulations of medication administration activities involving subjects interacting with real or simulated patients). Evaluations based on simulated clinical activities may allow for a high degree of experimental control while at the same time maintaining a high degree of realism in the situations presented to subjects during testing (i.e. a high level of fidelity). Simulations can be conducted in usability laboratories, however from experience we have found a number of limitations of this approach, including the issue that laboratories may not be able to have software or devices actually used in clinical setting easily brought into or accessed from a laboratory for testing purposes (including local interfacing technologies and local work stresses and organizational issues).

Furthermore, there may be circumstances where health professionals, patients or other subjects simply cannot be brought to a laboratory site. Simulations can also be conducted in actual clinical environments (e.g. in hospital wards or operating rooms after hours). The advantages of conducting simulations in real environments when they are available – i.e. in-situ, is that they are less costly to develop (as the physical environment does not need to be constructed or replicated) and they can lead to collection of data more representative of realistic environments and use of systems (as they can often be conducted in the actual environment systems will be used in, including all interfacing technology such as bar code scanning, imaging etc.) [14].

As an example of clinical simulations, in a number of reported evaluations of electronic patient records, physicians' interactions with the system under study can be recorded while the physician interviews a "simulated patient" (i.e. a collaborator playing the part of a patient) in an approach modified from the use of standardized patients in medical education. Kushniruk et al. [12] used this approach to evaluate the effects of usability on doctor-patient interviews. The researchers found that the layout and arrangement of content on the computer screen had considerable impact on the flow and questioning of patients during doctor-patient interviews, where the doctor was entering data into a computerized patient record at the same time as interviewing the patient [12-13]. Other forms of usability evaluations involving simulations at the level of job task/process (see Figure 1) could include the use of realistic mannequins, which serve as patients and can be used to assess use of information technologies in activities such as medication administration.

The advantage of evaluations at the level of simulated work activities can be used to predict the impact of health information systems on clinical activity *before* they are actually released into real clinical settings and used. For example, in our recent work we have examined the impact of medication order entry systems on clinician workflow using realistic clinical simulations conducted in real hospital rooms (with all interfacing technology) after hours [15]. This research involved 16 subjects, consisting of doctors and nurses, who were given instructions for interacting with a medication order entry system to administer medications to a simulated patient. The subjects interacted with both the computer system, the devices (i.e. workstation, bar code scanner) and the "patient", consisting of a standard mannequin. The study took place in a patient room in a hospital with all computer screens recorded using a screen capture program, along with all audio and video captured using a strategically place digital video camera. The simulation varied the number and complexity of medication orders and required the subjects to set up the medications as well as interacting with the computer system to carry out the tasks. From an analysis of the recordings of subjects carrying out the study tasks, it was observed that the system imposed a very sequential order of activities upon medication administration activities [15]. In addition to identifying potential sources of specific problems that would arise from implementation this change was characterized by a serialization and hard wiring of the workflow processes. For example, the nurse or physician would have to administer one medication at a time in a rigid order. Under normal conditions, this might lead to increased safety in medication entry by providing a structured and standardized procedure for medication entry. However, from our simulations it was clear that under certain test conditions (e.g. when there is a need to administer a number of medications under time pressure) the new system could easily result in cognitive overload and error, necessitating complete bypass of the system by users under emergency or stressful situations. It should be noted that such consequences were not anticipated but rather were determined through simulation study, which allowed for sufficient feedback to the system implementation team to mitigate the risk of such error once the system was released. From this and related work it has been argued that such simulation testing of new healthcare information systems (under varying conditions of complexity) may be necessary in order to ensure system safety prior to deployment in real clinical settings [15].

3.3. In-Situ Naturalistic Studies

At the far end of the continuum depicted in Figure 1 are studies involving observational and naturalistic monitoring approaches for observing real healthcare activities. From this perspective, activities and interactions with a system may be monitored or recorded using the same unobtrusive recording techniques that may be deployed in conducted in-situ simulations. The objective of this type of usability study is to determine the impact of systems in real healthcare contexts and to determine if predictions generated using laboratory or simulation based analyses (as described above) are confirmed in real settings. Here an unobtrusive approach is designed, with little or no experimental control [18]. This may involve video recording of user interactions with a system using the same type of screen recording software as is used in laboratory and simulation based studies. In addition, similar types of data analyses (e.g. qualitative coding and identification of usability problems, or medication errors) that are used for laboratory or simulation studies can also be conducted using recordings from "live" interactions of health professionals interacting with systems in real work contexts [19]. This approach more closely approximates the use of the "black box" in aviation safety.

The remote naturalistic evaluation of the use and usability of Web-based healthcare information systems and resources is also becoming recognized as being a critical area within health informatics. We have recently developed a tool that has evolved from our previous research for conducting remote user tracking and usability analysis, known as the Virtual Usability Laboratory (VULab) [19]. The VULab consists of 4 components: (1) a central tracking component for remotely tracking and logging use of Web-based information systems, (2) a component for controlling the presentation of sequenced on-line forms to assess the usability of Web sites remotely, (3) a component for collecting and integrating the results of on-line logging and the results of presentation of other forms of data, such as results from presentation of on-line forms, and (4) a researcher user interface component, designed for evaluators, where parameters control distance evaluations and can be easily set up by the evaluator. The approach allows for the automated integration of a wide range of sources of data, ranging from user logs, collection of on-line demographic questionnaires, collection of remotely recorded computer screens (including video and audio tracks of user interactions with systems) [20]. The data collected are stored in an integrated database system, allowing for subsequent data mining and ad-hoc querying of both quantitative and qualitative data by researchers. The VULab was designed to facilitate the researchers in setting up the parameters for studies and automatically monitoring users of systems. Our current work involves the application of the VULab in the evaluation of Web-based patient record systems, use of health related Web portals by patients and application of on-line clinical guidelines by health professionals (as they are accessed from any Web-accessible location). The automated analysis of a wide range and large amount of both qualitative as well as quantitative data is currently an emerging area in usability engineering and involves new methods borrowed from a number of areas including data warehousing and data mining. We are currently working on applying the approach to identifying the occurrence and frequency of technology-induced error in mining usage and usability data from a range of healthcare information systems.

4. Discussion

Over the past two decades, usability engineering has emerged as an essential approach to the evaluation of healthcare information systems. Based on our experience in conducting a range of usability studies in healthcare we have presented in this paper a framework for advancing usability studies for application in ensuring system safety. This framework considers usability studies along a continuum from laboratory-based studies to simulations of clinical activity (which may be conducted in the laboratory or alternatively conducted in-situ) and naturalistic studies, reflecting one trend in the application of usability engineering to healthcare. A number of other trends have occurred in healthcare usability engineering, including the development of low-cost in-situ approaches to evaluation that can be taken into local health care settings to ensure system safety prior to widespread release within a healthcare organization [11]. The complexity of healthcare as compared to other domains has led to a focus on conducting studies that attempt to capture the complex workflow of healthcare professionals. In addition, a focus on applying usability studies to assess the impact of healthcare information systems on health professionals' cognitive processes has emerged as another trend. Recent concerns about ensuring the safety of healthcare has led to a new wave of studies that have focused on the ability to *predict* and *prevent* technology-induced error.

Work in the application of usability engineering methods, in particular usability testing, now has a considerable history in healthcare IT spanning the past two decades. Much of the early work had involved analysis of user interactions to lead to more effective and efficient systems from the users' perspective. However, right from the beginning, much of this work has had implications for ensuring system safety through the identification of severe usability problems that might lead to medical error once a system is released. More recently, the importance of this has come to the fore in work that has indicated that healthcare information systems may lead to medical error. In our work we have termed such error as "technology-induced" error, which refers to a category of error different from typical software errors – where it is the complex interaction of the user (as a cognitive agent) with a non-optimal user interface design or work sequence that leads to an error. Indeed, our work has shown that there is a close and statistical relationship between specific usability problems and occurrence of technology-induced medical error [5], and that furthermore, such error may be prevented through application of methods involving usability testing and realistic clinical simulations.

References

[1] J. Preece, Y. Rogers, H. Sharp, *Interaction Design: Beyond Human-computer Interaction*, John Wiley & Sons, New York, 2002.
[2] A. Kushniruk, V. Patel, Cognitive computer-based video analysis: Its application in assessing the usability of medical systems, *Proc MED-INFO'95*, 1995, 1566-9.
[3] J. Nielsen, *Usability Engineering*, Academic Press, New York, 1993.

[4] R. Koppel, J.P. Metlay, A. Cohen, B. Abaluck, A. Localio, S.E. Kimmel, B.L. Strom, Role of computerized physician order entry systems in facilitating medication errors, *JAMA* **293** (2005), 1197–203.
[5] A.W. Kushniruk, M. Triola, E. Borycki, B. Stein, J. Kannry, Technology induced error and usability: The relationship between usability problems and prescription errors when using a handheld application, *Int J Med Inform* **74** (2005), 519–26.
[6] J.S. Ash, M. Berg, E. Coiera, Some unintended consequences of information technology in health care: The nature of patient care information system related errors, *J Am Med Inform Assoc* **11** (2004), 104–12.
[7] A.W. Kushniruk, V. L. Patel, Cognitive and usability engineering methods for the evaluation of clinical information systems, *J Biomedical Inform* **37** (2004), 56–76.
[8] P.L. Elkin, D.N. Mohr, M.S. Tuttle et al., Standardized problem list generation, utilizing the Mayo Cannonical Vocabulary embedded within the Unified Medical Language System, *AMIA Annu Symp Proc* (1997), 500–4.
[9] A.W. Kushniruk, V.L. Patel, J.J. Cimino, R.A. Barrows, Cognitive evaluation of the user interface and vocabulary of an outpatient information system, *AMIA Annu Symp Proc* (1996), 22–6.
[10] M. Beuscart-Zephir, S. Pelayo, F. Anceaux, J. Meaux, M. Degroisse, P. Degoulet, Simplifying the complexity surrounding ICU work processes – Identifying the scope for information management in ICU settings, *Int J Med Inf* **74** (2005), 491–503.
[11] A. Kushniruk, E. Borycki, Low-cost rapid usability engineering: designing and customizing usable healthcare information systems, *Healthcare Quart* **9** (2006), 98–101.
[12] A.W. Kushniruk, D.R. Kaufman, V.L. Patel, Y Levesque, P. Lottin, Assessment of a computerized patient record system: A cognitive approach to evaluating an emerging medical technology, *M.D. Computing* **13** (1996), 406–15.
[13] V.L. Patel, A.W. Kushniruk, S. Yang, J.F. Yale, Impact of a computer-based patient record system on data collection, knowledge organization and reasoning, *J Am Med Inform Assoc* **7** (2000), 569–85.
[14] E. Borycki, A.W. Kushniruk, Identifying and preventing technology-induced error using simulations: Application of usability engineering techniques, *Healthcare Quart* **8** (2005), 99–105.
[15] A. Kushniruk, E. Borycki, S Kuwata, J Kannry, Predicting changes in workflow resulting from healthcare information systems: ensuring the safety of healthcare, *Healthcare Quart* **9** (2006), 114–18.
[16] J. Zhang, R. Johnson, V. Patel, D. Paige, T. Kubose, Using usability heuristics to evaluate patient safety of medical devices, *J Biomed Inform* **36** (2003), 23–30.
[17] E. Borycki, A. Kushniruk, J. Anderson, M. Anderson, *Designing and integrating clinical and computer-based simulations in health informatics: From real-world to virtual reality*. In S. Cakaj (Ed.) *Modeling,* Simulation and Optimization: Focus on Applications, In-Tech Publishers, Vukovar, Croatia, 31–51, 2010.
[18] A.W. Kushniruk, C. Patel, V.L. Patel, J. Cimino, Televaluation of clinical information systems: An integrative approach to assessing Web-based systems, *Int J Med Inform* **61** (2001), 45–70.
[19] A.W. Kushniruk, R. Owston, F. Ho, K. Pitts, H. Wideman, C. Brown, S. Chu., Design of the VULab: A quantitative and qualitative tool for analyzing use of on-line health information resources, *Proc ITCH 2007*, 117–21.
[20] H. Wideman, R. Owston, C. Brown, A. Kushniruk, F. Ho, K. Pitts, Unpacking the potential of educational gaming: A new tool for gaming research, *Simulation & Gaming* **41** (2010), 607–29.

Patient Safety Informatics
V. Koutkias et al. (Eds.)
IOS Press, 2011

doi:10.3233/978-1-60750-740-6-57

ICT for Quality and Safety of Care: Beyond Interoperability

Zoi KOLITSI [1]
Informatics and Information Security Laboratory,
Aristotelean University of Thessaloniki, Greece

Abstract. Risk Management in healthcare is a particularly challenging task. From a health system perspective a systemic and person centered approach is needed. From an ICT perspective, continuity of care and sharing information for clinical purposes, research and care improvement can be supported though interoperable systems and services and concurrent ability of proper interpretation of this knowledge by different users. Research provides solutions to specific patient safety challenges. Supporting the dynamics of change will furthermore necessitate strategies to shorten the innovation cycle from research to implementation, deployment, adoption and routine use. Transferring research results to deployable solutions requires in addition a high degree of co-ordination at EU level, with strong links to the national competent organisations and stakeholder communities. The breadth and complexity of the issues that need to be addressed require that an appropriate, EU Collaborative Governance is set up.

Keywords. Patient safety, quality, standards, interoperability, European co-operation, eHealth, collaborative governance

Introduction

Risk Management in healthcare is a particularly challenging task, as it emerges from the interaction of a multitude of interlinked processes and activities that are constituent parts of complex dynamic systems. Healthcare integrated processes are composed of a multitude of interacting activities that exhibit particular characteristics in terms of inputs, processing and outputs. Their emergent properties arising from the interactions of several entities cannot be deduced simply by aggregating their properties. The understanding of risk emergence in healthcare processes is further complicated by the fact that such processes are often part of systems that are artificially separated by different environments and disciplinary boundaries.

From a health system perspective, "patient safety improvements demand a complex system-wide effort, involving a wide range of actions in performance improvement, environmental safety and risk management, including infection control, safe use of medicines, equipment safety, safe clinical practice and safe environment of care", according to WHO (World Health Organisation).

From an ICT perspective, complexity science methods have been applied to develop conceptual frameworks for understanding the dynamics and behaviours of

[1] Corresponding Author: kolitsi@vivodinet.gr

networked complex systems and model complete patient safety loops. A fundamental principle of continuity of care is that health professionals share information about and with patients as well as with other professionals across a number of disciplines, over the whole pathway of the care process. Sharing the necessary information, however, requires that information captured within a particular care episode in a given context by a healthcare professional can be interpreted in exactly the same way by another professional, often of a different professional discipline. This is probably one of the most challenging areas of interoperability as it reaches down into the heart of the clinical content and the interpretation of the medical knowledge.

The European Commission supports several projects focusing their efforts in health systems research. Remarkably, however, so far these projects and initiatives have not established any links with research projects funded under the ICT COOPERATION and PSP programmes, in Europe focusing on ICT enabled services for patient safety.

Experience shows that bringing research results to deployment requires a deeper understanding of the human factors involved. Safety culture must be viewed as a dynamic and multidimensional concept, influenced by a wide variety of individual and group-related personal and professional, organisational, ethical, social, and societal factors. European policy support actions focus on supporting innovation and reducing time from research and development to full service deployment. In these efforts, an interesting observation has emerged: while understanding the dynamics and behaviours of networked complex systems requires the application of conceptual frameworks to simulate their behaviours through *decomposition* and modelling of their individual components properties, proposing realistic and deployable solutions requires a *synthesis* to increasingly higher levels of abstraction bringing together, under a single co-ordinated mechanism, all aspects of our complex organisation of society and public administration [1]. This level of co-ordination will then permit prioritisation and a concrete action plan in order to make innovation a reality for European citizens.

1. Human Factors in Patient Safety

Several recent studies have documented an alarming deficiency of our current systems of care in preventing adverse events. Our current suboptimal ability to manage risk is not due to neglectfulness, but it rather stems from significant deficits in developing a safety oriented environment in healthcare. A substantial proportion of the adverse events which occur annually in healthcare settings in the EU are preventable and effective interventions can be introduced to reduce the effect of error on morbidity and mortality. National and international guidelines on patient safety converge to the need to address simultaneously and in a multidisciplinary way a number of priority areas [2]:

- to support the development of national policies and programmes for patient safety with a focus on the proactive design of safe healthcare systems;
- to develop a mindset for improving patient safety, focused on reducing the harm and suffering of patients and their families and a culture that is receptive to effective working relationships across disciplinary domains; the establishment of transparent, open and honest healthcare professional / patient relationships; and on the involvement, support and empowerment of citizens and patients in their health matters;

- to develop and maintain a culture for patient safety which begins at the time of initial professional training and continues throughout professional life, while patients must be similarly provided with information and education on patient safety and their rights to safe healthcare services and redress;
- to design healthcare systems that make a paradigm shift to focus on continuity of care and information flow across the different levels of care provision and the different actors involved;
- to enable healthcare environments to become learning organisations, encouraging openness and transparency around adverse events, shifting from a blame and shame culture to a supportive and learning paradigm of continuously improving by exploiting such knowledge.

In this area, the International Classification for Patient Safety (ICPS) has been developed under the WHO family of international classifications. While not yet taxonomy, it introduces a conceptual framework aiming to create an accurate view of a patient safety event, in order to gather detailed information for all relevant parameters, including categories to fully describe such events and the circumstances that lead to them.

One way of addressing this complexity in eHealth is through working and solving problems around specific use cases or integrated services. In order to put innovation to practice, a certain degree of re-engineering of processes and workflows across disciplines, organizations and jurisdictions will be necessary. Exploiting the full potential of ICT in healthcare will therefore call for a supportive role of ICT experts and these activities should be driven by the end users and beneficiaries of these services.

The greatest challenge in practice is however in managing the needed change and especially the organizational complexity of a multidisciplinary environment. While new technological challenges will need to be addressed, the focus is shifting more and more towards human factors and the cultivation of a trusted collaborative environment that will sustain an open and transparent dialogue and eventually make this change possible. The transition to a new way of working needs to be an informed decision of both healthcare authorities and the key players that will make it happen.

2. European Co-operation on Common Patient Safety Challenges

Patient Safety and Quality of care in an environment of increasing complexity of health systems, ageing societies and financial pressure are common challenges faced by European member states. The need for continuity of care and safety is also addressed by the Directive of the European Parliament on the application of patients' rights in cross border healthcare, voted by the European Parliament in January 2011, foreseeing that systematic and continuous quality and safety standards are improved following advances in medical science and good medical practices as well as taking into account new health technologies. To this goal, a Joint Action is currently in the pipeline aiming to support Member State collaboration, building on EUNetPaS (European Union Network for Patient Safety) which has been supported by the European Commission within its 2007 Public Health Programme.

Patient safety related ICT research is exemplified by major collaborative research efforts, such as the DebugIT (Detecting and Eliminating Bacteria UsinG Information Technology), PSIP (Patient Safety through Intelligent Procedures in Medication), and

EU-ADR (Exploring and Understanding Adverse Drug Reactions by Integrative Mining of Clinical Records and Biomedical Knowledge) integrated projects which focus on specific patient safety use cases however addressing complete, ICT enabled patient safety learning cycles. They also address semantic interoperability challenges by developing interoperable platforms and infrastructures, federated virtual distributed databases, ontologies, and knowledge management platforms; however, such results cannot be readily transferred to practice. Interoperability, in its extended concept encompassing legal, organisational, technical and semantic challenges is a prerequisite for sharing health information.

European policy support actions focus on improving integration and reducing time from research and development to full service deployment. epSOS[2] is such an action; it is a large scale pilot project (LSP) focusing on cross-border exchange of patient summaries and e-prescriptions, in order to improve safety of care when travelling abroad. epSOS has demonstrated a pragmatic approach to eHealth interoperability including an interesting approach to semantic interoperability and has proven the feasibility of this approach for these two epSOS use cases; epSOS service deployment would however depend on the sustainability of these semantic services. This in turn would require substantial revision of policy in several areas, such as establishing collaborative governance to co-ordinate international efforts towards building and maintenance of the infostructure, as well as funding policies for access and use of e-Heath standards.

The CALLIOPE[3] thematic network has taken these findings one step further by incorporating them into a global view of an *EU eHealth Interoperability Roadmap* describing possible "highways" and presenting a coherent factual basis for decision making. The CALLIOPE Roadmap is developed around four areas of interoperability: legal (including regulatory and ethics); standardisation / technical issues; semantics and identification and authentication. The document makes significant contribution in bringing all elements together into a workable model supporting a common understanding and eventually co-operation on eHealth policy in Europe. While this is not a political document itself, it is drafted with the intent to provide sufficient support in the planning of work and relevant decisions of the European eHealth Governance Initiative (eHGI) at strategic level in Europe. The eHealth Governance Initiative itself brings a new element to the European co-operation - that of a political layer - and presents a unique opportunity to pursue informed decisions on policy alignment in eHealth towards an integrated European health space. The aim remains to be able to boost deployment of eHealth services in Member States though co-operation in appropriate areas at EU level.

3. From Co-operation to Collaborative Governance

What is then necessary is strong co-ordination at all levels. Figure 1 attempts a graphical representation of the areas and levels of consolidation. Health systems and ICT research alike should be driven by common priorities for health policy in associated areas, if the goal of creating an infostructure that will permit re-usability of data in patient records for patient care, health system improvement and public health

[2] European Patients Smart Open Services: http://www.epsos.eu/
[3] CAll for InterOPErability: http://www.calliope-network.eu/

alike is to become possible. A first set of common priorities are by implication, the areas with relevance to cross border care set forward by the cross border care Directive. To these, common national priorities such as chronic disease management are to be added. These priorities shall then drive equally research and policy support actions in the near future.

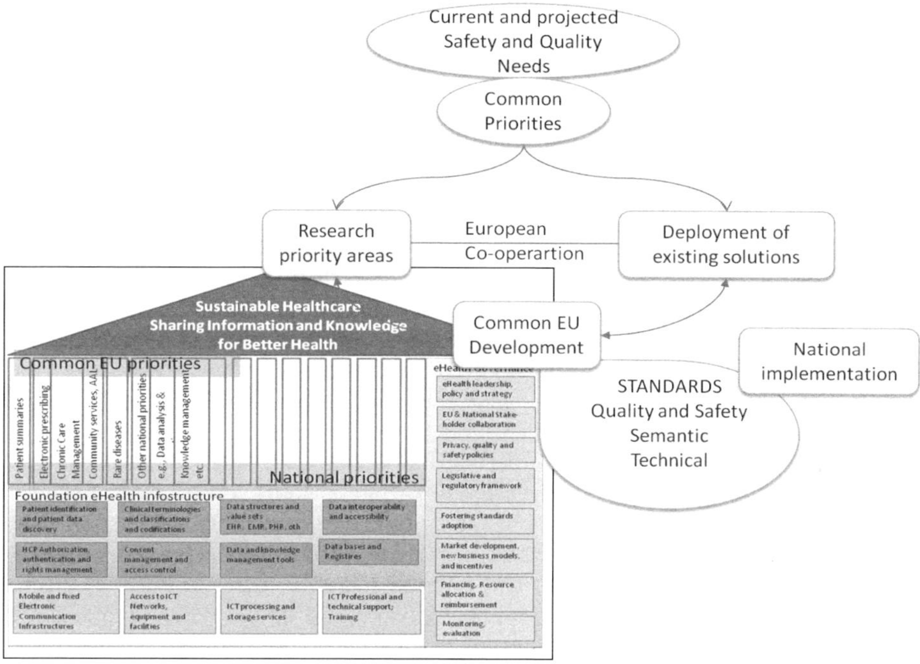

Figure 1. Co-ordinating policy, research and deployment for patient safety. Insert: from the CALLIOPE common working model [1]; the middle Foundation layer refers to eHealth Infostructure and shall benefit particularly from international co-operation.

Supporting the dynamics of change will furthermore necessitate strategies to shorten the innovation cycle from research to implementation, deployment, adoption and routine use. This involves the challenge to integrate research results that address real citizens' needs into health service provision faster and, in turn, provide immediate input to advanced research and development areas. The CALLIOPE Roadmap recommends actions to improve the capacity of healthcare to deal with disruptive innovation throughout the innovation chain. While this could result in better integration and reduced time from research and development to full service deployment, CALLIOPE has not made any recommendations in support of research policy as such.

Pooling resources to address interoperability challenges in common is especially relevant in the area of standards development. Typically, such common priority areas include the development of commonly accepted European quality and safety standards as well as standards to support technical and semantic interoperability. Furthermore, European added value exists in common implementation profiles integrating several components of standards to solve specific common European use cases. The epSOS successful approach has demonstrated how this can be achieved in practice and has unveiled the great challenge of "thinking globally and acting locally" in eHealth, exemplified around its semantic services. Further areas for EU collaboration include the use of open collaborative tools to jointly develop terminologies as well as the development of tools needed to deploy them; common approaches to testing, evaluation, quality assurance, maintenance of semantic resources are typical areas for joint efforts.

Naturally, this co-operation will need to be organized at EU level, however with strong links to the national competent organisations and stakeholder communities. This in turn involves facilitating effective collaboration between the policy, strategy and the operational levels. The breadth and complexity of the issues that need to be addressed as well as the imperative integrity for such a process require that an appropriate EU Collaborative Governance is set up. The establishment of "collaborative governance" is essential for ensuring interoperability, avoiding duplication, optimizing use of resources and ensuring coherent action in a range of crucial areas such as privacy and data protection.

Globally, at the policy level, the political process in the EU will be now driven by the High Level Governance Group (HLGG) at the level of Secretaries of State, that will come under EU governance, encompassing rules, processes and behaviour that affect the way in which powers are exercised at European level [3]. In addition, a scalable and sustainable pan-European organisational and governance process at the operational level is necessary to help ensure that electronic health record systems are optimised for patient care, public health and clinical research across healthcare systems and institutions.

The CALLIOPE Roadmap has particularly considered standards and semantic interoperability as key areas largely catering to multinational collaboration and has called for a priority to empower a collaborative governance framework that will facilitate collaboration of the various stakeholders, including international Standards Development Organisations (SDOs) and relevant industry bodies at all three layers: steering, providing a framework for collaboration and governing rules; strategic, deal with the business (use) cases for each of the stakeholders involved, and empirical, focusing on development around concrete, prioritised use cases in a narrow domain. Overall, there seems to be also consensus about the need for close collaboration with global players, in particular the USA and Canada.

In addition, the CALLIOPE collaborative platform itself has proven its process capability of delivering results of high level of integrity and broad acceptance and has communicated several lessons learned, especially on how clear governance, shared processes, sound expert work, commitments and collective engagement may be pursued and Trust and Confidence be maintained.

References

[1] "Sustainable Healthcare: Sharing Information and knowledge for better health", Common Interoperability Roadmap, CALLIOPE Network, http://www.calliope-network.eu/, last access on March 2011.

[2] Council Recommendation on Patient Safety, including the prevention and control of healthcare associated infection, COM (2008)837 final/2 Commission of the European Communities, Brussels, 2009.

[3] European Governance: a White Paper. (COM(2001) 428 final), Commission of the European Communities, Brussels, 2001.

Part C

Designing IT Systems for Patient Safety

Patient Safety Informatics
V. Koutkias et al. (Eds.)
IOS Press, 2011

doi:10.3233/978-1-60750-740-6-65

Four Principles for User Interface Design of Computerised Clinical Decision Support Systems

Anne Marie KANSTRUP [a], Marion Berg CHRISTIANSEN [b] and Christian NØHR [b,1]
[a] *Department of Communication, Aalborg University*
[b] *Department of Development and Planning, Aalborg University*

Abstract. The paper presents results from a design research project of a user interface (UI) for a Computerised Clinical Decision Support System (CDSS). The ambition has been to design Human-Computer Interaction (HCI) that can minimise medication errors. Through an iterative design process a digital prototype for prescription of medicine has been developed. This paper presents results from the formative evaluation of the prototype conducted in a simulation laboratory with ten participating physicians. Data from the simulation is analysed by use of theory on how users perceive information. The conclusion is a model, which sum up four principles of interaction for design of CDSS. The four principles for design of user interfaces for CDSS are summarised as four A's: All in one, At a glance, At hand and Attention. The model emphasises integration of all four interaction principles in the design of user interfaces for CDSS, i.e. the model is an integrated model which we suggest as a guide for interaction design when working with preventing medication errors.

Keywords. Computerised clinical decision support systems, patient safety, medication errors, human-computer interaction, design principles

Introduction

In this paper we present results from our research on design and evaluation of user interfaces (UI) for computerised clinical decision support systems (CDSS). The research is carried out in the European project Patient Safety through Intelligent Procedures in medication (PSIP), which aims to prevent medical errors through computerised clinical decision support [1]. For this reason our focus is medication errors and we have worked on design solutions for the prescription process.

Computerised decision support systems for the health care environment have been defined as 'computer programs that provide expert support for health professionals making clinical decisions' [2]. This is a quite broad definition, which is difficult to apply as direction for design solutions. Consequently, it has been an ambition to develop models and principles, which can guide design of clinical decision support. In this paper we present a model that summarises four design principles for UI-design derived

---

[1] Corresponding Author: cn@plan.aau.dk

from our design and evaluation of a CDSS prototype aimed to support health care professionals in clinical decisions and prevent medication errors in the prescription process.

First, we present the background of the study, which includes current instruments used for error prevention and the design challenge for UI design of CDSS. Second, we present the process and methods used in the design process. Third we present a theoretical model, which we employ in the analysis of the designed and evaluated prototype. The analytic results are discussed and a concluding model is presented.

1. Background

Computerised information systems are argued to contribute to clinical decision support alone by their ability to integrate information from various distributed information sources [3]. Integrated information is primarily laboratory systems, management systems, patient specific data from health records, medicine information, and clinical systems [3, p. 12 ff.]. Systems integrating information are called "simple" decision support systems [3]. Elsewhere [4] we have introduced this integrated accessibility to information as a "base level" for decision support. Inspired by Liaw et al. [5-6], we have worked with a four level model of decision support in our effort to systematise, design, and analyse CDSS.

1. A base level of categorised information for clinical decision support that require further processing and analysis by users before a decision can be made.
2. A second level we define as information on trends of patients changing clinical status, e.g. graphs or other visual presentations of laboratory results and alerts about out of range assessment results and intervention strategies.
3. A third level is system recommendations, deductive inference engines where diagnostic or intervention recommendations are based on changing patient clinical condition and knowledge and inference engines stored in a knowledge base.
4. Additional advanced solutions are complex knowledge management systems and inference models working with Bayesian networks, self-learning (e.g. neural networks), similarity measures, confidence level computation and the like.

In Denmark, which has been our empirical base, CDSS solutions can be categorised as level one and two. However, even level one is not realised fully. Danish health care systems consist primarily of a patchwork of proprietary information systems with low integration from one system to the other. A video recorded observation of the work practice of a physician and a nurse at a Danish cardiology ward that we carried out initially in the PSIP project, shows that consequences of this lack of integration are remarkable [7]. Analysis of the video observations focused attention on how many different information sources – various IT-systems as well as paper sheets – the physician and the nurse consult while making decisions medication for a patient. After the decision is made the computerised provider order entry (CPOE) system is used as a data entry system to perform the actual prescription [7].

At the second level Danish systems traditionally use alarms and gates as instruments in error prevention. These instruments are well known within medication procedures [3] and transferred to computer systems. Alarms vary in types from red bold text warnings, to pop-up windows which the user can remove with a mouse click on an "ok" button, to alarm pop up's where the user is required to type a text explaining why a warning is ignored. Gates are designed to secure a procedure. Gates are widely used within drug prescribing and it is argued that computerised systems can support gates [3]. In Danish CPOE systems gates are primarily seen where users are required to fill in text boxes before they are allowed to move on to the next level in the prescription process.

Evaluations of computerised decision support show that these commonly used instruments - alarms and gates - are important but also problematic solutions since they tend to slow down the clinical work, which results in alarm fatigue and work-arounds and naturally means that the design is not used as intended and errors are most likely not prevented as intended [3]. In our empirical work clinical professionals have raised these problems as most important [4] and our data material includes numerous accounts of work-arounds, ignored alarms, irritation regarding system use etc.

Since our first video observations and workshop activities with health care professionals it has been clear that designing computerised clinical decision support calls for finding a very fine balance between perceived affordance and perceived annoyance.

2. Methods and Material

The design and evaluation of a user interface for CDSS has been organised in an iterative design process with series of meetings between clinicians, researchers and software developers including workshops, interviews and simulations.

The first step was a design workshop. The outcome from the design workshop was a number of design principles for computerised decision support systems, which was implemented in a paper mock-up [4]. Second, a number of clinicians discussed and revised the mock-up, which in turn was further developed into a running prototype shell. This first prototype was tested in an authentic simulation environment to give the clinicians a hands-on experience with a possible realisation of their original ideas. Their feedback from the simulation provided the final input for the design and implementation of a real prototype integrated with the commercial CPOE system used in the regional hospitals.

The final prototype provides decision support to the physician during the prescription process. This is accomplished by embedding adverse drug events (ADE) responses from a decision support module on the prescription screen based on the choices of drug to be prescribed and the conditions of the patient. In the same screen a selection of additional information is presented to give the overview demanded by the clinicians. The screen used in the prescription process is shown in Figure 1. Panel ① corresponds to the patient identification data: name, unique personal identifier, birth date, and age. Drug allergies are listed in panel ②. Panel ③ present the observation diagnosis. Here the first physician who sees the patient can inform the later prescribing physicians about the hypothesis of the patient's main problem. The patients' confirmed earlier diagnoses are listed in panel ④. Test results, pulse, temperature, and blood pressure are presented in panel ⑤. A special feature allows the user to select specific test results to be presented graphically in a pop-up window as in Figure 2. The patient's current medication list is shown in panel ⑥. In panel ⑦ the new drug is selected. As soon as a drug is chosen the decision making mechanism is launched through the PSIP CDSS engine [8], and if any of the rules are triggered, the relevant alerting information will appear in panel ⑧. A double click on triggered rules will bring up elaborated information about the rule in a pop-up window illustrated in Figure 3.

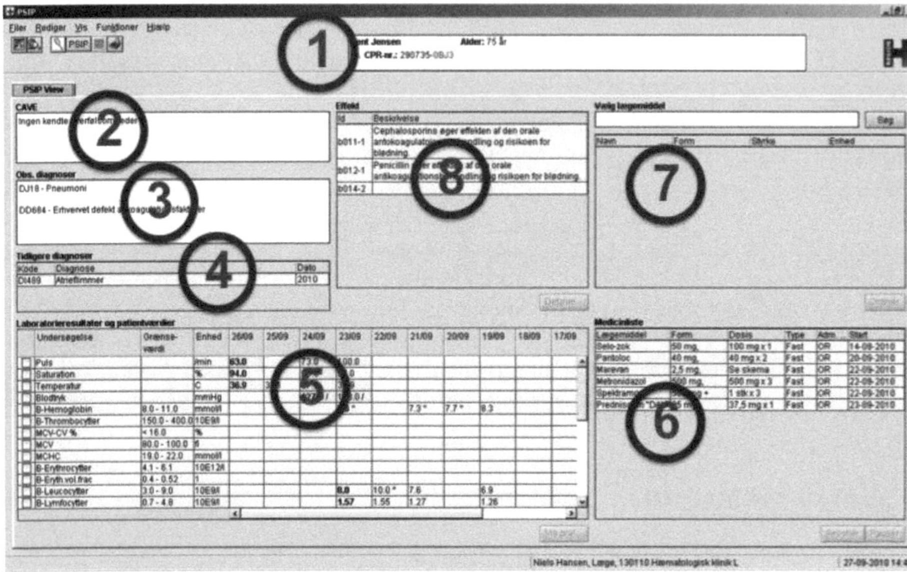

Figure 1. The panels in the main UI screen.

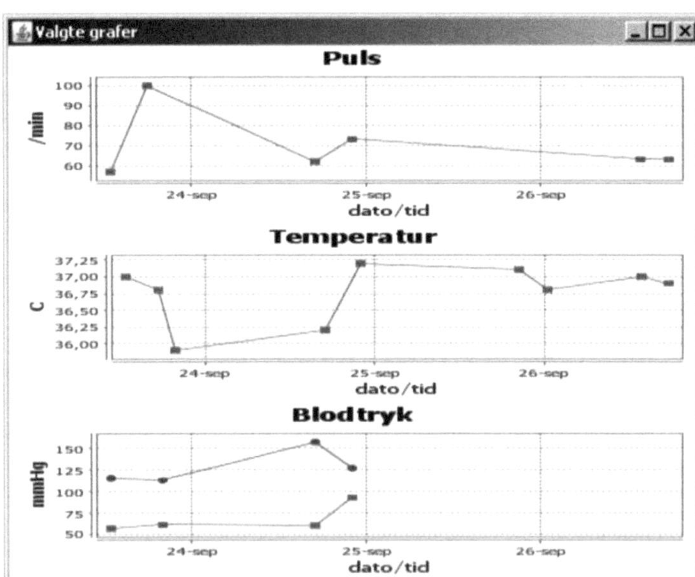

Figure 2. Pop-up window showing graphics of selected patient measurements.

The design of the final prototype balances the requirement of an efficient and straightforward prescription process with the requirement to inform the prescribing physician about ADE responses regarding patient safety.

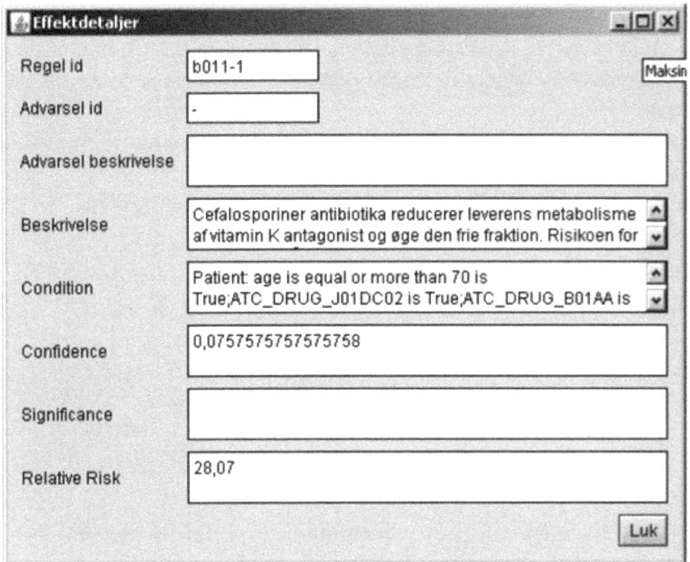

Figure 3. Pop-up window showing further details about a particular rule.

A primary goal for the prototype has been to place the response from the decision support module in focus of the healthcare professional during the prescription decision process. Placing the decision support in the central part of the application panel and placing other groups of information with a more immediate and natural interest of the physician around it accomplishes this.

The prototype has been tested in a simulation laboratory with ten participating physicians. Each physician had to go rounds in one of two bedrooms (B2 or B3) where they used the system to prescribe medicine to 2 or 3 patients. The patients were actors instructed to play the role of a particular patient with specific diseases [9]. The screens of the computers running the system were captured in a video file and the actions in the simulation was video recorded with ceiling mounted cameras as well as hand held cameras. After the test the physicians were interviewed, and the data from the interviews are analysed in the following.

3. A Model for Analysis

Our focus is on designing the human-computer interaction, i.e. the user interface, which the user interacts with. Consequently, we give attention to how users relate to information they perceive on the screen. From this perspective we have found and used Bates generic model of information search widely applied in information science [10].

The model focuses on users' ways of relating to information. It is a matrix model with:

- a horizontal column representing how users relate to information from the system, actively or passively, and
- a vertical column representing how information is provided by the system, as directed or undirected information.

Directed information is information, which users seek. Undirected refers to information that the user is more or less randomly exposed to.

'Active' and 'passive' refer, respectively, to whether the user actively acquires information or is passively available to absorb information, but does not seek it out by intentional effort.

Based on the level of directedness and action, the model comprises four basic types of information search:

- directed active, which is what we normally mean by 'search',
- undirected active, which is called 'browsing',
- directed passive called 'monitoring', and
- undirected passive called 'awareness'.

This is summarised in Figure 4.

Generic ways of relating to information	**Active**	**Passive**
Directed	Searching	Monitoring
Undirected	Browsing	Being aware

Figure 4. Bates model of four generic types of information related behavior [10].

4. Analysis

When Bates' model is applied to the PSIP prototype it is clear that the prototype supports the user to relate actively to the information provided by the system. The prototype relies on the users' active search and browsing for information. Main information i.e. laboratory data, drug information and prescriptions, are directed while allergies and information about effects, which appear when rules are fired, are undirected.

As mentioned in section 2, the prototype design was based on co-operation with health care professionals who especially were concerned about alarm fatigue. They emphasised their own professional competencies and abilities to make decisions, but expressed a need for integrated data as support to do so. The result is a portal-metaphor where the user searches for relevant information and browses for warnings. Figure 5 sums up how users from the simulation test relate to the PSIP prototype.

The physicians participating in the simulation of the PSIP prototype were primarily positive towards the interaction with the user interface. However, they called for additional information and in general broader information focus in the design of the user interface. This is summarised in the following.

In general the results are positive in relation to integrating central information sources in one screen. This is regarded as an overview where users can search and access information easily. Examples of positive reactions from users are: "*I think it is really nice. I think the fact that blood pressure and pulse and blood samples are in [the same window] I think it is great! I definitely think it is. That was really, really nice*" (senior physician).

"It is really, really nice that all this information is available at the same time. It is really... you know, normally I have five windows open at the bottom and that is quite awkward and annoying at ward rounds. I think it's really nice that it all shows here." When asked if it gives a better overview he says: *"Exactly! Yes, yes, because you can see everything at the same time and get it, right"* (junior physician).

Generic ways of relating to information	**Active**	**Passive**
Directed	Integrated information i.e. observation diagnosis, previous diagnosis, laboratory test results, and current medication	None
Undirected	Information on drug allergies and effect when rules are fired from the PSIP CDSS engine.	None

Figure 5. The PSIP prototype design in relation to the generic types of information.

Junior physicians received the effect window positively, while senior physicians argued that this was mainly of relevance to juniors. Examples of positive reaction from junior physicians are: *"As I see it now I regard it as a toy that is supposed to make me aware when there might be something to be aware of"* (junior physician).

"I'm sure it's very helpful if it works, because I don't know all the interactions and I wouldn't look every last one of them up, and I know some medications are troublesome and I might look those up, but when you have a medication list that long and you have a lot of patients you have to see to, you just don't have the time to do it." (junior physician).

Overview of data in one screen was a primary subject during the design process [4]. The simulation test rather emphasised a need for monitoring of developments in patients clinical status. Here it is especially emphasised that the presentation of data is essential. Keyhole access to data where frequent scrolling is required to see all the data is not acceptable. The users require an easy access and informative picture of development. Consequently, data and their organisation are important. Examples of calls from the users are:

"We have for some time asked for this interface where we have more information, but working especially with this [PSIP system]... *first of all, some of the patients were very hard to get an idea of their total medication because you had to scroll up and down. And I had some problems with the laboratory results because things move and I had to get the left side back (...) It was a bit difficult to scroll up and down. I lost track sometimes."* (senior physician).

"I have difficulties getting an overview of the medication, because I have to scroll that much up and down I lose overview." (junior physician).

Alarm fatigue was a primary subject during the design process [4]. The simulation test rather emphasised a need for awareness support – that the system warns the user, i.e. from active users seeking information to passive users relying on system warnings. Examples of statements from the users on how they perceived the PSIP prototype where warnings called for active users are:

"I didn't get any warning I'm supposed to think of it myself (...) I have to realise it myself, because I tried to order Pinex [Danish trade name for paracetamol] *and I actually could do that without it telling me that I wasn't supposed to* [the patient had allergies to paracetamol]. *I think that is dodgy*" (junior physician).

"That's dangerous! I think that's dangerous because we're used to the other part, we're used to warnings" (junior physician).

The results from the test and analysis of human factors issues are summarized in Figure 6.

Generic ways of relating to information	**Active**	**Passive**
Directed	The main interface with the most used and relevant data is perceived as a good overview. It is stressed that several parts of the interface could be smaller. The main point is to get the overview and from this entry be able to access further details, i.e. open new windows.	The laboratory data and medicine lists are too small for the users to be able to follow developments. It is stressed that especially these two types of information must be designed so they support the users in 'at a glance' see developments in patient data, i.e. no scroll.
Undirected	The effect is perceived as a nice tool especially for junior physicians. If the information is informative this also saves time to look up information elsewhere.	Warnings must call for the users' attention. It is perceived as too dangerous to rely on the physician to look up this information.

Figure 6. Results from analysis of human factors issues of the PSIP prototype.

5. Conclusion

The results from the simulation of the PSIP test have emphasised a perspective on several but integrated types of information and interaction. Consequently, we conclude on a need for an integrated perspective on design of computerised clinical decision support. Our results point out four principles of interaction for design of CDSS. The four principles include:

- Directed active information where focus is on search. Important is that the user gets an overview. We call this interaction principle <u>All in one</u>.
- Undirected active information where focus is on browsing. Users are able to unfold information and browse along in the search for knowledge. Important is that information is accessible. We call this interaction principle <u>At hand</u>.
- Directed passive information where focus is on monitoring. Important is that the user easily can follow developments. We call this <u>At a glance</u>.
- Undirected passive information where focus is on awareness. Important is that the system warns the user. We call this interaction type <u>Attention</u>.

Following these conclusions, Figure 7 sums up the four principles for design of user interfaces for CDSS as four A's: All in one, At a glance, At hand and Attention. The model emphasises integration of all four interaction principles in the design of user interfaces for CDSS, i.e. the model is an integrated model which we suggest as a guide for interaction design when working with preventing medication errors.

User is: / Information is:	**Active**	**Passive**
Directed	**All in one** The user gets an overview. Support searching.	**At a glance** The user can easily follow developments. Support monitoring.
Undirected	**At hand** The user has access to information. Support browsing.	**Attention** The user is warned. Support awareness

Figure 7. The four A's model of interaction design for CDSS.

Acknowledgements

The research leading to these results has received funding from the European Community's Seventh Framework Programme (FP7/2007-2013) under grant agreement n° 216130 – the PSIP project.

Thanks to the participating clinicians from hospitals in the Capital Region in Copenhagen, the colleagues from the PSIP project and "patients" participating in the simulation. For pointing us to Bates model we thank our colleague at Aalborg University: Ellen Christiansen.

References

[1] http://www.psip-project.eu/, last access on March 2011.

[2] S. Phansalkar et al., A review of human factors principles for the design and implementation of medication safety alerts in clinical information systems, *J Am Med Inform Assoc* **17** (2010), 493–501.

[3] Dansk Selskab for Patientsikkerhed & Dansk Lægemiddel Information A/S: *Beslutningsstøtte til elektronisk medicinordination* (Decision support for electronic medicine prescription). Copenhagen, Denmark, April 2005.

[4] A.M. Kanstrup, C. Nøhr, Gaming against medical errors: methods and results from a design game on CPOE, *Stud Health Technol Infor* **148** (2009), 188–96.

[5] S.T. Liaw, P. Schattner, Electronic decision support in general practice. What's the hold up?, *Aust Fam Physician* **32** (2003), 941–44.

[6] NICT: Report of the electronic decision support governance workshop. Melbourne: National Institute of Clinical Studies, November 2001.

[7] C. Nøhr, M. Sørensen, A. Kushniruk, Method for testing a CPOE system in the medication process in a cardiology ward, *Stud Health Technol Inform* **160** (2010), 183–7.

[8] V. Koutkias et al., A knowledge engineering framework towards clinical support for adverse drug event prevention: the PSIP approach, *Stud Health Technol Inform* **148** (2009), 131–41.

[9] K. Lawton, K. Binzer, P. Skjot, S. Jensen, Lessons learnt from conducting a high fidelity simulation test in health IT, *Stud Health Technol Inform* **166** (2011), 217–226.

[10] M.J. Bates, Toward an integrated model of information seeking and searching, *New Review of Information Behaviour Research* **3** (2002), 1–15.

Patient Safety Informatics
V. Koutkias et al. (Eds.)
IOS Press, 2011

doi:10.3233/978-1-60750-740-6-74

Implementation of a Taxonomy Aiming to Support the Design of a Contextualised Clinical Decision Support System

Stéphanie BERNONVILLE [a,1], Romaric MARCILLY [a], Radja MESSAI [b], Nicolas LEROY [a], Emma PRZEWOZNY [b], Nathalie SOUF [b] and Marie-Catherine BEUSCART-ZÉPHIR [a]

[a] *INSERM CIC-IT Evalab, CHU Lille, UDSL EA2694, Univ Lille Nord de France, F-59000 Lille, France*

[b] *Centre d'Etude et de Recherche en Informatique Médicale, UDSL EA2694, Univ Lille Nord de France, F-59000 Lille, France*

Abstract. Clinical Decision Support Systems (CDSS) are recently implemented in hospital settings to improve the reliability of drug ordering. However, such systems have limited effects due to their tendency to over-alert. To healthcare professionals consider alerts, it is necessary to adapt the CDSS to their activity. Thus, it is necessary to consider contextualisation aspects in the system design. In this article, we propose a taxonomy integrating contextualisation elements issued from an activity analysis to guide the design of a contextualised CDSS. This taxonomy has been developed within the framework of the European project PSIP (Patient Safety through Intelligent Procedures in medication) aiming to make easier the identification and the prevention of Adverse Drug Events.

Keywords. Taxonomy, contextualisation, clinical decision support system, design, medical informatics

Introduction

To improve the reliability of the medications' use process in hospital, Clinical Decision Support Systems (CDSS) are coupled with Computerised Physician Order Entry (CPOE). Thus, CDSS provide healthcare professionals or patients with computer-generated clinical knowledge and patient-related information, intelligently filtered or presented at appropriate times, to enhance patient care [1].

However, the way of alerting got limits. Indeed, alerts often interrupt healthcare professionals' activity by being not displayed at the right time and/or at the right actor (inadequate display); moreover, they are often too numerous and most of them are considered as irrelevant by healthcare professionals. Together, those problems lead to "alert fatigue" and therefore to an overriding of the alerts

---

[1] Corresponding Author: stephanie.bernonville@univ-lille2.fr

or a deactivation of the CDSS. To fix the "inadequate display" and the "over alerting" problems, the CDSS behavior must be adapted to the healthcare professionals' activity and needs. Consequently, the context of the alert must be taken into account in the design of the system [2]. The definition we apply for context is the one proposed by Dey [3], i.e. context is "all the information which can be used to characterize an entity situation (person, physical or computer object); and globally, all the elements which can affect a system behavior".

To guide the design of Contextualised CDSS (CX-CDSS), it is necessary to identify relevant and useful information to be considered. To that end, we elaborated a taxonomy gathering all relevant information and integrating contextualisation elements derived from an activity analysis. This approach allowed extracting interesting *context,* then identifying *contextualisation elements* in the taxonomy and focusing on corresponding necessary real data to be considered for the design of CX-CDSS (Figure 1).

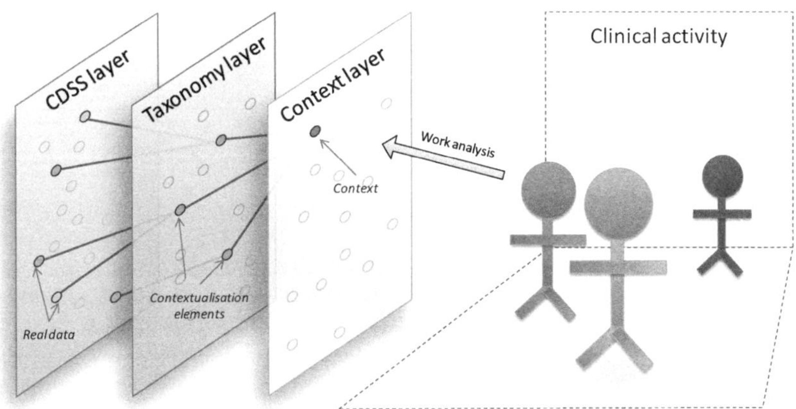

Figure 1. Contextualisation principle in the taxonomy.

The taxonomy presented in this paper is based on the PSIP project experience. The European project PSIP (Patient Safety through Intelligent Procedures in medication - http://www.psip-project.eu/) aims at developing and demonstrating innovative tools so as to generate and provide relevant knowledge to healthcare professionals and patients for Adverse Drug Event (ADE) prevention by means of Information and Communication Technologies (ICT) and data/semantic mining techniques [4-5].

The PSIP taxonomy has been elaborated from the PSIP data model developed to structure medical data issued from hospital databases. The objectives of this data model are to (1) make easier their use in data-mining process to detect potential ADEs and (2) to support a data architecture usable in the PSIP prototypes. Now, this data model contains only relevant information for the detection of potential ADEs and does not take into account context elements (as uses or decision making contexts). Thus, it has been decided to improve the data model and to turn it into a model usable to guide the design of CX-CDSS.

This paper presents the PSIP taxonomy and particularly the process leading to its design and the integration of contextualisation elements. First, the origin of the PSIP taxonomy is described followed by a description of its overall structure. Then an application example is presented just before a discussion.

1. Origin and Development of the PSIP Taxonomy

The PSIP taxonomy comes from a collaborative work between PSIP project's partners: ergonomists, computer scientists and medicine/pharmacology experts worked together to ensure that every element it contains is relevant and that its structure is coherent. All along the development of this taxonomy, each kind of professional provided its point of view: "design" point of view for computer scientists, "medical knowledge" point of view for medicine/pharmacology experts and "actual work" point of view for ergonomists.

The starting point of the collaborative work was the PSIP data model and meeting after meeting, several kinds of elements (namely existing taxonomy elements, work analysis elements, reference data and terminology specific to PSIP) has progressively been added to develop the more exhaustive possible taxonomy. At each work meeting, a free mind-mapping software, called "Freemind©" (http://freemind.sourceforge.net/wiki/index.php/Main_Page) has been used to make easier the discussion and the organisation of the ideas through a tree structure.

1.1. The PSIP Data Model

The PSIP data model [6] is made up of information about "stays", "steps of the stay", "diagnosis", "medical procedure" "drug prescriptions", "lab results", "reports" and "semantic mining"[2]). This data model has been the starting point for the development of the PSIP taxonomy. It allows ensuring the structuring of medical data issued from hospital databases that are used to detect the ADEs' cases.

1.2. Elements Issued from Existing Taxonomies

The incorporation of an existing ADEs' taxonomy was mandatory to get already structured and large knowledge about this topic. However, before using elements from an existing taxonomy to design the PSIP one, we had to select amongst those dealing with the ADEs' issue, the most in agreement with the PSIP project's aims. To this end, seven international taxonomies (or reports' forms on medications errors) have been compared to PSIP data model:

- NCC-MERP [7]: National Coordinating Council for Medication Error Reporting and Prevention, http://www.nccmerp.org
- AAQTE [8]: Association for Quality Assurance in Therapeutics and Evaluation, http://adiph.org/aaqte/index.html

[2] In some hospitals, semantic mining techniques are used to extract ICD10 codes (International Classification of Diseases) and ATC codes (Anatomical Therapeutic Chemical classification) from medical reports. A specific table allows the storage of these codes.

- USP-ISMP [9]: US Pharmacopeia (USP) - Institute for Safe Medication Practices, https://www.ismp.org/orderForms/reporterrortoISMP.asp
- MedWatch: US FDA, http://www.fda.gov/medwatch
- ICPS [10]: International Classification for Patient Safety (ICPS), http://www.who-icps.org/
- DPSD - Danish Patient Safety Database Danish National Board of Health, http://www.dpsd.dk/
- JCAHO [11]: Joint Commission on Accreditation of Healthcare Organisations (US).

Two comparison criteria have been used:

- The focus of the taxonomy: all taxonomies compared were not specifically dedicated to ADEs. Thus, we had to ensure their composition was compatible with the PSIP project's aim.
- The two key-points of the PSIP data model are the administered medications and the lab tests results. Thus, it was mandatory that both points were contained in the compared taxonomy.

Figure 2 presents the result from the comparison among existing taxonomies and the PSIP data model.

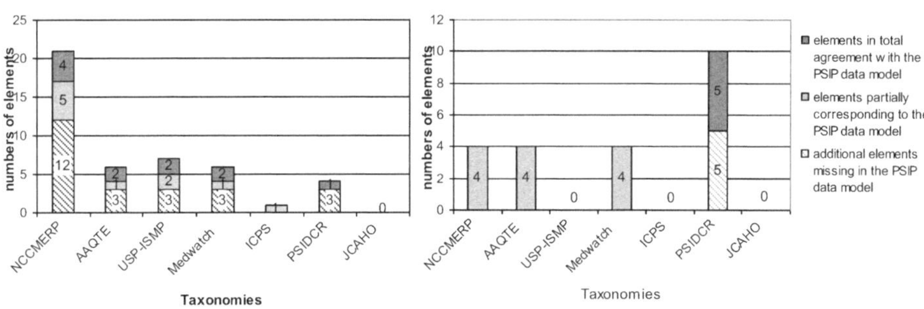

Figure 2. Numbers of elements dealing with the medications (left) and the lab tests (right) in the compared taxonomies according to those present in the PSIP data model.

This comparison reveals that NCC-MERP fits the most to PSIP data model as regards to the medication's items and that PSIDCR fits the most as to the lab test's items. However, only NCCMERP is dedicated to the ADEs' report: thus, it is the taxonomy that suits most to the PSIP project. So, its structure and components have been used to feed the PSIP taxonomy.

1.3. Elements from a Work Analysis of the Patient Care Process

To know which elements of context constraining healthcare professionals' works, an ergonomics work analysis has been carried out [12]: ergonomists proceed to observations of actual work healthcare professionals taking in charge patients in hospital. Results allowed identifying key points to which the CX-CDSS should adapt [13]. For example, a key-point in the making of the therapeutic decision is that the physician needs to have not only the medications previously ordered but also relevant lab test results in mind. Indeed, since the patient's condition is evolving naturally and under the effect of the medications, each lab tests results has its own validity duration. Thus, for their results to be pertinent and useful for the therapeutic decision, they must be regularly ordered and performed anew. So, those elements have been included in the PSIP taxonomy.

1.4. Reference Data

Reference data are elements to which a CX-CDSS should refer to have a standard and common description of medical data. Indeed to ensure the PSIP taxonomy is interoperable with Hospital Information System PSIP taxonomy integrates a set of existing national and international reference data terminologies for common identification of medical data (e.g. ATC[3] codes, IUPAC[4] codes), basic medical information (for example, standard name of lab analysis). For the CX-CDSS to be compliant with the PSIP project results and innovation in term of ADEs' detection and prevention, references specific to the PSIP context have also been embedded in the PSIP taxonomy. For example, for the CX-CDSS to support healthcare professionals' activity; relevant set of information such as "action's suggestions to be undertaken to manage an ADE" have been added.

1.5. Specific terms derived from the PSIP Context

To integrate the whole knowledge created in the PSIP project, specific terms have been defined and included in the PSIP taxonomy. For example, data-mining techniques have been used to generate a set of ADE detection rules[5]; a work analysis has been performed. This knowledge has been integrated thanks to our own specific terms as "data-mining rules", "use context".

2. Results

2.1. Overview of the PSIP Taxonomy

The PSIP taxonomy is represented through a tree-structure composed with categories and sub-categories of terms. Figure 3 represents an overall view of the PSIP taxonomy[6]. The entire PSIP taxonomy is available at the following Web address: http://www.psip-project.eu/index.php?q=node/843.

The PSIP taxonomy is organised according to four categories:

- **"Operational Knowledge"** category gathers all the terms dealing with the knowledge production. According to their origin, the elements have been sorted into two sub-categories: "PSIP knowledge" and "Other knowledge".
- **"Patient record"** category gathers all relevant terms for the PSIP project dealing with medical data that can feed the CX-CDSS. For this

[3] Anatomical Therapeutic Chemical
[4] International Union of Pure and Applied Chemistry
[5] Association of drugs and patient characteristics for which ADEs can be triggered.
[6] For clarity sake, only main categories and sub-categories are displayed.

reason, the category contains the PSIP data model. The elements are sorted into six sub-categories: "drug", "other products", "administrative information", "physiological parameters", "observations" and "laboratory techniques and procedures".

- **"Setting"** category gathers all the relevant terms for the PSIP project dealing with the hospital organisation. It is based on a work analysis of the patient care process. The elements are sorted into four sub-categories: "environment", "time", "agents" and "management of patient care process".
- **"Reference data"** category aims at gathering elements issued from existing standards. It is subdivided into "general reference data" (i.e. raw elements from existing standards, e.g. it is useful to use common terminologies as ICD10 to ensure the system be interoperable) and "specific reference data" (new organisation of standards elements to make them useful in the PSIP context, e.g. suggestions' base to monitor or counter an ADE).

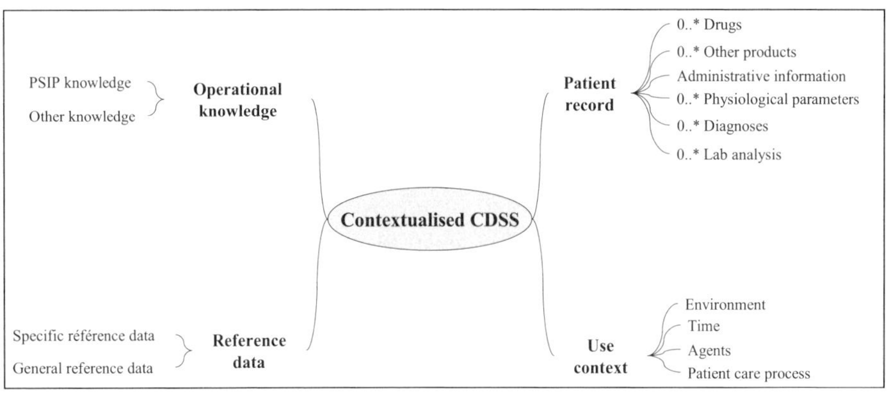

Figure 3. Overview of the PSIP taxonomy.

2.2. Application Example of the PSIP Taxonomy

To show an application example of the PSIP taxonomy, especially the integration of contextualisation elements, we chose to focus on an example of context identification derived from the activity analysis of patient care process performed by ergonomists involved in the PSIP project. This specific context concerns the making of the therapeutic decision is that the physician needs to have not only the medications previously ordered but also relevant lab test results in mind. Indeed, the performed work analysis revealed that, during the medical round, for 83% of the patients for whom he is looking at the medications, the physician looks also at lab tests results for they are informing about the medications' effect. The intertwinement between medications and lab test results has an impact on the healthcare professionals' work.

This constraint on the healthcare professionals' work has been embedded in the PSIP taxonomy into the categories "use contexts" and "PSIP knowledge" (cf. 2.3.). Firstly, figure 4 represents the integration of the context key point in the PSIP taxonomy. Thus, the "Reading of lab results reports" element is represented in the "use context" category. Now, this "use context" element have to be linked with other elements of the PSIP taxonomy to determine which information are relevant and useful for the CX-CDSS.

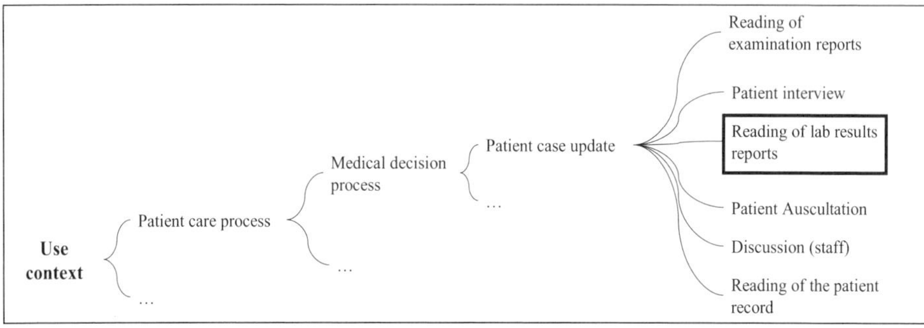

Figure 4. Excerpt of the representation of the PSIP taxonomy focusing on the context element "reading of lab test results".

Four contextualisation elements determining the state of the lab results report and consequently its use have been identified and included in the PSIP taxonomy. They allow defining the context in which the physician is ordering medications (by answering the questions linked to the elements) in terms of relevant and useful information for the CX-CDSS. The four contextualization elements are the following:

- **Availability** of the lab results to monitor:
  Is the lab test result linked to the potential ADEs detected is available?
- **Normality of** the lab test result to monitor:
  Is the lab test results linked to the potential ADEs detected into acceptable threshold?
- **Recency** of the lab test result to monitor:
  Is the lab test results linked to the potential ADEs detected recent enough to be considered?
- **Order** of the lab test whose result should be monitor:
  Is the lab test already ordered?

Figure 5 represents the integration of those four contextualisation elements into the "Operational knowledge" category of the PSIP taxonomy.

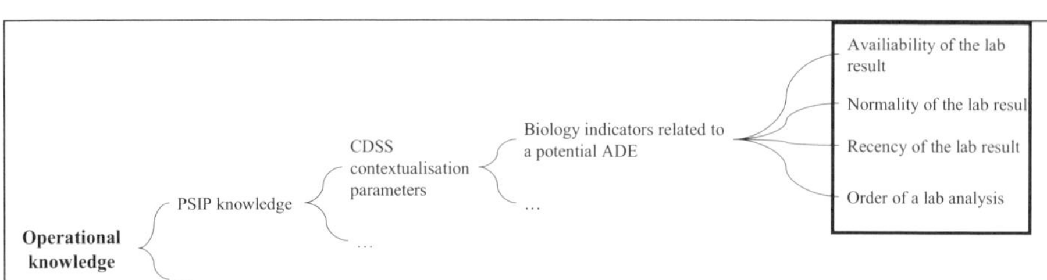

Figure 5. Excerpt from the PSIP taxonomy focusing on the four contextualisation elements.

The identification of relevant and useful information made, it is necessary to focus on the corresponding real data to be considered in the design of the CX-

CDSS. The figure 6 focuses on the specific context concerning the intertwinement between medications and lab test results for the making of the therapeutic decision derived from the work analysis. This context has been identified by the "Reading of lab results" use context element in the taxonomy and more precisely by the "order of the lab test", "recency of the lab result", "availability of the lab result" and "normality of the lab result" contextualisation elements. Then for each contextualisation element real data to be considered in the design of the CX-CDSS can be identified. For example, the "order of the lab test" information can be localised in the lab orders list from the CPOE system eventually connected to the CDSS system. The "recency of the lab result" information can be computed thanks to the date of the lab results and the date of the current day. Finally, the consideration of those four elements in the design of the CX-CDSS will allow adapting the display of alerts. For example, the physician has already ordered a monitoring of the biological parameter and the last result is normal. Thus, the CX-CDSS identifies the following context: there is a result of lab test linked to the identified ADE that is recent enough and normal. The case is under control, thus, the physician should not be bothered with an intrusive alert.

In conclusion, the PSIP taxonomy provides relevant elements allowing the design of a CX-CDSS, especially as regards the display of alerts and avoiding the over-alerting issue thanks to the consideration of contextualisation aspects.

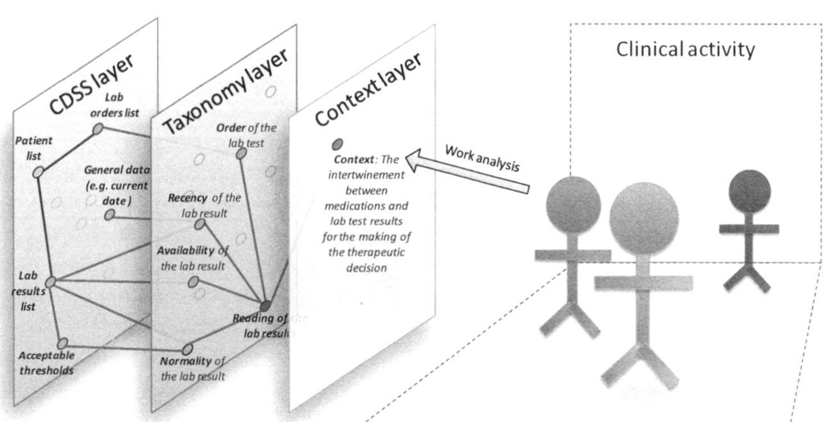

Figure 6. Example of integration of contextualisation elements in the PSIP taxonomy.

3. Discussion and Conclusion

This paper presents a taxonomy aiming at guiding the design of a CX-CDSS for ADE prevention. The taxonomy has been developed through a collaborative work from several sources of existing data as ADE taxonomy, a medical data model developed in the PSIP project, standards to take into account the interoperability and an activity analysis of the patient care process to take into account contextualisation aspects.

The particularity of the PSIP taxonomy is the integration of contextualisation aspects, which will allow guiding the design of a CDSS corresponding to healthcare professionals' needs. Indeed, the activity analysis allowed highlighting more precise contextualisation elements (for instance, cognitive elements) useful for healthcare professionals to make their therapeutic decision.

The PSIP taxonomy has been design to be the more exhaustive possible about the ADEs' detection and prevention issue. It targets also an ideal implementation of context elements into a CX-CDSS. Now, this ideal implementation is still not reached for reason of data collection from the HIS and knowledge availability. Indeed, some data are not easily retrievable from the HIS. For instance, the fact that a lab test has been ordered requires that the CX-CDSS seeks for the concerned lab test code in the prescription. Even if the IUPAC codes have been included in the taxonomy, some HIS are using other others kinds of codes. Thus it is always not possible to retrieve whether the lab test has been ordered or not. Moreover, the taxonomy allows that the severity of the potentially encountered ADEs be used to display the alert and that the alert include action's advices for the healthcare professionals. Now, those two kinds of information are medical knowledge that is still not defined because they are very complex.

In sum, through its sufficiency aim, the PSIP taxonomy is not yet completely implementable. However, by targeting an ideal contextualisation of the alert display, it allowed detecting knowledge challenges that remain to be overcome.

Acknowledgements

The research leading to these results has received funding from the European Community's Seventh Framework Programme (FP7/2007-2013) under grant agreement n° 216130 – the PSIP project.

References

[1] J.A. Osheroff, E.A. Pifer, J.M. Teich, D.F. Sittig, R.A. Jenders, Improving outcomes with clinical decision support: an implementer's guide, Health Information Management and Systems Society, 2005.

[2] N. Bricon-Souf, C.R. Newman, Context awareness in health care: a review, *Int J Med Inform* **76** (2007), 2–12.

[3] A. Dey, G. Abowd, D. Salber, A conceptual framework and toolkit for supporting the rapid prototyping of context-aware applications, *Human-computer Interaction* **16** (2001), 97–166.

[4] E. Chazard, G. Ficheur, B. Merlin, M. Genin, C. Preda, PSIP consortium, R. Beuscart, Detection of adverse drug events detection: data aggregation and data mining, *Stud Health Technol Inform* **148** (2009), 75–84.

[5] S. Pereira, B. Plaisantin, M. Korchia, N. Rozanes, E. Serrot, M. Joubert, S.J. Darmoni, Automatic construction of dictionaries, application to product characteristics indexing, *Stud Health Technol Inform* **150** (2009), 512–16.

[6] E. Chazard, B. Merlin, G. Ficheur, J.C. Sarfati, PSIP Consortium, R. Beuscart, Detection of adverse drug events: proposal of a data model, *Stud Health Technol Inform* **148** (2009), 63–74.

[7] National Coordinating Council for Medication Error Reporting and Prevention, NCC MERP: The First Ten Years "Defining the Problem and Developing Solutions", Available at: http://www.nccmerp.org/, last access on March 2011.

[8] Association for Quality Assurance in Therapeutics and Evaluation, Available at: http://www.adiph.asso.fr/aaqte/FormulaireREEM.pdf, last access on March 2011.
[9] U.S.Pharmacopeia (USP) - Institute for Safe Medication Practices (ISMP), Available at: https://www.ismp.org/orderForms/reporterrortoISMP.asp, last access on March 2011.
[10] World Alliance for Patient Safety, International Classification for Patient Safety (ICPS), Available at: http://www.who.int/patientsafety/taxonomy/ICPS_Statement_of_Purpose.pdf, last access on March 2011.
[11] A. Chang, P.M. Schyve, R.J. Croteau, D.S. O'Leary, J.M. Loeb, The JCAHO patient safety event taxonomy: a standardized terminology and classification schema for near misses and adverse events, *Int J Qual Health Care* **17** (2005), 95–105.
[12] C. Riccioli, N. Leroy, S. Pelayo, The PSIP approach to account for human factors in adverse drug events: preliminary field studies, *Stud Health Technol Inform* **148** (2009), 197–205.
[13] R. Marcilly, S. Pelayo, S. Bernonville, N. Leroy, J. Forrierre, Prise en compte du contexte pour la conception d'un Système d'Aide à la Décision Médicamenteuse, 45ème congrès de la Société d'Ergonomie de Langue Française 2010, Liège.

Patient Safety Informatics
V. Koutkias et al. (Eds.)
IOS Press, 2011

doi:10.3233/978-1-60750-740-6-84

Medication Related Computerized Decision Support System (CDSS): Make it a Clinicians' Partner!

Romaric MARCILLY [a,1], Nicolas LEROY [a], Michel LUYCKX [b,c], Sylvia PELAYO [a], Costanza RICCIOLI [d] and Marie-Catherine BEUSCART-ZÉPHIR [a]

[a] *INSERM CIC-IT, Lille, CHU Lille; UDSL EA 2694; Univ Lille Nord de France; F-59000 Lille, France*

[b] *Faculté des Sciences Pharmaceutiques et Biologiques, UDSL2, Univ Lille Nord de France, F-59000 Lille, France*

[c] *Centre Hospitalier de Denain, France*

[d] *Kite Solutions, SNC, Via Labiena 93, 21014 Laveno Mombello (Va), Italy*

Abstract. Medication related Computerized Decision Support System (CDSS) are known to have a positive impact on Adverse Drug Events (ADE) prevention but they face acceptance problems due to over alerting and usability issues. We present here a Human factors approach to the design of these Clinical Decision Support (CDS) functions and to their integration into different Electronic Health Record (EHR) / Computerized Physicians Order Entry (CPOE) systems, so that the resulting CDSS corresponds to the users needs and fits clinical workflows and cognitive processes. We used ethnographic observations completed with semi-structured interviews to analyse existing work situations and work processes. These were then described in detail using the SHEL (Software, Hardware, Environment & Liveware) formalism, which enables a structured description of the work system and provides an appropriate classification of human errors potentially leading to ADEs. We then propose a Unified Modelling Language (UML) model supporting the characterization by the CDSS of the drug monitoring and clinical context of patients at risk of ADE. This model combines the status of the lab test orders on the one hand with the validity and normality of the lab results on the other hand. This makes the system able to catch the context of the monitoring of the drugs through their corresponding lab tests and lab results (e.g. kalemia for potassium) and also part of the context of the clinical status of the patient (actual lab values, but also diseases and other pathologies that are identified as potential causes of the ADE e.g. renal insufficiency and potassium). We show that making the system able to catch the monitoring and clinical contexts opens interesting opportunities for the design of the CDS information content and display mode. Implementing this model would allow the CDSS to take into account the actions already engaged by the healthcare team and to adapt the information delivered to the monitoring and clinical context, thus making the CDSS a partner to the clinicians, nurses and pharmacists.

Keywords. Computerized decision support systems, clinical decision support, human factors engineering, adverse drug events, system design

[1] Corresponding Author: romaric.marcilly@univ-lille2.fr

Introduction

Adverse Drug Events (ADE) are the most common Adverse Events occurring during the care process [1]. These ADEs result in human costs in terms of patients' deaths or injuries and economic costs in terms of hospital prolonged stays or lawsuits. Therefore, many countries consider ADEs to be a major public health issue and currently invest a lot of resources in patient safety programs aiming at identifying, characterizing and preventing ADEs. One way among many to prevent ADEs is to implement medication related Clinical Decision Support (CDS) functions, usually integrated in or interfaced with Computerized Physicians Order Entry applications (CPOE). These systems support physicians' therapeutic decision by checking the orders against a medication knowledge base providing alerts or suggestions to the prescribers. As a result, physicians can adjust their decision according to the known side effects of the drugs, their interactions and potential contra-indications. Kuperman et al. [2] identify two categories of medication CDS. Basic CDS includes drug-allergy checking, basic dosing guidance, formulary decision support, duplicate therapy checking, and drug–drug interaction checking, while advanced CDS includes dosing support for renal insufficiency and geriatric patients, guidance for medication-related laboratory testing, drug–disease contraindication checking, and drug–pregnancy checking. Despite some acceptance and usage problems [3], the implementation and use of medication related CDSS have been found to be beneficial in improving the quality of clinicians' prescriptions and reducing medication errors [4-5] and ultimately preventing ADEs [6]. Therefore it seems worth pursuing the efforts in designing and developing acceptable, user centred advanced medication CDSS applications.

1. Background

1.1. Scope of the Study

The present study is part of the European project entitled "Patient Safety through Intelligent Procedures in medication-PSIP". The first goal of the PSIP project is to automatically generate knowledge about ADEs, therefore providing reliable numbers about ADEs per country, region, hospital or medical unit, describing their type, consequences and probable causes. This knowledge about ADEs helps identify situations at risk in each context of care, depending on the patients' characteristics, i.e. medical history and current symptoms, and on the care place, for instance the type of hospital / medical specialty. The second goal of the PSIP project is to deliver to the healthcare professionals and to the patients who find themselves in these risky situations, the contextual knowledge that can help them characterize the problem and adapt the treatment to avoid potential ADEs.

PSIP addresses a particular subset of preventable ADEs, which according to the NCCMERP taxonomy [7] may be characterized as "medication monitoring errors", with a specific focus on faulty monitoring of clinical or laboratory values. As a consequence the advanced CDS functions developed in PSIP result mainly in Drug-Laboratory alerts and Drug-Condition/Disease/Age alerts.

The project adopts a user centred / user driven approach to the design of these CDS functions and to their integration into different EHR (Electronic Health Record) /

CPOE systems, so that the resulting CDSS corresponds to the users needs and fits clinical workflows and cognitive processes.

1.2. Human Factors Limitations of Current Medication CDSS

In spite of their known positive impact, medication CDSS applications remain difficult to implement and face acceptance problems [3, 8]. These difficulties are due to a combination of human factors related drawbacks of current systems.

The major drawback of existing systems is undoubtedly their poor signal-to-noise ratio [9-10]. This problem generates a well known "over-alerting" syndrome due to too many false positives which in turn engenders "alert fatigue" for the prescribing physicians. Alert fatigue is "the mental state that is the result of too many alerts consuming time and energy" [9]. Moreover, the fact that a number of "alerts" are clinically irrelevant [11] diminishes the clinicians' confidence in the system. Reducing over-alerting is therefore one of the major challenges for the design of a medication CDSS. This question points at the quality and the completeness of the knowledge implemented in the knowledge base of the medication CDSS and at its ability to catch and take into account the clinical context of the patient at hand. The PSIP system partly addresses this issue by contextualizing the alerts depending on the probability of occurrence of the ADEs per hospital, per clinical unit or medical specialty [12]. However, it is unreasonable to think that a CDSS might incorporate a "perfect" (*i.e.* accurate and exhaustive) knowledge so that it would be able to identify and take into account all relevant characteristics of the clinical case at hand and eradicate the over alerting. Ultimately, only the clinician is able to gather the relevant clinical information, assess it and finally make the therapeutic decision. Therefore, no medication CDSS will ever be "perfect" enough so as to act as a substitute to the clinicians and fully automate the therapeutic decision making. As a consequence, it is necessary that the CDS functions support and not replace the clinician's decision and act as a partner to her/his medical reasoning and decision making cognitive process.

The second drawback of many existing systems is their poor usability [13]. On a fundamental level, the model of work and the model of clinicians' reasoning incorporated in the systems are often inadequate. This usability weakness issues "compatibility" problems defined as a lack of match between users' and task characteristics on the one hand, and the organisation of the output, input, and dialogue for a given application, on the other hand [14]. As a consequence, alerts are too often disruptive of the clinical workflows and of the cognitive processes inherent to medication decision making and monitoring, due to wrong timing, wrong display mode and wrong/weak content of the information delivered. For example, it is not wise to suggest to the physician an action s/he is just about to carry out [15], or to alert him/her on a potentially dangerous situation for which s/he has just taken action by ordering the corresponding lab tests. All physicians dislike such alerts which they find unnerving. Moreover, most of the systems fail to make available upon request short or extended versions of the scientific justifications of the CDS recommendations, which are necessary to allow the physicians properly assessing their clinical relevance and the resulting cost-benefit of the medication order for the patient under consideration.

Given the nature of the difficulties and usability issues, a Human Factors Engineering [16] approach to the design of advanced medication CDS functions would help solve a part of those problems and contribute to the design of applications acting as effective and reliable clinicians partners.

1.3. The Human Factors Engineering (HFE) Approach to the Design of Advanced Medication CDS Functions

A Human Factors Engineering approach to healthcare work systems aims at optimizing the relationships between the users, their tasks and the technologies they use to carry out these tasks in various work environments and organizations. It requires a user-centred approach to the design of the IT applications, taking into account the needs, expectations and characteristics of the end users, who need to be actually involved in the design process. This approach would help design effective and usable medication CDSS. The most important phase in the HFE approach is the initial one, i.e. the observation, analysis and modelling of the existing work system. It is therefore important to retrieve and use the knowledge on the work system accumulated in previous HF studies on the medication use process in hospital settings [17-18]. These studies have already provided valuable insights on the intangible characteristics of the clinical workflows and of the healthcare professionals' decision making process. The results emphasize the fact that therapeutic decision making is a dynamic process [19]: the patient's condition evolves depending on the healthcare professionals' actions but also spontaneously by itself. At each encounter with the patient, clinicians have to update their knowledge about the patient's status and his/her evolution, especially as regards new important elements in the situation, e.g. new lab results or unexpected clinical evolution of the patient [20]. Moreover, the medication use process is characterized as a complex distributed work situation: the information is distributed across the minds of the members of the clinical team but also across physical media, such as the EHR, the CPOE or the CDSS [21]. These disparate pieces of information should then be integrated, completed, and interpreted. From the users' point of view, the collection, documentation, communication, and retrieval of information are critical activities.

In the present study, we elaborated on this existing knowledge and completed previous field studies and analyses by focused observations and modelling of the monitoring process of patients' therapeutic treatments based mainly on corresponding lab values. The objectives of this research are to:

- Identify the relevant indicators of the context of lab values based monitoring of the drug,
- identify the relevant indicators of the context of the clinical status of the patients that may have an impact on the considered ADE, i.e. actual lab values and eventually other diseases inferred from lab results such as renal insufficiency, and
- elaborate a model supporting the implementation in the CDSS of functions able to reflect these clinical and monitoring contexts.

2. Methods

2.1. Study Site

The study took place in a 416-bed hospital, the Hospital Center of Denain in northern France. The hospital has a Patient Care Information system (PCIS), the commercial product DxCare® from the MEDASYS Company. It includes an EHR equipped with a

CPOE which in this version has very limited CDS functions (e.g. alerts in case of duplicates). The PCIS is interfaced with a pharmacy system, which allows the pharmacists to check the medication orders and send physicians alerts when they suspect improper orders. The analyses were carried out in two medicine departments: the "cardiology" department (medicine A) and the "internal medicine and infectious diseases" department (medicine B).

2.2. HFE Methods

2.2.1. On Site Observations and Interviews

Over a period of one month (May-June 2009), four HF experts observed all tasks related to the medication process carried out by 4 physicians, 6 nurses, 2 pharmacists and 2 assistant pharmacists, with a special focus on all actions related to lab values monitoring. Observation time amounted to 53 hours and concerned 101 different patients. Observations were completed with debriefings and semi-structured interviews to clarify actors' goals, thought processes and information needs while monitoring lab values and patients' treatments. Detailed description of methods can be found in [22].

2.2.2. Structured Analysis of Data and Modelling

We used the SHEL (Software, Hardware, Environment & Liveware) formalism to describe the data collected. Originally developed for the aviation domain [23], SHEL aims at representing working contexts and main actors while specifically identifying existing barriers against errors. It enables a structured description of the work system and provides an appropriate classification of human errors potentially leading to ADEs. Given the objective of the project, i.e. to design medication CDS functions, this formalism is particularly appropriate because it helps designing a system enhancing and completing existing barriers thus acting as a professional's partner.

We also used Unified Modelling Language (UML) to express the HF recommendations as this language has been shown to facilitate the dialogue between HF experts and computer scientists (designers and developers) [24].

3. Results

3.1. Results of the Analysis of the Work Situation

The analysis of the data collected during the field observations issued twelve SHEL descriptions of the various tasks performed by all actors during the medication use process or related to it. For illustration purposes Figure 1 provides a SHEL overview of the survey by the physicians of the patient therapeutic treatment during the daily medical round, focused on information gathering activities.

Once the main SHEL elements have been identified, it is possible to describe the interactions between the four dimensions, in order to get a full picture of the work system. SHEL also allows identifying existing barriers to errors. For the example described above, barriers would help the physician not to overlook important information that should be taken into account to adapt the patient's treatment.

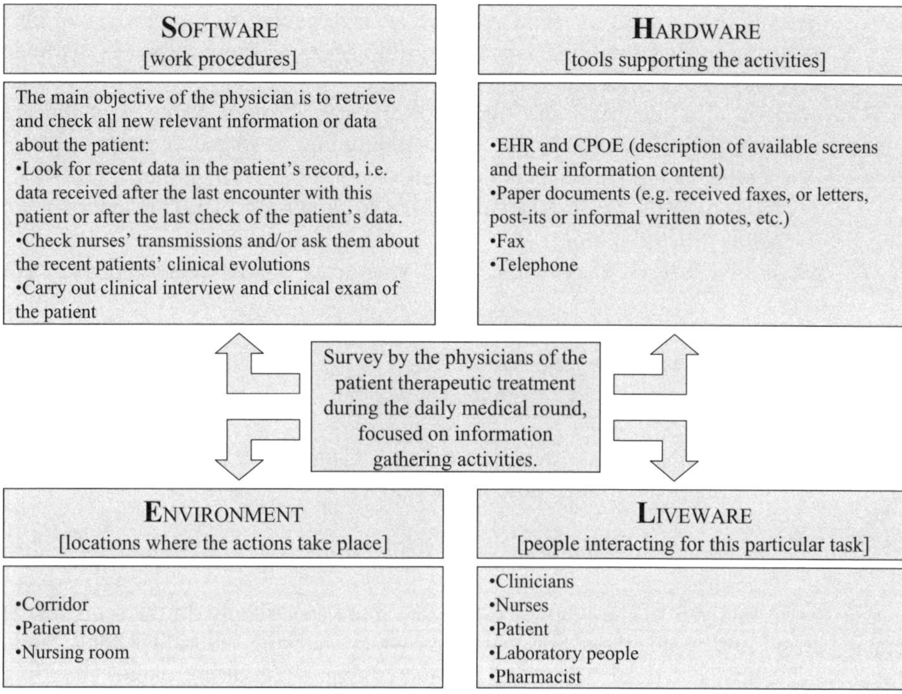

Figure 1. SHEL overview of the work situation - survey of the patient therapeutic treatment during the daily medical round.

Examples of such barriers are:

- Doctor-nurse communications and nurses' reminders to physicians
- Phone calls or faxes from the laboratory in case of abnormal results. Those calls are usually received by nurses who then pass on the information to the physicians
- CPOE alerts on new available lab results, i.e. results that have not been yet acknowledged by a clinician
- Patients' complains

The analysis highlights the close intertwinement between the medications' use process and the laboratory ordering and reporting cycle. The dependency between the drugs administered to the patient and the biological indicator of their effect (*i.e.* the lab test result) is time dependant and strongly impacts the work procedures of the nurses and physicians:

- Lab results must be retrieved on time for the physician to be able to decide how best to adapt the treatment to the patient's condition.
- For certain drugs (e.g. anticoagulant VKA – Vitamine K Antagonist) nurses need to check the last corresponding lab values (e.g. INR-International Normalized Ratio) before administration. When this information is missing, nurses may have to take initiatives such as taking a new sample of blood and ask for urgent results, ordering reconciliation being performed later by the physician in the CPOE system.
- The patient's state evolving as a result of the medications' effect but also on its own, the lab results are valid only for a given time period. This period

depends on the type of medication whose effect must be monitored and also on the patient's conditions. Once the validity period elapsed, the lab test must be re-ordered to get a new (valid) lab result.

The analysis also identifies the fundamental steps through which a healthcare professional goes when s/he relies on lab values to monitor the impact of a drug:

- Check whether the lab result is available or not:
  - In case the lab result is not available: check whether the corresponding lab test is ordered or not
- When the lab result is available, check whether it is recent enough to be valid or not:
  - In case the result is not recent enough, check whether the corresponding lab order has been renewed or not
- When the lab result is available, check whether it is normal (within acceptable limits) or not:
  - In case of abnormal results, consider adapting the treatment (modifying the drug prescription / administration)

3.2. Characterization of the Monitoring and Clinical Context

Relying on the analysis of the work situation and more specifically on the sequence of actions carried out by healthcare professionals when checking lab values for a given drug, we identified typical situations characterizing the current status of drug monitoring. These situations result form the combination of the status of the lab tests orders on the one hand and the validity and normality of the available lab values on the other hand. For each typical situation we can identify whether the monitoring procedure is appropriate or not, and whether the patient's clinical status, assessed by the lab value, is alarming or not (yet). Therefore, these situations characterize the lab value-based monitoring context and a part of the clinical context for the patient under consideration.

Figure 2 presents the UML model of the classification process to be performed by the Contextualized Computerized Decision Support System (Cx-CDSS), leading to the identification of the monitoring and clinical context for the patients identified by the system as being at risk of an ADE.

For example, Context 3 corresponds to a situation under control: the drug is properly monitored because the required lab values are available and recent enough to be considered valid indicators of the patient's clinical status, and these lab results are in normal range.

On the contrary, Context 2 corresponds to a situation which is not properly monitored, because the required lab values are not available and the system cannot find any corresponding lab test order.

Context 7 is perhaps even more alarming as the system can identify that the last available lab value was abnormal, but this value is not recent enough to be considered a valid indicator of the current patient's clinical state, and the corresponding lab test order has not been renewed. In this context, the probability of appearance of the potential ADE is higher but the effect is not likely to be prevented as it is not properly monitored.

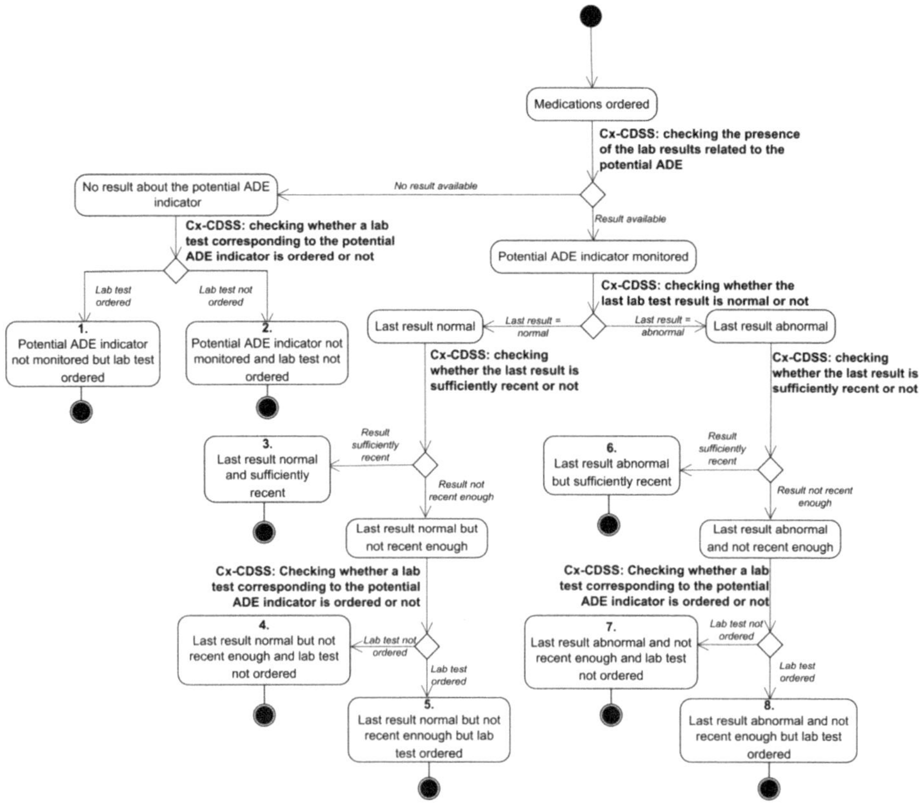

Figure 2. UML model supporting the classification of the situations leading to the identification of the eight relevant monitoring and clinical contexts.

3.3. Recommendations for the Design of the CDS Information Delivered to Healthcare Professionals

Making the system able to catch the monitoring and clinical contexts opens interesting opportunities for the design of the CDS information content and display mode.

It is for instance possible to group the contexts in terms of urgency of the situations and to reflect this degree of urgency in the display mode of the CDS information. All contexts for which the last lab result available is abnormal (i.e. contexts 6, 7 and 8) should be considered a priority and given a high "urgency" indicator. Contexts 2 and 4 correspond to situations that are not properly monitored but where no alarming results have been received yet. For these contexts the information delivered by the CDSS should be given a medium "urgency" indicator. Finally, contexts 1, 3 and 5 correspond to situations that are properly monitored because the lab tests have been ordered and when these lab results are available they are not (yet) abnormal. Therefore, the information delivered in these situations should be given a low "urgency" rating. The designers may choose the most appropriate way of indicating the "urgency" rating in the Human Computer Interface, depending for example on the design chart of the application (CPOE, EHR) in which the system is integrated.

It is also possible to adapt the content of the information delivered to the clinicians depending on the context. It is recommended that the CDSS not only displays an alert but also makes suggestions [2]. In contexts 2, 4 and 7 corresponding to situations that are not properly monitored, and in addition to the display of the rule leading to the identification of the case as being at risk of ADE, the CDSS could suggest that the clinician orders the required lab test and eventually propose a short cut to the lab tests ordering page. On the contrary context 6, in which a new (recent and valid) lab value came in abnormal, the system could alert the physician on the increasing negative side effect of the drug and invite him/her to reassess the cost benefit ratio of the incriminated drug(s).

Finally advanced parameterization functions based on the identification of the context could be offered to clinicians, pharmacists and nurses to let them upgrade the level of urgency if needed for specific ADEs, or to take advantage of the monitoring protocols adopted in the department

4. Discussion

Making a CDSS able to catch elements of the clinical context is highly desirable goal. The model proposed in this paper is operational and seems simple enough to be implemented in any medication CDSS integrated in a CPOE or an EHR. However it requires the incorporation in the system of specific knowledge, as is illustrated in the case below.

Example: a patient is identified by the PSIP system by triggering the following rule:

- CDSS rule b011: vitKantagonist + cephalosporin → high_inr;
- Text of the rule for the physician: "An increased effect of the oral anticoagulant can occur in an infectious context. Cephalosporins by themselves may increase hemorrhagic risk. Ref.: Thesaurus AFSSAPS 2009".

In this case the characterization of the monitoring and clinical context would require the following knowledge to be integrated in the system.

4.1. Identify the Targeted Lab Value

The system has to know what the targeted lab value is for this ADE risk. This knowledge may be retrieved from the rule itself, i.e. INR (International Normalized Ratio). However, although international guidelines recommend monitoring VKA (Vitamin K Antagonist) effect through INR, a number of physicians / laboratories / hospital departments still rely on other lab values such as aPTT (activated Partial Thromboplastin Time). This knowledge has to be incorporated to improve the accuracy of the system and make it able to check for alternative lab tests / values when the search for INR fails.

4.2. Assess the Lab Value Normality

The system has to know whether the retrieved INR values are "normal" or not. This knowledge is usually available in the Laboratory Information System as results are delivered along with normality thresholds and special marks for abnormal results.

4.3. Assess the Lab Value Validity

Finally, the system has to know whether the last available INR value is recent enough to be considered valid. The knowledge necessary to answer this question is more complex. For example, chronic patients who have long been on VKA and are stabilized do not require frequent monitoring (once every two weeks or once a month). But as soon as the clinical status changes (e.g. infection), or if a new drug is introduced, a closer monitoring is required, and this is often the case for hospitalized patient. Similarly, when the VKA treatment is first introduced, a close monitoring is required until the patient is stabilized. By default, it is usually recommended to test the INR every 2 days, and this corresponds to the most common VKA monitoring protocol in hospital departments. This simple, by default knowledge, could be used by the system. Ultimately a more elaborated knowledge based on the drug's pharmacodynamics (elimination half-life of the product) would be more accurate and allow adaptation to the type of VKA actually prescribed.

This example shows that a basic, operational knowledge based on by default values and protocols running in the hospitals could be used to support the characterization of the monitoring and clinical context of patients at risk of ADE. But further research could progressively elaborate a more accurate and sophisticated knowledge, therefore improving the efficiency and accuracy of the system.

5. Conclusion

The characterization of the monitoring and clinical context and the advanced functions they make possible are not currently available in medication related CDSS. Their implementation would allow the system to take into account the actions already engaged by the healthcare team and to adapt the information delivered to the monitoring and clinical context thus making the CDSS a partner to the clinicians, nurses and pharmacists. They would also probably lessen the burden of over alerting by allowing the clinicians to identify at a glance the urgency and type of problem addressed by the alerts.

Acknowledgments

The research leading to these results has received funding from the European Community's Seventh Framework Programme (FP7/2007-2013) under grant agreement n° 216130 – the PSIP project.

References

[1] Committee on Identifying Medication Errors, *Preventing Medication Errors: Quality Chasm Series*, National Academies Press, 2006.

[2] G.J. Kuperman et al., Medication-related clinical decision support in computerized provider order entry systems: a review, *J Am Med Inform Assoc* **14** (2007), 29–40.

[3] R. Koppel, D.A. Kreda, Healthcare IT usability and suitability for clinical needs: challenges of design, workflow, and contractual relations, *Stud Health Technol Inform* **157** (2010), 7–14.

[4] D.C. Classen, S.L. Pestotnik, R.S. Evans, J.P. Burke, Computerized surveillance of adverse drug events in hospital patients, *Qual Saf Health Care* **14** (2005), 221–5.
[5] P.M. Kilbridge, U.C. Campbell, H.B. Cozart, M.G. Mojarrad. Automated surveillance for adverse drug events at a community hospital and an academic medical center, *J Am Med Inform Assoc* **13** (2006), 372–7.
[6] E. Ammenwerth, P. Schnell-Inderst, C. Machan, U. Siebert, The effect of electronic prescribing on medication errors and adverse drug events: a systematic review, *J Am Med Inform Assoc* **15** (2008), 585–600.
[7] National Coordinating Council for Medication Error Reporting and Prevention, NCC MERP: The First Ten Years "Defining the Problem and Developing Solutions", Available at: http://www.nccmerp.org/, last access on March 2011.
[8] E. Ammenwerth et al., Impact of CPOE on mortality rates--contradictory findings, important messages, *Methods Inf Med* **45** (2006), 586–93.
[9] S.H. van der Sijs, J. Aarts, A. Vulto, M. Berg, Overriding of drug safety alerts in computerized physician order entry, *J Am Med Inform Assoc* **13** (2006), 138–47.
[10] J.F. Peterson, D.W. Bates, Preventable medication errors: identifying and eliminating serious drug interactions, *J Am Pharm Assoc* **41** (2001), 159–60.
[11] S.M. Handler et al., A systematic review of the performance characteristics of clinical event monitor signals used to detect adverse drug events in the hospital setting, *J Am Med Inform Assoc* **14** (2007), 451–8.
[12] E. Chazard, G. Ficheur, B. Merlin, M. Genin, C. Preda, PSIP consortium, R. Beuscart, Detection of adverse drug events detection: data aggregation and data mining, *Stud Health Technol Inform* **148** (2009), 75–84.
[13] R. Khajouei, M.W. Jaspers, The impact of CPOE medication systems' design aspects on usability, workflow and medication orders: a systematic review, *Methods Inf Med* **49** (2010), 3–19.
[14] J.M.C. Bastien, D. Scapin, Ergonomic criteria for the evaluation of human-computer interfaces, *Institut National de recherche en informatique et en automatique*, France, 1993.
[15] R.A. Miller, R.L. Waitman, S. Chen, S.T. Rosenbloom, The anatomy of decision support during inpatient care provider order entry (CPOE): empirical observations from a decade of CPOE experience at Vanderbilt, *J Biomed Inform* **38** (2005), 469–85.
[16] M.C. Beuscart-Zéphir, P. Elkin, S. Pelayo, R. Beuscart, The human factors engineering approach to biomedical informatics projects: state of the art, results, benefits and challenges, *Yearb Med Inform* (2007), 159–77.
[17] M.C. Beuscart-Zephir et al., Impact of CPOE on doctor-nurse cooperation for the medication ordering and administration process, *Int J Med Inform* **74** (2005), 629–41.
[18] M.C. Beuscart-Zephir, S. Pelayo, F. Anceaux, D. Maxwell, S. Guerlinger, Cognitive analysis of physicians and nurses cooperation in the medication ordering and administration process, *Int J Med Inform* **76** (2007), S65–77.
[19] M.C. Beuscart-Zephir, S. Pelayo, S. Bernonville, Example of a human factors engineering approach to a medication administration work system: potential impact on patient safety, *Int J Med Inform* **79** (2010), e43–57.
[20] S. Pelayo, M.C. Beuscart-Zéphir, Organizational considerations for the implementation of a computerized physician order entry, *Stud Health Technol Inform* **157** (2010), 112–7.
[21] T. Cohen, B. Blatter, C. Almeida, E. Shortliffe, V. Patel, A cognitive blueprint of collaboration in context: Distributed cognition in the psychiatric emergency department, *Artif Intell Med* **37** (2006), 73–83.
[22] C. Riccioli, N. Leroy, S. Pelayo, The PSIP approach to account for human factors in adverse drug events: preliminary field studies, *Stud Health Technol Inform* **148** (2009), 197–205.
[23] F.H. Hawkins, *Human Factors in Flight*, Aldershot, UK, Gower, 1987.
[24] S. Bernonville, C. Kolski, N. Leroy, M.C. Beuscart-Zephir, Integrating the SE and HCI models in the human factors engineering cycle for re-engineering Computerized Physician Order Entry systems for medications: basic principles illustrated by a case study, *Int J Med Inform* **79** (2010), 35–42.

Patient Safety Informatics
V. Koutkias et al. (Eds.)
IOS Press, 2011

doi:10.3233/978-1-60750-740-6-95

Information Contextualization in Decision Support Modules for Adverse Drug Event Prevention

Julie NIES [a,1], Vassilis KOUTKIAS [b], Vassilis KILINTZIS [b], Bertrand GUILLOT [a], Nicos MAGLAVERAS [b], Henrik Gliese PEDERSEN [c], Anna-Lis BERG [c] and Peter SKJOET [d]

[a] *MEDASYS, Gif-Sur-Yvette, France*

[b] *Aristotle University, Medical School, Lab of Medical Informatics, Thessaloniki, Greece*

[c] *IBM Global Business Services, Healthcare, Denmark*

[d] *Region Hovedstaden, Copenhagen, Denmark*

Abstract. This paper presents an analysis of hospitals' organization and Hospital Information Systems' features which can contribute in contextualization of Clinical Decision Support Systems (CDSS) for Adverse Drug Event (ADE) prevention. We identified four categories of contextualization: ENVIRONMENT, TASKS, USERS and TEMPORAL ASPECTS. Based on this analysis, we studied the technical possibilities at the architectural level to determine which component(s) of a standalone knowledge platform could technically handle contextualization. The results impact three types of components of this platform: (1) a CDSS providing decision support based on ADE signals mined in large data repositories; (2) a Connectivity Platform providing transformation and routing services (enabling any application to connect to the CDSS); (3) three prototype applications for accessing the decision support services realized within an industrial Computerized Physician Order Entry, an industrial Electronic Health Record and in an independent Web prototype, respectively. In each of the above components we present the dimension(s) of contextualization that has/have been determined to cope with and the design followed in the implementation phase.

Keywords. Adverse drug event (ADE) prevention, clinical decision support system (CDSS), contextualization, computerized physician order entry (CPOE), electronic health record (EHR)

Introduction

The project "Patient Safety through Intelligent Procedures in medication" (PSIP) involves a Consortium of 13 partners (universities, hospitals and industries) and aims at preventing medication errors [1]. In particular, its objectives are (1) to facilitate the systematic production of epidemiological knowledge on Adverse Drug Events (ADE) and (2) to improve the entire medication cycle in a hospital

[1] Corresponding Author: julie.nies@medasys.com

environment. The first sub-objective is to produce knowledge on ADE: to know, as exactly as possible, per hospital, per medical department, their number, types, consequences and causes, including human factors [2]. Data mining techniques applied on structured hospital data repositories and semantic mining of free-texts have provided a list of observed ADE, with frequencies and probabilities, thus giving a better understanding of potential risks [3]. The second sub-objective is to develop innovative knowledge, based on the mining results and to deliver professionals and patients contextualized knowledge fitting the local risk parameters, in the form of alerts and decision support functions. This knowledge is incorporated in an Information Technologies platform: the PSIP platform, which is a standalone knowledge service, independent of Hospital Information System (HIS) existing applications.

The notion of context takes a central place in the PSIP project. The initial idea was that ADEs do not occur with the same probability in a surgery unit, in a cardiology unit, or in an Internal Medicine unit. They can also be different among hospitals, due to different prescription protocols, and even to cultural characteristics. This could be one of the reasons why alerting systems linked with Computerized Physician Order Entry (CPOE) systems are so often disregarded by physicians and not even consulted by junior doctors. This idea was confirmed by the results of data mining, i.e. whatever their origin, the ADE rules obtained by data mining do not have the same statistical significance everywhere [3].

The aim of this paper is to describe the concept of 'information contextualization' as conceived in the PSIP project and what it means for the hospitals participating in the project in terms of elements which could be handled by the PSIP platform.

1. State of the Art

1.1. Definitions of 'Context'

A first definition of 'context' was proposed by experts from the Consortium as a response to the questions rose during Workshops about the characteristics of context. Our experts agreed on a broad definition. "Contextualization process helps to give:

- The right information (= for the right patient);
- At the right time;
- To the right person;
- At the right place;
- In the right format."

Dey defines context as "any information that can be used to characterize the situation of an entity" [4]. This is a general, broad definition of context that can be easily transposed in applications in Computer Science and Medical Informatics.

From a "Human Factors" (sociological) viewpoint, as described by Schmidt et al. [5], the main elements of relevance for the description of contexts can be structured into 3 categories:

- the USER (expertise, knowledge of habits, emotional state, bio-physiological conditions, etc.);

- the user's ENVIRONMENT (co-location of others, social interaction, group dynamics, etc.), and
- the user's TASKS (spontaneous activity, engaged tasks, general goals, etc.).

ADE prevention involves a lot of knowledge, tasks, users, etc. To face this complexity, a Human Factors based analysis of the existing work systems has been performed. As previous works [6-8], this analysis pointed out the importance of TEMPORAL ASPECTS. Those aspects describe the sequences between TASKS (time when the different actions are performed, time delays between prescription and administration, time delay between the administration of the drug and the occurrence of a potential ADE, etc.) or describe some aspects of the physical ENVIRONMENT (time-shift, workload, etc.) that could lead to ADEs.

1.2. Contextualization as a Way to Improve CDSS Impact

Clinical Decision Support Systems (CDSS) are defined as applications that integrate clinical data from several sources to generate alerts and recommendations on the basis of pre-established rules [9]. When CDSS are integrated into CPOE, they become a component for CPOE evaluation [10, 11]. This evaluation must address both the technical quality of the systems and the extent to which their use can improve medical practices.

A lot of articles have been published from 70's on CDSS. Many efforts have been made to synthesize the results of these studies in terms of reviews of CDSS impacts on clinical practices or patient outcomes [12-14] and to help healthcare organizations to use such systems [15, 16]. These works concluded that CDSS could improve medical practices but their effects on clinical outcomes are not yet well established.

Despite those works, no clear typology of effective CDSS was described; but several works pointed out that the integration of CDSS into HIS is a key point in the CDSS efficiency [12, 14]. It is thus mandatory to evaluate the possibilities of a HIS before setting up a CDSS into its architecture.

1.3. Contextualization as a Way to Improve CDSS Adoption

Alerts and point-of-care reminders have been shown to be the most effective form of decision support in many studies [12, 17]. Appropriate integration of those decision support interventions are key factors of their impact on clinical practices or patient outcomes [12, 13]. Their setup requires prudence about the condition of their triggering and mainly about their relevancy. Examples of "fatigue" could appear against the CDSS, when it is triggered in manners too frequently inappropriate [18]. A reflex behavior could be induced to the user who will systematically ignore the alert and thus will not read its content. Thus, there is a risk that a really relevant alert could be hidden by the huge amount of information transmitted to the user and consequently not taken into account.

There is a consensus in all evaluation studies about the critical importance of human and organizational factors and usability of the application (either CPOE or CDSS) for its acceptance and ultimate efficiency [12, 19]. It is thus important to study local organization before setting up a CDSS, so as to also take this aspect into account in the decision support process and design.

2. Methods

Our analysis has been focused on organizational aspects in the hospitals involved in the PSIP project and on the technical environments available in these hospitals where HIS and CPOE are installed. We used two frameworks for data collection which were sent to all hospitals involved in the Consortium. They were filled by administrative, medical and technical people.

We studied the technical possibilities at the architectural level to determine which component(s) could technically handle contextualization.

2.1. Analysis of Organizational Environment

2.1.1. Description of the Population Treated

We analyzed the patient hospitalizations during year 2007 to have a broad picture of the hospitals environments (e.g. which population is treated? are there some particular risk factors? are there particular environmental or sociological particularities?). We used data collected to fulfill the first PSIP sub-objective and we analyzed them for our specific purposes.

2.1.2. Hospital Organization Description

Each hospital partner had to describe their organization in terms of:

- eventual dependencies existing between hospitals;
- medical departments and medical specialties available;
- roles and responsibilities of each medical profession.

2.2. Analysis of Technical Environment

2.2.1. Data available in the HIS

A grid, based on the PSIP data-model [20], was provided to each hospital partner to help them describe their HIS/CPOE capabilities. They could have provided additional details, if needed. They could also send complete description of the technical characteristics of their Information Systems.

2.2.2. HIS Processes Description

Each hospital partner had to describe the use of their HIS, and more specifically, the use of their CPOE system by the medical users. Three minimum documentations were needed:

- Physician prescription process;
- Pharmacist dispensation process, and
- Nurses administration process.

2.3. Technical Possibilities for Handling Contextualization

The PSIP platform architecture consists of three types of components (Figure 1):

- a CDSS providing decision support services for ADE prevention;
- a Connectivity Platform providing transformation and routing services (enabling the prototypes or any other application to connect to the CDSS);
- three prototypes respectively embedded into an industrial CPOE, an industrial EHR and an independent Web prototype [21].

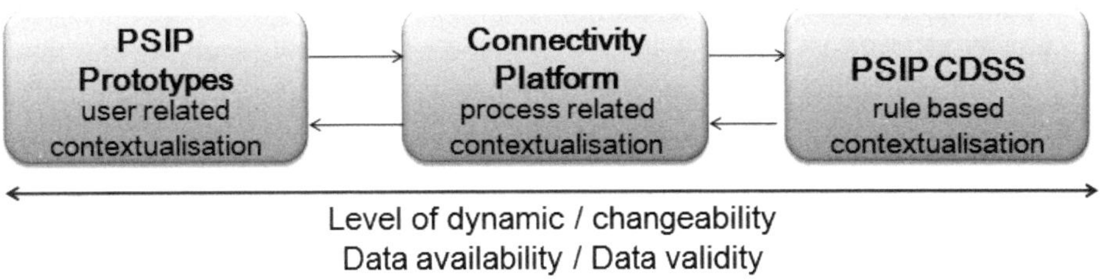

Figure 1. Different ways of contextualization depending on the PSIP components' functionalities.

According to the level of dynamic, changeability and the data availability or validity, the contextualization processes could be handled by each component of the PSIP platform. Contextualization can be handled:

- when implementing rules in the CDSS, as contextual attributes can be added to each rule, in order to identify the relevant context. This form of contextualization is based on the availability of data revealing context-related difference in rule's content, rule's relevance and need for feedback. Additionally, contextualization can be implemented in the CDSS by applying, not only per rule but also per context, configurable post-process alert filtering procedures.
- by the Connectivity Platform, where a process-based behavior can be implemented. This kind of contextualization is based on context-related need for data collection, filtering and communication, and is based on the availability and implementation of context-based process diagrams.
- by the prototypes, as user-related based on each user's profile. User-related contextualization is based on organizational decisions about system access, on personal decisions about the use of decision support services, on the detail level of information awaited in alerts or decision supports, etc.

3. Results

3.1. Environment Analysis

Our analysis organized the environment parameters according to the nature of the contextualization parameters (Figure 2):

- ENVIRONMENT: Country and Language Characteristics (France, Denmark, and English as a pivot language); Epidemiological environment (geography, population, risk factors); Hospital organization characteristics at the Hospital and Medical Unit levels (type of hospitals and medical unit; differences in the healthcare roles);
- TASKS: For the PSIP project the main tasks considered are Prescription, Dispensation, Administration and Information, according to the technical use of the HIS/CPOE and the available data;
- USERS: Hospital organization characteristics at healthcare profession level, i.e., junior and senior physicians, nurses, pharmacists, other healthcare professionals; and
- TEMPORAL ASPECTS: Description of sequences involving the three other descriptors of contextualization that could lead/contribute to ADE.

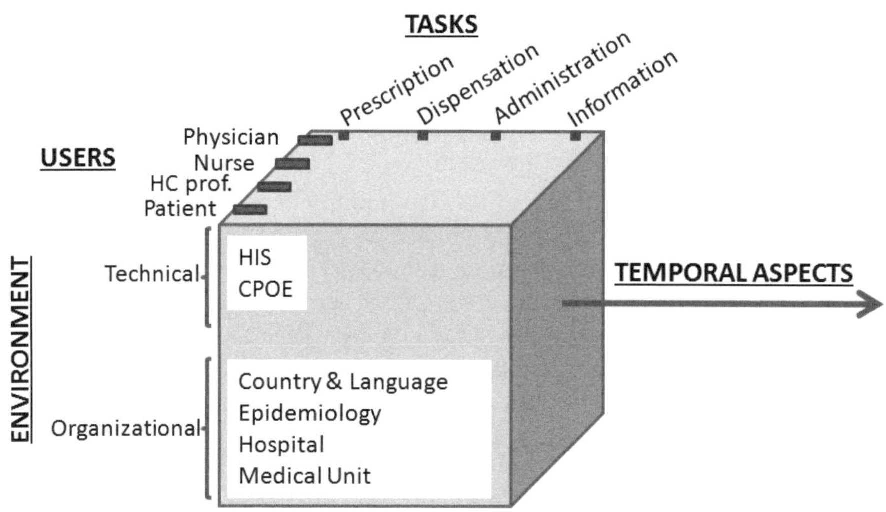

Figure 2. Summary of the results from the environment analysis.

3.2. Technical Principles and Realization of Information Contextualization

3.2.1. Contextualization Handled by the Connectivity Platform

The two industrial prototypes embedded into existing CPOE or EHR, and the independent Web prototype exchange information through the Connectivity Platform. In order to keep its connectivity role intact, this component was preferred to handle simple routing and data translation and not contextualized communication and/or data collection, although technically feasible as described in section 2.3.

Contextualization is thus handled according to the intrinsic functions of the other components.

3.2.2. Contextualization Handled by the CDSS

The most cited definition for CDSS is the one proposed by Wyatt and Spiegelhalter: "active knowledge systems which use two or more items of patient data to generate case-specific advice" [22]. A more recent, industrial source defined CDSS as a system which gives physicians structured (rule-based) information to help make decisions on diagnoses, treatment plans, orders and results [9].

In the PSIP project, the ability of data mining to detect ADE rules that may fire differently based on context parameters should be seen as the key argument to place the handling of that context parameter in the CDSS or elsewhere. Furthermore, data should be persistent, due to the static nature of the information held in CDSS. A CDSS is generic for TASKS/USERS aspects and sends information for every task and user.

But the results from data mining suggest that the CDSS could take into account parameters for ENVIRONMENT aspects like language and geographical data in the following format: Region H = Danish; Denain Medicine A = French… It could also manage epidemiological parameters (list of rules, thresholds…).

A significant challenge in the application domain of PSIP constitutes handling time-dependent clinical data and information. In this regard, several concepts have been included in the data-model, such as 'stay', 'duration_of_stay', 'delay_drug', etc., and implemented in the CDSS [23]. In this regard, the CDSS does not explicitly define time-dependent information on its own, but rather implicitly encapsulates this TEMPORAL ASPECTS dimension for the implementation of rules. It is noted that the formalism of the CDSS adopted is suitable to implement such approaches. This was proved via the implementation of meta-rules, i.e. procedures or instructions about how to apply the main ADE rules. In addition, wherever applicable, time-related decisions made in the data mining phase can be re-assessed upon each contextual setting, e.g. the time threshold in days before which the input data shall not be taken into account by the CDSS which is defined as a local parameter.

3.2.3. Contextualization Handled by the PSIP Prototypes

The work on the data available in the data-model has not revealed information that makes it possible to instantiate rule sets having the attributes of the USERS dimension to be a decisive factor in the CDSS. Simply said, the criteria that leads to fire rules in the CDSS are independent of the USERS dimension, i.e. a parameter indicating profession will not change the set of rules that fires. But, as recommended by the human factor analysis, the CDSS provides different information according to the user.

This work also revealed that the attributes of the TASKS dimension are not yet linked with the instantiation of decisive rule sets in the CDSS. Put simply, the criteria that lead to fire the rules in the CDSS are independent of the identified parameters in the TASKS dimension, i.e. a parameter indicating Prescription, Dispensation, Administration or Information will not change the set of rules fired in the CDSS. Thus the response is independent of the tasks parameter.

However, some parts of decision support presented to the end user, when a rule fires, need to be according to the user's profession. That is, a message explaining the potential ADE to a Physician might not be suitable as explanation to a Nurse and vice versa. But other information such as statistics on the potential ADE risk is identical regardless of the user's profession. This clinical need leads to the request to implement a relation between the rule and the presented explanatory message that is dependent of the profession of the user.

In the same way, parts of response presented to the end user when a rule fires might need to be aware of the Task. That is, a message explaining the potential ADE might be different during a prescription process from the message suitable to explain the potential ADE during dispensation. Other information such as statistics on the potential ADE risk is identical regardless of the task.

The close relation between profession and task should also be noticed, as the relation between profession and task is dependent on country, but constant in a same country. This can be used to provide task specific information embedded in the profession specific information.

In summary, the prototypes are then able to handle the USER and TASK dimensions as they know which type of medical practitioner is logged in, and performing which tasks of the Prescription, Dispensations, Administration or Information processes.

4. Discussion

The main results about information contextualization are depicted in Figure 3, i.e.:

- the CDSS handles ENVIRONMENT and some TEMPORAL ASPECTS of contextualization;
- the three prototypes (respectively embedded into an industrial CPOE, an industrial EHR and an independent Web prototype) handle TASKS and USERS contextualization.

Contextualization can be handled in many ways and at many different levels depending on its inherent dynamic nature, as well as the availability of verification based on structured data. As we found no golden solution, principles for contextualization handling described in this paper are first approaches which have been tested by the first prototypes implementation [21].

Our description of contextualization aspects involved in ADE apparition is made from computable data. Other aspects are known as influencing ADE apparition but are very difficult to compute [24]: workload, bed occupancy rate, duty hours, staffing, interruptions and stress.

However, all hospitals:

- have data on staffing including turnout-plans/roster;
- have data on how many inpatients there are at the hospital/ward on a quite detailed level, which can potentially express the bed occupancy rate over time;
- register when members of the staff are ills or absents of other reasons and when they are working in double shift.

If those data could be integrated into HIS, they could add value in data mining and thus in CDSS intervention.

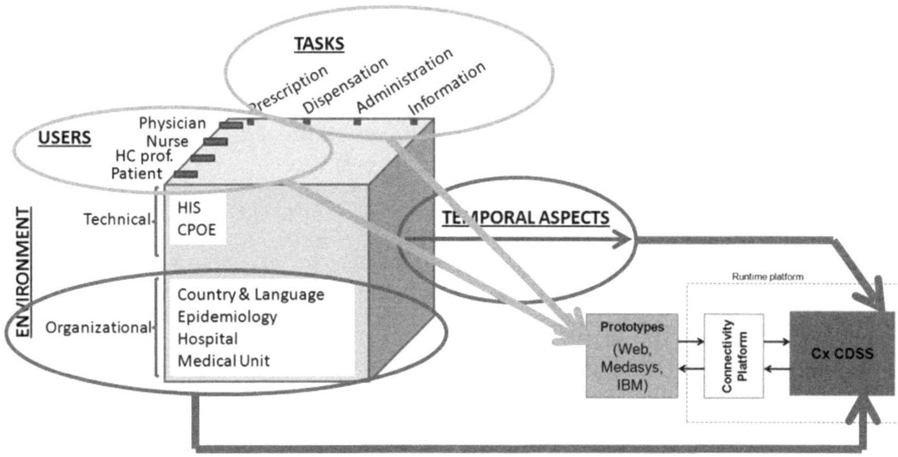

Figure 3. Summary of the information contextualization in the PSIP decision support services.

Other aspects which could explain ADE apparition (actual working conditions for the nurses and physicians: interruptions and disturbances, changes in the scope of treatment, day- and night shift, communication and coordination between staff concurrent use of HIS and patient record, clinical guidelines, paper forms, etc.) are not computable and could only help to explain why an ADE occurred but could not be taken into account in a computerized intervention.

Acknowledgements

The research leading to these results has received funding from the European Community's Seventh Framework Programme (FP7/2007-2013) under grant agreement n° 216130 – the PSIP project.

References

[1] R. Beuscart, P. McNair, J. Brender, Patient safety through intelligent procedures in medication: the PSIP project, *Stud Health Technol Inform* **148** (2009), 6–13.

[2] M.C. Beuscart-Zephir, C. Nohr, Human factors engineering for computer-supported identification and prevention of adverse drug events, *Stud Health Technol Inform* **148** (2009), 14–24.

[3] E. Chazard et al., Adverse drug events prevention rules: multi-site evaluation of rules from various sources, *Stud Health Technol Inform* **148** (2009), 102–11.

[4] A.K. Dey, G.D. Abowd, Towards a Better Understanding of Context and Context-Awareness, 1st International Symposium on Handheld and Ubiquitous Computing 1999.

[5] A. Schmidt et al., There is more to Context than Location, *Computers & Graphics Journal* **23** (1999), 893–902.

[6] J.H. Jahnke et al., Context-aware information services for health care, Modeling and retrieval of context 2004 - CEUR workshop proceedings **114** (2004), 73–84.

[7] D. Zhang et al., Context-aware infrastructure for personalized healthcare, *Stud Health Technol Inform* **117** (2005), 154–63.

[8] A. Soylu et al., Context and Adaptivity in Pervasive Computing Environments: Links with Software Engineering and Ontological Engineering, *Journal of Software* **4** (2009), 992–1013.

[9] HIMSS, *HIMSS Dictionary of Healthcare Information Technology Terms, Acronyms and Organizations*. 2006, Chicago, IL: HIMSS.
[10] P.M. Kilbridge, E.M. Welebob, D.C. Classen, Development of the Leapfrog methodology for evaluating hospital implemented inpatient computerized physician order entry systems, *Qual Saf Health Care* **15** (2006), 81–4.
[11] D.C. Classen, A.J. Avery, D.W. Bates, Evaluation and certification of computerized provider order entry systems, *J Am Med Inform Assoc* **14** (2007), 48–55.
[12] A.X. Garg et al., Effects of computerized clinical decision support systems on practitioner performance and patient outcomes: a systematic review, *JAMA* **293** (2005) 1223–38.
[13] K. Kawamoto et al., Improving clinical practice using clinical decision support systems: a systematic review of trials to identify features critical to success, *BMJ* **330** (2005), 765.
[14] J. Niès et al., Determinants of success for computerized clinical decision support systems integrated in CPOE systems: a systematic review, *AMIA Annu Symp Proc* (2006), 594–8.
[15] J.A. Osheroff et al., Improving Outcomes with Clinical Decision Support: An Implementer's Guide. 2005, Chicago, IL: HIMSS.
[16] J.M. Teich et al., Clinical decision support in electronic prescribing: recommendations and an action plan: report of the joint clinical decision support workgroup, *J Am Med Inform Assoc* 12 (2005), 365–76.
[17] K.G. Shojania et al., The effects of on-screen, point of care computer reminders on processes and outcomes of care, *Cochrane Database Syst Rev* **3** (2009), CD001096.
[18] H. van der Sijs et al., Overriding of drug safety alerts in computerized physician order entry, *J Am Med Inform Assoc* **13** (2006), 138–47.
[19] Z. Niazkhani et al., The impact of computerized provider order entry systems on inpatient clinical workflow: a literature review, *J Am Med Inform Assoc* **16** (2009), 539–49.
[20] E. Chazard et al. Detection of adverse drug events: proposal of a data model, *Stud Health Technol Inform* **148** (2009), 63–74.
[21] S. Bernonville et al., Three different cases of exploiting decision support services for adverse drug event prevention, *Stud Health Technol Inform* **166** (2011), 180–188.
[22] J. Wyatt, D. Spiegelhalter, Field trials of medical decision-aids: potential problems and solutions, *Proc Annu Symp Comput Appl Med Care* (1991), 3–7.
[23] V. Koutkias et al., Constructing clinical decision support systems for adverse drug event prevention: a knowledge-based approach, *AMIA Annu Symp Proc* (2010), 402–6.
[24] National Board of Health, Working Environment and Unintended Events in Healthcare (report in Danish). 2009: Copenhagen.

Patient Safety Informatics
V. Koutkias et al. (Eds.)
IOS Press, 2011

doi:10.3233/978-1-60750-740-6-105

Designing, Implementing and Evaluating e-Prescription: A Field Study and Comparison with PSIP Results

Costanza RICCIOLI [a,1], P. Carlo CACCIABUE [a], Mauro CAMPANINI [b] and Martin JUNG [c]
[a] *KITE Solutions, SNC, Via Labiena 93, 21014 Laveno Mombello (Va), Italy*
[b] *Ospedale Maggiore della Carità, Corso Mazzini 18, 28100 Novara, Italy*
[c] *University for Health Informatics and Technology Tyrol (UMIT), Innrain 98, 6020 Innsbruck, Austria*

Abstract. E-prescription is amongst the most widespread medical electronic support functions. However, several studies reported acceptance and utilisation rates not as high as expected. This paper performs firstly an analysis of the literature on e-prescription characteristics and functionalities especially with respect to their actual usage. Then a specific field study was conducted in an Internal Medicine ward, to investigate human factor issues associated to the introduction of an e-prescription system. Finally, the findings of the field study are framed within the actual implementation of various electronic support outputs resulting from the European Project "Patient safety through intelligent procedures in medication" (PSIP). The results show the importance of a systemic view when designing, implementing and evaluating medical support systems, as the pre-existing structures and tools largely influence the impact of those systems and their effects.

Keywords. e-Prescription, medical support systems, field studies, human factors, usability

Introduction

E-prescription can be defined as "clinicians' computerized ordering of specific medication regimens for individual patients" [1]. It is one of the longer-lasting and more widespread medical e-function. It was one of the basic requirements of a medical information management system according to the 1970 study of Collen [2]. In 70s and 80s the majority of implementation attempts of such systems met failures of varying nature and degree, while in the 90s the advances in information technology and the decrease of hardware prices led to a renewed interest and a growing diffusion of the technology [3]. Nevertheless, recent studies have shown that despite the wide diffusion, e-prescription acceptance and utilisation rates are not as high as expected.

In the recent study of Wang et al. [4], 37% of e-prescribing users reported using the system for all the prescriptions, 46% only for some prescriptions, and 17% reported that they were no longer using the system. Also Pagán et al. found a relatively low

[1] Corresponding Author: costanza.riccioli@kitesolutions.it

physician utilisation rate of electronic prescription [5]. These studies did not investigate the causes of this failure, that could be possibly related not only to IT systems technical limitations (slowness, inefficacy, inefficiency) but also to an inadequate integration with the actual medical workflows, communication and ward organisations, as various studies have highlighted [3] [6-8].

Nowadays, the landscape seems to be quickly changing: electronic prescribing nearly tripled in 2009 over 2008 and the number of physicians and other prescribers using electronic prescribing more than doubled [9]. These results can be partially due to the adopted incentives and penalties [9] [10].

The goals of this paper are: a) to analyse the literature on e-prescription characteristics and functionalities related to their use/non use; b) to investigate human factor aspects by means of a field study conducted in a Internal Medicine ward, before and after implementation of an e-prescription system; c) and to compare the findings with the actual implementation of various electronic supports output of the European Project "Patient safety through intelligent procedures in medication" (PSIP).

1. e-Prescription Systems: A Brief Review of Benefits and Disadvantages

The acronym CPOE (Computerised Physician Order Entry) usually indicates a great variety of systems. There are no clear and universally accepted boundaries of CPOE: some definitions include e-prescription, electronic medical records, alert functionalities, decision-making supports. Some studies of the literature refer to "CPOEs" even if no electronic medical records are present, or vice versa they refer to "e-prescriptions" when also advanced functions are implemented. The presence/absence of decision support mechanisms is more easily assessable, even if no standard definitions of "advanced" or "basic" decision support functionalities exist.

In this section we define and analyse three possible alternative systems with regard to e-prescription, in order of decreasing complexity:

1. systems with decision support features (Computerised Decision Support System, CDSS), e.g., advanced alerts, drug formulary knowledge, advanced dosing guidance, advanced guidance for medication-associated laboratory testing, advanced checking of drug-disease interactions and contraindications, advanced drug-pregnancy alerting, etc.;
2. systems where e-prescription is integrated with electronic medical records (Computerized Physician Order Entry, CPOE);
3. e-prescriptions as a stand-alone function.

In the last two types of system some kinds of basic and interaction alerts can be present.

1.1. e-Prescriptions with CDSS

There are no univocal conclusions about e-prescription systems with "advanced decisional features". However most of the studies report quite positive effects. Johnston et al. [11] found that advanced features as clinical decision-support tools (i.e., alerts and reminders based on patient's clinical conditions and/or allergies) and electronic medical records (i.e., a complete medication list and a recent medication history for each patient) could greatly expand clinical and financial benefits of e-prescribing. Hunt et al. [12] in a systematic review of studies of computerised decision supports found improved clinical care in nine of fifteen studies on computerized drug dosing. Evans et al. [13] describe the positive effects of an advanced clinical decision support system for antibiotic prescribing: it decreased costs, days of unnecessary therapy and adverse events. However, compliance with dosing suggestions in other studies is not high [14-16].

Wang et al. [4] investigated e-prescribing users and non-users perceptions regarding prescription safety and workload and two e-prescribing standards, one for medication history, that can be considered a quite basic function of e-prescription, and a more advanced decisional function (formulary and benefit standard). E-prescribing users reported patient safety benefits but no perceived benefits from the two standards taken into account by the study.

Some advanced e-prescribing systems assist prescribers listing the medications that are indicated for particular diagnoses. According to the panel members of the Bell et al. [17] study, this feature, though important, should not force the assignment of a diagnosis. The physician could enter a fake diagnosis to access the medications they want to prescribe. In addition, the diagnostic codes used for billing often do not take into account clinically important distinctions [18]. "Diagnosis-based medications menus" is however one of the four e-prescribing core capabilities individuated by the Bell et al. study [1].

In their review, Kuperman et al. [19] distinguish between advanced and basic decision support features. Regarding the advanced dosing guidance, Nebeker et al. [20] found that preventable ADEs (Adverse Drug Events) remained common with a CPOE that lacked decision support for drug selection, dosing, and monitoring. Advanced guidance for medication-associated to laboratory testing can have, on the contrary, positive effects, in particular in decreasing the rate of inappropriate ordering [21] [22]. In advanced drug-pregnancy alerting, despite the efforts in minimizing the number of alerts, the acceptance rate was very low [23].

The systematic review by Ammenwerth et al. [24] analysed systems with no decision support, limited decision support (evidence-based patient-specific recommendation of a drug, dosing, frequency, etc.) and advanced decision support (drug-allergy, drug-drug or other patient-specific alerts). The advanced decision support studies showed a relatively greater reduction of risk of ADE than limited decision support or no decision support studies. However, a possible limit of such results is the fact that most studies with limited support were compared to computer-based ordering, and the studies with advanced decision-support or no support were compared to paper ordering.

1.2. e-Prescriptions and CPOE

Positive effects have been reported about e-prescriptions within various kinds of CPOEs, in particular in reducing the risk for medication errors and ADEs [24].

However, the Kuperman et al. [19] analysis of basic decision support features pointed out also some possible problems related to the use of alerts. In particular, drug-allergy alerts are often excessive, clinically irrelevant, disruptor of clinicians workflows, not presented in effective and appropriate ways [25], and therefore widely overridden [26], modified and removed [27] [23]. Duplicate therapy alerts can interrupt clinicians' workflow and cause frustration if they are not clinically relevant [19]. Miler [28] for example, found that they had been even inactivated. Similarly, drug-drug interaction alerts can be clinically insignificant. Payne et al. [29] found that 11% of medication orders caused some kind of alert(s) and clinicians overrode them in 88% of the cases, even if the alert referred on a critical drug-drug interaction.

Doolan & Bates [30] identified four barriers to the use and diffusion of CPOEs: a) physicians' work practices; b) current level of technology; c) status of commercial systems; d) lack of financial incentives.

1.3. e-Prescriptions as a Stand-alone Function

Lawrence [9] claims that even hospital organizations without Electronic Medical Records (EMR) are observing gains in clinician workflow and patient safety by the use of e-prescriptions. The opinion of a CMIO (Chief Medical Informatics Officer) on e-prescribing alone was that the improvement of the quality of care is due to the fact that general physicians logging onto the hospital's portal are able to check the prescription that the hospital has on patients. In addition, the hospital can always fax a clear print out of the prescription to the physician office.

According to the expert panel recommendations of the Bell et al. study [17], e-prescribing systems should on the contrary include also some CPOEs and CDSSs functions (access to patient's historical data, patient education, prescriber-level feedback, diagnosis-based medication menus). However, Wang et al. [31] made a comparison between different e-prescribing systems and the Bell et al. recommendations and found that most of the recommended functions were not implemented, and not for technical feasibility limits.

In the Tierney et al. study [32], randomised controlled clinical trial inpatient medical teams assigned to CPOE generated 12.7% lower charges and a 0.89 day shorter length of stay than teams using handwritten orders.

In a recent study by Lapane et al. [33], 64% of the participants rated e-prescribing as very efficient and only 3% as very inefficient. Clinicians were more likely than non-clinicians to rank it as very efficient. E-prescribing was considered in general "time-saving": the perceived efficiencies have little to do with the actual amount of time required to actually writing a prescription. Perceived efficiency gains were related to: 1) decreased errors, time to resolve errors and prescription clarifications; 2) refill processing; 3) more efficient workflow; 4) formularies knowledge and prior authorisation at the point of prescribing saves time. Perceived inefficiencies were: 1) time consuming, especially during busy times; 2) repeated alarms being incorrect or distracting; 3) prescriptions not being received or received with delay by the pharmacy.

A study by Hollingworth et al. [34] showed no increase in the total amount of time that prescribers spent on computer and writing tasks, while a recent study [35] demonstrated that e-prescribing takes longer than handwriting.

According to Bell et al. [1], e-prescribing can originate some problems. "Slips" [36] can be common: when selecting from menus, the wrong patient may be inadvertently selected. Using menus decreases wrong-dose errors by disallowing invalid combinations and enabling alerts [14] [21], but can also introduce new errors, as for example the selection of an adjacent name on an alphabetised list [37] [38], very difficult for pharmacists to recognise. Furthermore, e-prescription can require longer times [39] [40], even if experience improves prescription speed [41].

Alerts can reduce ADEs [21] [13], but highly sensitive systems can generate a large number of false positive alerts. This could lead users to ignore all alerts [26], even if they are considered as a beneficial support to patient safety [42]. There can also be a problem of integration with other e-systems, if present, that could cause the generation of incorrect or inaccurate alerts.

In some cases the factors that caused e-prescription failures or increased hazards were not identified [43] [44].

Grossman et al. study [45] found gaps between advocates' vision of e-prescribing and how physicians use commercial e-prescribing systems. Even if their perception of e-prescribing was positive, they found difficulties in achieving some activities (e.g., maintaining patient medication lists, using clinical decision support, obtaining formulary data and electronically transmitting prescriptions to pharmacies). Those problems according to the study were due to product limitations, external implementation challenges and physicians' preferences about using specific product features.

2. A Field Study

The Azienda Ospedaliera-Universitaria "Maggiore della Carità" di Novara is a 818-bed hospital located in the North of Italy. It employs more than 2,000 people and in 2009 treated 41,278 hospitalisations. The Internal Medicine 2 ward employs 9 physicians including the head physician. It was chosen for this study as recently an e-prescriptions system connected with the drug deposit of the pharmacy has been installed.

The system (not tailored to the specific needs of the Novara hospital) is called BUSTERMED™. It is not coupled with a decision support and no electronic records are in place, for the time being. It provides automatic alerts on drug-allergy interaction and on the drug entry process (e.g., duplicated drugs or active principle) but not on the diagnostic process. There is additional information on drugs and on drug-drug interactions, but not presented as automatic alerts, the physician has to access the system section. This kind of information does not present thresholds nor likelihood, therefore rare and common interactions are presented in the same way.

2.1. Participants and Methodology

The study was conducted in two phases, before and after the implementation of an e-prescription system made at the end of 2008.

The first phase of the study took place in early 2008. The goal of the field study was to identify possible supports to the ward activity of physicians, and therefore the structure of the ward system was deeply investigated. Seven exploratory semi-structured interviews (to head physicians, substitute head nurse and 5 physicians) were run. Based on the results of the interviews, an in-depth questionnaire was designed and administrated to 8 physicians.

The second phase of the study was conducted at the end of 2010. The objective was to investigate the impact of the new e-prescription system on the ward organisation: possible workflow and communication flow changes, advantages and disadvantages. Two physicians, the head nurse and head physician were interviewed. Data from a questionnaire on e-prescription alerts [46], part of the PSIP Project and administrated to 6 physicians of the ward, were also analysed.

2.2. Results and Discussion

2.2.1. The Ward Structure and Information Sharing Processes

The ward is composed of two sections and the day hospital section. Patients arrive mostly from the emergency department (90-92%). Currently there are 8 physicians (they were 13 in 2008, when the ward was dealing also with emergencies).

As an Internal Medicine ward, the diagnosis emerged as the most important outcome of the physicians activity. Therefore, the sharing of information and the distributed cognition [47] are fundamental. During the first phase of the study, two kinds of information sharing were identified: *longitudinal* and *transversal*. The first one is due to the shifts organisation of the physician's activity, that causes a longitudinal distribution of the activities and therefore of the diagnostic process. For example, a first physician requires a laboratory test, and the physician of the following shift receives the results and integrates them in the diagnostic hypothesis. In 2008, the tools utilised for this kind of communication were a paper with patient summaries and emergencies, and the paper medical records.

The *transversal* information sharing process concerns the collaboration between various physicians at the same time. For example, this occurs during shifts overlapping, or medical round or when asking for advise or clarifications.

Table 1. Perceived benefits and disadvantages of the BUSTERMED™ system reported during the interviews.

Benefits	**Disadvantages**
	There is no integration with the other software (e.g., laboratory, radiology, chemotherapy prescriptions, etc.)
Communication between nurses and physician greatly improved	According to certain physicians, they are more prone to errors (the process is longer, and therefore there are more error opportunities); while nurses are less prone to errors (communication with physicians is highly improved)
Less transcription errors/clarification requests	There are some error prone contexts (e.g., once the dosage of a drug has been confused with the number of tablet)
More safety: all the administrations are clearly traced	
Copying e-prescriptions to the paper medical records is a barrier to possible errors	Copying e-prescriptions to the paper medical records can be another error prone situation
User friendly and clear interface	Some stiffness of the system has been pointed out (e.g., if two different dosages of a drug have to be entered in the system, the drug has to be entered twice)
E-prescriptions require more time: prescriptions have to be done more carefully and diagnostic reasoning is more accurate	E-prescriptions require more time than the paper procedure, especially at the entrance of the patient when a new medical record is compiled
	Only 2 or 3 laptops are available; otherwise the physicians have to use the system in their offices

2.2.2. The Introduction of an e-Prescription System

The BUSTERMED™ e-prescription system was introduced at the end of 2008. The head physician and the head nurse are very satisfied of this system. The interviewed physicians pointed out also some disadvantages of the system (see Table 1).The results of the questionnaire show that physicians agree on the fact that the BUSTERMED™ system can improve prescribing quality. Alerts and additional information on the detected interactions are in fact considered useful according to almost all the physicians. However, there is no consensus whether the system could provide information that they do not know already, nor that it could influence their decisions, even if they all agree that the system does not limit their decisions. Alerts are not seen as a waste of time, even if there is no consensus on the fact that reacting to them could be not time-consuming. Finally, there is no consensus on the fact that alerts should or not interrupt clinical workflows.

In general, e-prescription with the new system is not considered more time-consuming than handwriting; some actions require more time, others less. Even if more steps could mean more error-prone situations, the lengthening of some passages is considered even positive, since it leads to less automatic prescriptions and diagnostic reasoning. It could therefore improve the *transversal* sharing of information. In fact, the satisfaction level about the system has been reported as minor in other hospital wards that have implemented it, as for example the Surgery ward, where diagnosis is a less central activity.

An important limit of the system is the fact that it is not integrated with the other software (e.g., laboratory, radiology, chemotherapy prescriptions, etc.). Physicians have to remember many different passwords and closing and opening several applications at the same time. This could cause additional cognitive workload and waste of time. Different applications could also mean more possibilities to loose information (for example, duplicate information on the paper medical records could help in identifying errors but also create new transcription errors). The integration could in fact be useful also in order to optimise communication. In particular, it could improve the *longitudinal* sharing of information: the paper with the patient problems and emergencies, as suggested during the interviews, could be integrated in the system, and therefore more easily shared. The system has already greatly improved the communication between nurses and physician. In 2008, because of the lack of dedicated nurses-physicians briefings, that physicians apparently did not consider fundamental, this kind of communication emerged as potentially improvable. Now the new system makes actions and therefore sharing of information and communications univocally clear, nominative and traceable and thus greatly improved.

Finally, alerts did not emerge as a problematic aspect of the e-prescription system; the well known problem of overexposure is not present as the system provides only automatic allergy related alerts that are less common than other kinds of alerts. Drug-drug interaction information are present "on demand"; this does not cause overexposure but has several limits: a) physicians could not have the time to consult it; b) physicians could not know that this information is available; c) since this kind of information is not filtered/weighted by relevance, rarity, etc, physicians have to refer to their medical knowledge in order to value it, and thus they risk to take into account only information that they already know (*confirmation bias* [48]).

It is therefore possible to conclude that the e-prescription system could be better integrated with the other ward software and adapted to improve general communication and sharing of information; however the field study has shown that its introduction has not worsen the pre-existing situation, on the contrary it has introduced communication advantages in particular for nurses, but also regarding the physicians diagnostic process.

3. A Comparison with Some Outputs of the European Project PSIP

Within the PSIP Project, the design of the PSIP CDSS [49] and tools followed a user-centred process and led to a set of recommendations. Some of them are "high level recommendations" that can be applied also to similar support systems, as e-prescription systems. They are consistent with the findings from the literature on e-prescription limits and our field study:

- Integrate systems in the clinical workflows (for example filtering/parameterisation of alerts, supporting dialog with the user and feedbacks);
- Support the elaboration and maintenance of a shared mental model of the patient therapeutic plan for all the involved healthcare professionals;
- Support the access to systems information by patients;
- Support monitoring of system use for further improvement and maintenance of knowledge;
- Support parameterisation of the systems per hospital, per department, and, eventually, per physician (speciality).

The necessity of *integration of the systems* is considered fundamental, since it improves communication between the different professionals involved, and also with patients. Furthermore, it leads to *avoid additional waste of time* that could be also pursued by means of alerts filtering and parameterization/contextualization of systems.

The PSIP project, besides the CDSS module, has produced several support tools prototypes. The results of the human-centred design and usability analysis highlight the actual implementation of the recommendation and other findings, consistent with the above remarks.

The **Scorecards tool** presents the statistical results on the occurrence of Adverse Drug Events (detected by data mining of hospital databases) in order to support the discussion with healthcare professionals. Besides some minor usability problems, the tool appears as an effective implementation of the idea of parameterization/contextualization of supports per hospitals and of the monitoring and upgrading of the supports knowledge.

The **MEDASYS DxCare® prototype** objective is to integrate PSIP alerts and information with the MEDASYS DxCare®, a system that combines the functions of a CPOE and a patient record. Integration of systems is a recommendation emerged also from our field study. However, it can be difficult to implement, especially if some technical rigidness are present. In this case, some problems were noticed: the PSIP information is difficult to access from the main page; there is no way to know whether the alert has been "seen" or not; finally, the format of the PSIP information is difficult to read and to understand. The format of the PSIP information should be consistent in every output tool of the Project. The tool is based on the concept of "information on demand" since PSIP alerts deal mostly with risks that are not urgent to counteract. However, as emerged in our field study, information on demand is a positive feature since it does not interrupt clinical workflows, but could be easily ignored.

By utilising the **Support tool for healthcare professionals**, different professionals, in particular physicians and pharmacists, can manually enter prescriptions and verify the presence or absence of PSIP alerts. It can also integrate other kinds of knowledge and alerts. This tool is especially conceived for situations in which full integration is technically impossible, as electronic medical records are not available. However, as usability evaluations have shown, it is a very user friendly and easily utilisable tool; this kind of "information on demand" appears useful and not time-consuming and does not present many of the disadvantages pointed out in previous sections.

These examples from the PSIP project are consistent with the results from our study. This is a further demonstration that the activity carried out in a project like PSIP, where supports are designed on the basis of human factors analyses and integrated with the actual clinical activities and, more in general, the development of accurate and dedicated support systems in the medical environment has eventually found, after many years of R&D efforts and studies, an efficient and effective way forward for the actual improvement of safety in health care and decision making process at all levels of the patient safety process.

4. Conclusions

The implementation of electronic support systems in medical environments is very rapidly diffusing and the improvements resulting from their application is clearly demonstrated both at quantitative and qualitative level. However, as several studies reported, acceptance and utilisation rates are not always as good as expected. This is probably due to the impact of the new tools on pre-existing situations and workflows that are not always adequately accounted for when designing medical support tools and functions. The field study presented in this paper was conducted in order to investigate some of those human factors and organisational aspects before and after the introduction of an e-prescription system. The results from the study show very similar results with respect to the findings of the PSIP Project on the development and usability evaluation of other forms of electronic medical support tools: the importance of systems integration in actual clinical workflows and with other software; communication improvement as support of shared mental models for all healthcare professionals; parameterisation of alerts and systems knowledge. These findings confirm the importance of a systemic view when designing, implementing and evaluating medical support systems, as the pre-existing or collateral structures and tools largely influence the impact of those systems and their effects.

Acknowledgments

The research leading to these results has received funding from the European Community's Seventh Framework Programme (FP7/2007-2013) under grant agreement n° 216130 – the PSIP project.

References

[1] D.S. Bell, S. Cretin, R.S. Marken, A.B. Landman, A conceptual framework for evaluating outpatient electronic prescribing systems based on their functional capabilities, *J Am Med Inform Assoc* **11** (2004), 60–70.

[2] M.F. Collen, General requirements for a medical information system (MIS), *Comput Biomed Res* **3** (1970), 393–406.

[3] D.F. Sittig, W.W. Stead, Computer-based Physician Order Entry: The state of the art, *J Am Med Inform Assoc* **1** (1994), 108–23.

[4] C.J. Wang et al., Perceptions of standards-based electronic prescribing systems as implemented in outpatient primary care: A physician survey, *J Am Med Inform Assoc* **16** (2009), 493–502.

[5] J.A. Pagán, W.R. Pratt and J. Sun, Which physicians have access to electronic prescribing and which ones end up using it?, *Health Policy*, **89** (2008), 288–94.

[6] C. Riccioli, N. Leroy, S. Pelayo, The PSIP approach to account for human factors in Adverse Drug Events: Preliminary field studies, *Stud Health Technol Inform*, **148** (2009), 197–205.

[7] T.A. Massaro, Introducing physician order entry at a major academic medical center: I. Impact on organizational culture and behaviour, *Academic Medicine*, **68** (1993), 20–5.

[8] A.N. Healey, S. Olsen, R. Davis, C.A. Vincent, A method for measuring work interference in surgical teams, *Cognition Technology and Work* **10** (2008), 305–12.

[9] D. Lawrence, Steps forward on e-prescribing. As e-prescribing becomes more widespread, even hospital organizations without full EMR implementation are seeing gains in clinician workflow and patient safety, *Healthc Inform* **27** (2010), 24–6.

[10] S.N. Weingart et al., Assessing the value of electronic prescribing in ambulatory care: A focus group study, *Int J Med Inform* **78** (2009), 571–8.

[11] D. Johnston, E. Pan, J. Walker, The value of CPOE in ambulatory settings, *J Healthc Inf Manag* **18** (2004), 5–8.

[12] D.L. Hunt, R.B. Haynes, S.E. Hanna, K. Smith, Effects of computer-based clinical decision support systems on physician performance and patient outcomes: A systematic review, *J Am Med Inform Assoc* **280** (1998), 1339–46.

[13] R.S. Evans et al., A computer-assisted management program for antibiotics and other antiinfective agents, *N Engl J Med* **338** (1998), 232–8.

[14] J.M. Teich, P.R. Merchia, J.L. Schmiz, G.J. Kuperman, C.D. Spurr, D.W. Bates, Effects of Computerized Physician Order Entry on prescribing practices, *Arch Intern Med* **160** (2000), 2741–47.

[15] G.M. Chertow et al., Guided medication dosing for inpatients with renal insufficiency, *J Am Med Inform Assoc* **286** (2001), 2839–44.

[16] B. Killelea, R. Kaushal, M. Cooper, G.J. Kuperman, To what extent do pediatricians accept computer-based dosing suggestions?, *Pediatrics* **119** (2007), 69–75.

[17] D.S. Bell, R.S. Marken, R.C. Meili, C.J. Wang, M. Rosen, R.H. Brook, RAND Electronic Prescribing Expert Advisory Panel, Recommendations for comparing electronic prescribing systems: results of an expert consensus process, *Health Aff (Millwood)* **W4** (2004), 305–17.

[18] C.G. Chute, Clinical classification and terminology: some history and current observations, *J Am Med Inform Assoc* **7** (2000), 298–303.

[19] G.J. Kuperman et al, Medication-related Clinical Decision Support in Computerized Provider Order Entry systems: a review. *J Am Med Inform Assoc* **14** (2007), 29–40.

[20] J.R Nebeker, J.M Hoffman, C.R. Weir, C.L. Bennett, J.F. Hurdle, High rates of adverse drug events in a highly computerized hospital, *Arch Intern Med* **165** (2005), 1111–16.

[21] D.W. Bates et al., A randomized trial of a computer-based intervention to reduce utilization of redundant laboratory tests, *Am J Med* **106** (1999), 144–50.

[22] P. Chen, M.J. Tanasijevic, R.A. Schoenenberger, J. Fiskio, G.J. Kuperman, D.W. Bates, A computer-based intervention for improving the appropriateness of antiepileptic drug level monitoring, *Am J Clin Pathol* **119** (2003), 432–8.

[23] N.R. Shah et al., Improving acceptance of computerized prescribing alerts in ambulatory care. *J Am Med Inform Assoc* **13** (2006), 5–11.

[24] E. Ammenwerth, P. Schnell-Inderst, C. Machan, U. Siebert, The effect of electronic prescribing on medication errors and Adverse Drug Events: A systematic review, *J Am Med Inform Assoc* **15** (2008), 585–600.

[25] R.A. Miller, L.R. Waitman, S. Chen, S.T. Rosenbloom, The anatomy of decision support during inpatient Care Provider Order Entry (CPOE): empirical observations from a decade of CPOE experience at Vanderbilt, *J Biomed Inform* **38** (2005), 469–85.

[26] S.A. Abookire et al., Improving allergy alerting in a Computerized Physician Order Entry system, *Proceedings/AMIA Annual Symposium* (2000), 2–6.

[27] E. Resetar, R.M. Reichley, L.A. Noirot, W.C. Dunagan, T.C. Bailey, Customizing a commercial rule base for detecting drug-drug interactions, *Proceedings/AMIA Annual Symposium* (2005),1094.
[28] A.S. Miler, Pharmacy issues: Clinical screenings and discharge prescriptions, *Hospital Pharmacy* **36** (2001), 1290–95.
[29] T.H. Payne, W.P Nichol, P. Hoey, J. Savarino, Characteristics and override rates of order checks in a practitioner order entry system. *Proceedings/AMIA Annual Symposium* (2002), 602–6.
[30] D.F. Doolan, D.W. Bates, Computerized Physician Order Entry systems in hospitals: Mandates and incentives, *Health Aff (Millwood)* **21** (2002), 180–8.
[31] C.J. Wang, R.S. Marken, R.C. Meili, J.B. Straus, A.B. Landman, D.S. Bell, Functional characteristics of commercial ambulatory electronic prescribing systems: A field study, *J Am Med Inform Assoc* **12** (2005), 346–56.
[32] W.M. Tierney, M.E. Miller, J.M. Overhage, C.J. McDonald, Physician inpatient order writing on microcomputer workstations. Effects on resource utilization, *J Am Med Inform Assoc* **269** (1993), 379–83.
[33] K.L Lapane, R.K. Rosen, C. Dubé, Perceptions of e-prescribing efficiencies and inefficiencies in ambulatory care, *Int J Med Inform* **80** (2011), 39–46.
[34] W. Hollingworth et al., The impact of e-prescribing on prescriber and staff time in ambulatory care clinics: A time motion study, *J Am Med Inform Assoc* **14** (2007), 722–30.
[35] E.B. Devine et al., Electronic prescribing at the point of care: a time-motion study in the primary care setting, *Health Serv Res* **45** (2010), 152–71.
[36] J. Reason, *Human error*, Cambridge University Press, New York, 1990.
[37] B.L Lambert, S.J. Lin, K.Y. Chang, S.K Gandhi, Similarity as a risk factor in drug-name confusion errors: The look-alike (orthographic) and sound-alike (phonetic) model, *Med Care* **37** (1999), 1214–25.
[38] B.L. Lambert, K.Y Chang, S.J. Lin, Effect of orthographic and phonological similarity on false recognition of drug names, *Soc Sci Med* **52** (2001), 1843–57.
[39] D.W. Bates, D.L. Boyle, T.M. Teich, Impact of computerised physician order entry on physician time, *Proceedings of the Annual Symposium on Computer Application in Medical Care* (1994), 996.
[40] W.M. Tierney, J.M. Overhage, C.J. McDonald, F.D. Wolinsky, Medical students' and housestaff's opinions of computerized order-writing, *Acad Med* **69** (1994), 386–9.
[41] J.M. Overhage, S. Perkins, W.M. Tierney, C.J. McDonald, Controlled trial of direct physician order entry: Effects on physicians' time utilization in ambulatory primary care internal medicine practices, *J Am Med Inform Assoc* **8** (2001) 361–71.
[42] K.L. Lapane, M.E. Waring, K.L. Schneider, C. Dubé, B.J. Quiliam, A mixed method study of the merits of e-prescribing drug alerts in primary care, *J Gen Intern Med* **23** (2008), 442–6.
[43] D.W. Bates, J.M. Teich, J.Lee, D. Seger, G.J. Kuperman, N. Ma'Luf, D. Boyle, L. Leape, The impact of computerized physician order entry on medication error prevention, *J Am Med Inform Assoc* **6** (1999), 313–21.
[44] N.G. Leveson, C.S. Turner, An investigation of the Therac-25 accidents, *IEEE Computer* **26** (1993), 18–41.
[45] J.M. Grossman, A. Gerland, M.C. Reed, C. Fahlman, Physicians' experiences using commercial e-prescribing systems, *Health Aff (Millwood)* **26** (2007), w393-404.
[46] M. Jung, *Prioritization of Computerized Physician Order Entry system alerts using the clinical context: Integrating the results of an international physician survey into the technical architecture of the PSIP-project*, Master Thesis, UMIT: 2011.
[47] E. Hutchins, *Cognition in the Wild*, MIT Press, Cambridge, Massachusetts, 1995.
[48] T.S. Wallsten, Physician and medical student bias in evaluating diagnostic information, *Med Decis Making* **1** (1981), 145–64.
[49] V. Koutkias et al., Constructing clinical decision support systems for adverse drug event prevention: A knowledge-based approach, *Proceedings/AMIA Annual Symposium* (2010), 402–6.

Part D

Methods and Technologies for Developing Patient Safety Systems

Patient Safety Informatics
V. Koutkias et al. (Eds.)
IOS Press, 2011

doi:10.3233/978-1-60750-740-6-119

Shallow Medication Extraction from Hospital Patient Records

Svetla BOYTCHEVA [1]
Institute of Information and Communication Technologies, Bulgarian Academy of Sciences, 25A Acad. G. Bonchev Str. Sofia, Bulgaria
and University of Library Studies and Information Technologies

Abstract. This paper presents methods for shallow Information Extraction (IE) from the free text zones of hospital Patient Records (PRs) in Bulgarian language in the Patient Safety through Intelligent Procedures in medication (PSIP) project. We extract automatically information about drug names, dosage, modes and frequency and assign the corresponding ATC code to each medication event. Using various modules for rule-based text analysis, our IE components in PSIP perform a significant amount of symbolic computations. We try to address negative statements, elliptical constructions, typical conjunctive phrases, and simple inferences concerning temporal constraints and finally aim at the assignment of the drug ACT code to the extracted medication events, which additionally complicates the extraction algorithm. The prototype of the system was used for experiments with a training corpus containing 1,300 PRs and the evaluation results are obtained using a test corpus containing 6,200 PRs. The extraction accuracy (f-score) for drug names is 98.42% and for dose 93.85%.

Keywords. Information extraction, automatic patient record processing, patient treatment information

Introduction

Huge amount of clinical narratives are produced allover the world every day; free text is convenient for expressing details about patients but is difficult for automatic processing. One of the most important challenges in biomedical informatics nowadays is to find efficient methods for information extraction from unstructured texts. The main difficulties are due to the specific medical language: large amount of terms, variety of expressions describing clinical events, rich temporal information, negations of various kinds, much explicit and tacit knowledge needed for proper interpretation and so on. In particular the Bulgarian medical texts contain a specific mixture of terminology in Latin, Cyrillic and Latin terms transcribed with Cyrillic letters. The lack of nomenclatures, corpora, and electronic dictionaries for medical terminology in Bulgarian language makes the task of automatic text processing even harder.

We have developed automatic procedures for analysis of free texts in hospital patient records in order to extract information about drug names, dosages, modes, frequency and treatment duration, and to assign the corresponding ATC code to each medication event. We deal with hospital PRs which are anonymized by the hospital

[1] Corresponding Author: svetla.boytcheva@gmail.com

information system of the University Specialized Hospital for Active Treatment of Endocrinology "Acad. I. Penchev" (USHATE) at Medical University – Sofia.

This paper is organized as follows. Section 1 presents an overview of related work. Section 2 describes the resource bank used in our prototype. Section 3 discusses the system architecture and some examples; it presents our approach and the main problems that need to be solved. Section 4 summarizes the experiment results and the evaluation. Section 5 contains the discussion and sketches ideas for further work.

1. Background and Related Works

Natural language processing (NLP) is viewed as the most promising technology for capturing information from free text documents. Here we briefly overview the major NLP approaches which focus on automatic identification of drugs and adverse drug events in the text. During the Third i2b2 Shared Task and Workshop "Challenges in Natural Language Processing for Clinical Data: Medication Extraction Challenge" [1] several semi- and un-supervised systems for medical information extraction were presented, e.g. [2]. The most popular approaches for solving this task are:

- ***Information Extraction*** (IE) - simple pattern matching techniques and partial shallow analysis are widely used in biomedical text processing, see a recent review of systems which extract information from textual documents in the electronic health records [3].
- ***Rule-based methods*** recognize well the regular configurations of text entities. For instance, the NLP system CLARIT extracts drug-dosage information from clinical narratives using pattern matching based on regular expressions [4]. Text analysis is accomplished in five steps: tokenization, stemming, syntactic category assignment, semantic category assignment and pattern matching.
- ***Machine learning*** is another popular NLP technique. For instance, the article [5] presents a cascade approach for extracting medication information. The implemented system recognizes medication events by combining machine learning and a rule-based approach. Two machine learners were used, namely the Conditional Random Field (CRF) and Support Vector Machine (SVM). The authors report high recall (91.44% for medication and 93.49% for dosage), high precision (91.35% for medication and for 96.36% dosage) and correspondingly high f-measure (91.40% for medication and 94.91% for dosage). Another SVM-based named entity recognition system for extraction of medication related entities achieves best f-score of 90.05% [6].
- ***Statistical hybrid methods*** combine machine learning and rule-based modules. The article [7] presents a hybrid system performing medication information extraction. With only a handful of template-filling rules, the system's core is a cascade of statistical classifiers for field detection. This system did not participate in the i2b2 Challenge but it achieves good results that match the top i2b2 systems: recall for medication 88.5% and for dosage 90.8%; precision for medication 91.2% and for dosage 96.6%; f-measure for medication 89.9% and for dosage 93.6%.
- ***Event driven approaches***: the extraction of adverse drug events and effect relations from clinical records is presented in [8]. The authors propose a method

to extract adverse–effect relations using a machine learning technique with dependency features.

- ***Semantic mining*** comprises a set of ontology-based techniques which extract relevant information from medical letters and reports, using the main health terminologies [9]. Semantic mining applies NLP to capture information which is not included or is missing in the Hospital Information Systems and CPOE databases. Semantic mining provides for each medical letter or report relevant terms from different terminologies with their meaning and relations between them. Semantic Mining is closely related to various Natural Language Processing tools, therefore it addresses documents in specific languages.

The evaluation results cited above show that no contemporary NLP system provides extraction with 100% precision and recall. However, despite all difficulties to process automatically the narrative texts in the medical domain, the interest in the development of fundamental and applied NLP methods for medical text analysis is constantly growing. This is due to the fact that NLP is viewed as the only means for (partial) automatic understanding of medical documents [10]. Comparing the methods listed in this section we see that CRF delivers better results than the Rule-based approach, and the latter performs better than SVM.

2. Resource Bank

Unfortunately, the presented IE techniques cannot be directly adapted to our project, because we deal with documents in Bulgarian and major language-processing activities start from scratch. First we need to cope with the morphological variants (drug names might occur in various wordforms due to the inflectional Bulgarian language). Phrasal patterns are acquired manually, to enable shallow sentence analysis by pattern matching with cascading applications of regular expressions. We partly use available linguistic resources but they support extraction of diagnoses and patient status [11]. Thus, the medication IE started by the development of lexicons and training corpora.

UNIQUE ID	ATC code	Pharmacy code	Drug Name in Bulgarian	Pharmacy Unit	Dose	Dose Unit	Drug Name in EN
52	A10AB01	01000054	Инсулин актрапид МС	амп	300,000	I.U.	Insulin actrapid MC
53	A10AB01	01000055	Инсулин актрапид НМ	амп	300,000	I.U.	Insulin Actrapid HM
448	A10AB01	01000560	Хумулин R 40Е 10Ммл	бр	400,000	I.U.	Humulin R 40

Figure 1. Excerpts of drugs-related records in the USHATE Hospital Pharmacy.

The list of registered drugs in Bulgaria is provided by the Bulgarian Drug Agency [12]; it contains about 4,000 drug names and their ATC codes. The main reference list uses the Latin drug names and the Bulgarian translations are provided in additional pdf-files. However, the patient records in USHATE use mostly Bulgarian drug names, so we needed to compile a Bulgarian lexicon of drug names. The Hospital Pharmacy (HP) supports names in two languages (HP entries in Figure 1): ATC code, drug names in Bulgarian and English, pharmacy code, dose, etc. Currently the HP operates with 1,537 medications because USHATE is specialized mostly for treatment of diabetic patients.

By matching lists of Bulgarian drug names, compiled from various sources including informal public sites in the Internet, we have found 304 drugs that are mentioned in the USHATE hospital PRs but are not prescribed via the Hospital Pharmacy. These drugs occur in the free PR texts because they are taken by the patients to cure additional (chronic) illnesses while USHATE HPs contain records of drugs curing the diabetes. For instance, hypertony is a typical accompanying disease, and normally the patients arrive to USHATE bringing the medications prescribed by their GPs. In this way our present system processes 1841 drug names in Bulgarian and their ATC codes.

The Defined Daily Dose (DDD), associated to the ATC-classification, helps to assign default dosages when they are not explicitly mentioned in the PR texts. Lists of measurement units (both in English and Bulgarian) and various abbreviations support the recognition of text fragments discussing medication events. Our resources also contain several regular expressions and rules for (phrasal) pattern matching.

3. System Architecture

The length of PR texts in Bulgarian hospitals is usually 2-3 pages. The document is organized into the following sections: *(i)* personal details; *(ii)* diagnoses of the leading and accompanying diseases; *(iii)* anamnesis (personal medical history), including current complains, past diseases, family medical history, allergies, risk factors, and medical examiners comments; *(iv)* patient status, including results from physical examination; *(v)* laboratory and other tests findings; *(vi)* medical examiners comments; *(vii)* discussion; *(viii)* treatment; *(ix)* recommendations. Medication information is contained in sections *(iii)* anamnesis, *(vii)* discussion, *(viii)* treatment, and *(ix)* recommendations. Practically we need to process almost all text fragments in the PR.

Figure 2 presents the typical occurrences of medication descriptions in the PR texts. There are more than 50 different patterns for matching text units discussing medication name, dosage and frequency; five of them are illustrated at Figure 2.

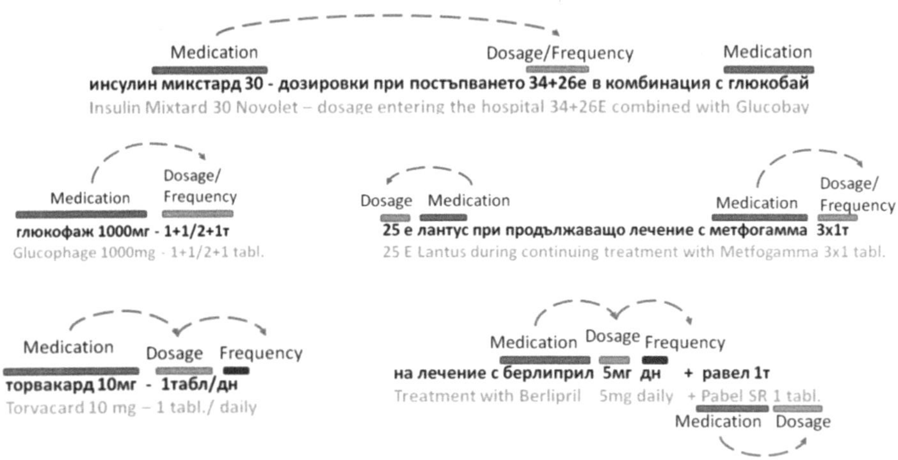

Figure 2. Sample patterns for recognition of text units expressing medication, dosage and frequency.

In some cases the dosage precedes the name: see e.g. the 3rd example, *'25E Lantus'*, while in other cases the dosage follows after the name e.g. in the 3rd example, *'Metfogamma 3x1 tabl.'*. Sometimes the drug name contains the unit signature without separators – e.g. the 2nd example – *'Glucophage 1000 mg'* and *'Torvacard 10 mg'*, but the dosage is given after a separator *'–'*. In other cases the number in the drug name does not show the unit but refers to the active substance – for instance, in the 1st example *'Mixtard 30'*, the number *'30'* means 30% Insulin Rapid.

The remaining patterns describe all variants of appearance of drug names, dosages, frequency and route and their combinations. These expressions are learnt from the training corpus.

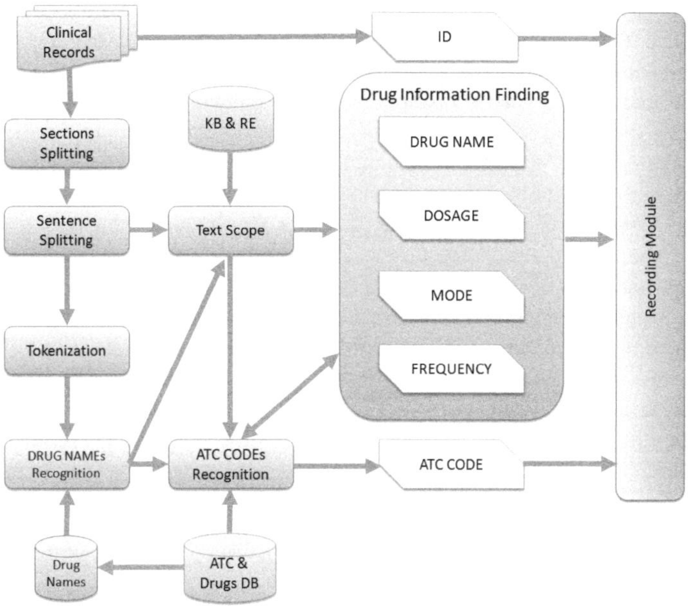

Figure 3. System Architecture: main components, resources and workflow.

The architecture of the system, which extracts medication information from hospital PRs in Bulgarian language, is shown in Figure 3. It contains eight modules:

<u>*Sections splitting*</u> – this module separates the PR texts into standardized sections. The splitting is not trivial due to varying section names, various abbreviations used to name the sections, missing sections in the PRs or missing section names, and swapped sections. The PRs summarize major patients' diseases and their treatment; the system searches medications in the whole PRs and the correct section splitting enables capturing of some temporal relations: the current treatment is presented in the anamnesis – esp. medical examiners comments, discussion, treatment and recommendations. The information about accompanying diseases and drugs which are not prescribed by the Hospital Pharmacy is given in the anamnesis section, as well as the discussion of allergies and risk factors, so it is important to fix the section boundaries correctly.

<u>*Sentence splitting*</u> – this module separates the sentences in each PR section which facilitates the further text analysis. Missing delimiters are the major difficulties in this task. Usually the PR sentences end with a period, a colon, or the end of the line, but due to several abbreviations and formatting styles additional rules for sentence splitting are needed.

<u>*Tokenization*</u> – the input PR text is split into words, digital literals and punctuation.

<u>*Drug names recognition*</u> – this module matches the 1,841 items of the drug list to the words in the PR sections. Some drug names occur several times in the text. The

resulting list contains PR drug names without duplications. The main difficulties in this task are due to the fact that *(i)* many drug names in the list have names longer than one word and *(ii)* there is a huge variety of drug descriptions in PR text: names given in Latin or in Latin transcribed with Cyrillic letters; names given by abbreviations; short names or generic descriptions given instead of full brand names. For instance: "*витамин с*" (*vitamin C*) in the PR text has to be recognized as the brand name "*Вит Ц 100мг 40бр*"; "*хумулин н*" (*Humulin N*) in PR text has to be matched to "*Хумулин N*"; "*лтироксин*" (*L-Thyroxin*) or "*л тироксин*" in the PR text is actually "*Л-тироксин 50 мг.*"; "*апидра солостар*" (*Apidra*) or "*апидра*" in the PR text has to be recognized as the brand name "*Апидра Солустар*". The algorithm first tries to match the full names, if this fails different matches of name variations are tried and finally, skipping or swapping some of the words is tried.

Text scoping – this module finds the text fragment which contains the actual information about dosage and frequency for each drug name. We assume that the last drug name's occurrence contains the actual treatment information. Sometimes the dosage and frequency are mentioned together with the previous drug name occurrences, and the last one contains only information that the previously prescribed dosage needs to be increased, decreased, doubled or remain unchanged. In this case the system finds the previous occurrence of the same drug name and captures the dosage from there, and then refines the dosage and frequency information according to last occurrence. However, as it was shown in Fig. 2, the scope of the text conveying drug names and dosage can be quite wide; this text can also contain elliptical constructions with other drugs with equivalent dosage and frequency. The text scope is determined by a cascade approach for regular expressions matching onto the PR text. The text scoping algorithm uses names of measures and a lexicon of abbreviations for dosage units' detection.

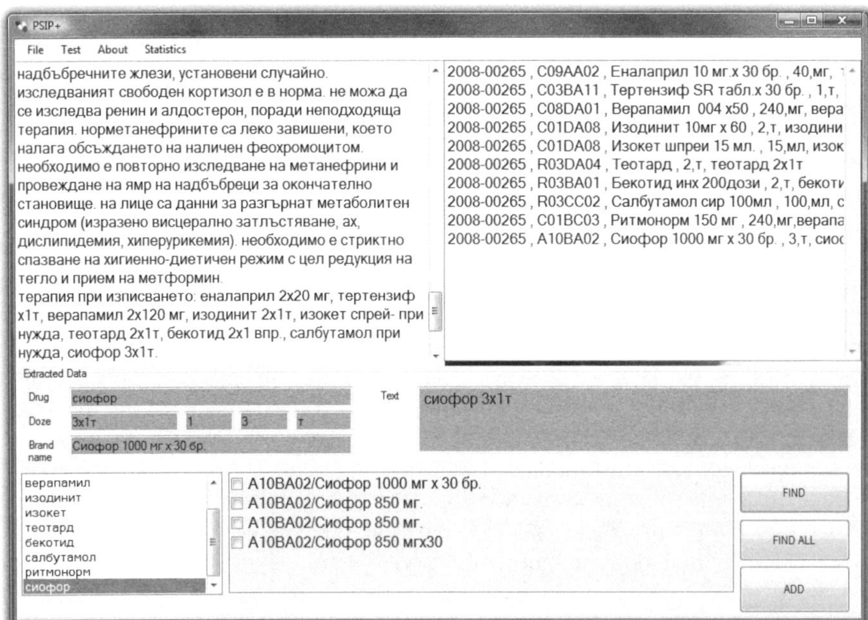

Figure 4. The user interface presenting the extracted medication data from a particular Patient Record.

Drug information finding – this module captures information about drug name, dosage, mode and frequency from the scoped text using regular expressions. If it succeeds, the result is given to the next module. If the dosage, frequency or mode/route are not recognized (because explicit details are missing in more than 30% of the PR descriptions), the drug name is passed to the next module for assignment of an ATC code and then the DDD is selected as a default value.

ATC code recognition – after the identification of drugs in the text the system finds the appropriate brand name and the corresponding ATC code. For instance, in the case of "*еналаприл 2x20 мг*" (*Enalapril*) there are two options: "*Enalapril tabl. 10 mg x 30*" and "*Enalapril tabl. 20 mg x 30*" with the same ATC code C09AA02. According to the dosage 20 mg the system chooses "*Enalapril tabl. 20 mg x 30*". If no information about the dosage is available the algorithm chooses ATC code from the generated list, according to associated priority.

Recording module – this module collects all data extracted by the previous modules and saves them in different formats – XML, ASCII or MS Excel table.

The system presented here can process PRs in *(i)* automatic mode – analyzing all PRs from a chosen folder and producing a file with the extracted medication data and *(ii)* single mode – analyzing PRs separately and presenting the results at the user interface. A sample from a single-mode analysis of one PR is shown at the screenshot in Figure 4. The PR contains information about 10 drugs; the system is ready to propose their ATC codes, dosage, mode and frequency. The last processed drug name is "*сиофор*" (*Siofor*); an ATC code and brand name from 4 options is chosen. In this way the user can test the system and evaluate its performance.

4. Evaluation Results

The experiments were made with a training corpus containing 1,300 PRs and the evaluation results are obtained using a test corpus, containing 6,200 PRs. In the test corpus there are 5,859 PRs with prescribed drugs during the hospitalization. The remaining 341 PRs concern patients hospitalized for clinical examinations only; these 341 PRs are excluded from the evaluation.

Figure 5 shows the number of drugs taken by patients during their hospitalization in USHATE. The maximal number of drugs is 27, the minimal number is 1 and the average number of drugs per patient is 5.43. Most often the patients take 2-4 drugs.

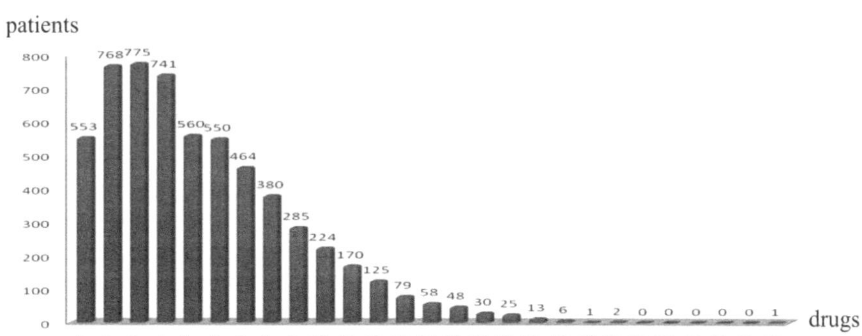

Figure 5. Number of drugs per patient.

The performance accuracy is measured by the *precision* (percentage of correctly extracted entities as a subset of all extracted entities), *recall* (percentage correctly extracted entities as a subset of all entities available in the corpus) and their harmonic mean $F=2*Precision*Recall/(Precision+Recall)$. The evaluation figures presented here summarize the IE performance for extraction of 667 different drugs (brand names) which were juxtaposed 346 different ATC codes. Evaluation results (Table 1 & Table 2) shows high percentage of success in drug name recognition in PRs texts. False negatives in Table 1 are mainly due to misspelling or too strict rules in the algorithm for recognition of drug names used in different context. False positives are mainly caused by some negation detection. We consider the negated descriptions as one expressing, following a study of negative forms in Bulgarian medical patient texts [13]. The true positive percentage is very high for drug names (30,987 true positive out of 31,853 records extracted from the test corpus, Table 1).

Table 1. Number of extracted medication events in 5,859 PRs.

	All extracted	True positive	False positive	False negative
Drug Name	31,853	30,987	836	127
Dose	26,827	24,750	2,077	1,163

Table 2. Extraction sensitivity according to the IE performance measures.

	Precision	Recall	F-Score
Drug Name	97.28%	99.59%	98.42%
Dose	92.25%	95.51%	93.85%

Below we discuss the major reasons for incorrect recognition. Errors come from:

(i) Misspelling of drug names, such as "*лтироксин*" (*LThyroxin*) or "*л тироксин*" (*L Thyroxin*) instead of "*Л-тироксин*" (*L-Thyroxin*).

(ii) Drug names occurring in the contexts of other descriptions, such as: Diagnosis e.g. "*Vitamin D deficiency*"; Examination results – such as Calcium, Kalium; Hormones – such as Testosteron and Progesterone.

(iii) Undetected descriptions of drug allergies – we have found 392 unrecognized cases, among them 316 for allergies, 25 for sensibility, 15 for intolerance and 36 for side effects.

(iv) Drug treatment described by (exclusive) *OR* – we have found about 30 cases of incorrect recognition in such kind of phrases, e.g. "*in case of deterioration the treatment should be replaced by Glucobay 3x100 or Amaryl 2mg*". In these cases both drugs are recognized and inserted in the resulting extracted records.

(v) Negations and temporally-interconnected events of various kinds:

- Undetected descriptions of canceled medication events – we have found 205 incorrect cases where the extracted drugs need to be excluded from the resulting records, e.g. "*the therapy with biguanides preparation (Glucophage) was stopped and Gliper was replaced by Diaprel*".
- Undetected descriptions of changes or replacements in therapy – we have found 234 unrecognized phrases. In this case both drugs are extracted and the previous one is not deleted from the result records.
- Undetected descriptions of insufficient treatment effect and change of therapy.

As seen in Table 1 and Table 2, the dosage recognition is less successful than the recognition of drug names. About 30% of the medication events in the test corpus were described without any dosage, e.g. "*to continue the treatment with Flarex and Azopt in the eyes*". Lack of explicit descriptions occurs mostly for treatment of accompanying diseases (because the attention of USHATE's medical expert is focused on the specialized hospital treatment, disregarding drugs that are prescribed by other clinicians beforehand). After applying the recognition algorithm and using the default DDD dosage, the number of records lacking dosage was reduced to 5,026 or 15.7% in the final result containing 31,853 records. For the PRs with explicitly declared dosages, the main sources of errors are the following ones:

- Mismatch between the PR text and the content of the respective Hospital Pharmacy/ATC values – for instance, "*C07AB0 / Atenolol 50 mg x 30*" in the Hospital Pharmacy and "*Atenolol 2x25 mg*" in the PR text. In this case the system recalculates the dosage according to the closest Pharmacy/ATC value;
- Unfixed dosage – for instance "*recommend treatment with Metformin from 3x850mg to 3x1000 mg / daily under control of the blood sugar profile*";
- Ambiguous dosage – "*treatment with Siofor 3x1 tabl.*" but in Pharmacy we have "*Siofor 1000 mg*" and "*Siofor 850 mg*".
- Partial or incomplete information about the therapy scheme or mixing dosage as part of the brand name, e.g. "*Siofor 850 mg*" etc.

Despite all complications listed in this section, the precision and recall in the automatic recognition of drug dosage are relatively high as well (see Table 2). At present we complete the evaluation of the extraction procedures which recognize drug mode/route and frequency. Our present results are comparable to the performance of advanced systems such as MedEx [14]. We try to address negative statements, elliptical constructions, typical conjunctive phrases, and simple inferences concerning temporal constraints and finally aim at the assignment of the drug ACT code to the extracted medication events, which additionally complicates the extraction algorithm.

5. Discussion and Further Work

The system presented in this article was developed and applied in the PSIP project for the preparation of an experimental USHATE's repository for PSIP validation. Actually the system enables extraction of drug-related information about drugs which are mentioned in the PR texts as accompanying medications but are not prescribed by the Hospital Pharmacy. This system is a pilot prototype performing extraction of drugs and medication events from Bulgarian medical texts. The promising results support the claim that the Information Extraction approach is helpful for obtaining of specific medication information from free patient record texts. The performance cannot be directly compared with other results reported in the literature, because of the language specific analysis techniques and the specific hospital personal records in Bulgarian language, but nevertheless the accuracy is relatively very high.

The article [15] presents French Multi-Terminology Indexer (***F-MTI***), which indexes documentation in several health terminologies. ***F-MTI*** is applied for automatic detection of Adverse Drug Events in discharge letters. The authors have developed a detailed evaluation scenario in two French hospitals (Rouen University hospital and Denain General Hospital) where the extracted entities are compared to the suggestions by human experts or the information available in the EHR (which is already encoded). The extraction of ATC codes from the free text of French discharge letters is performed with f-measure 88% when compared to the manual extraction; however, compared to the CPOE content, the f-measure is 49%. We note that the discharge letters in French seem to have no predefined structure, which is available in Bulgaria and is often (more or less) kept and significantly helps to recognize events.

When designing our solutions for processing PR texts in Bulgarian language, we keep in mind the lessons learned about other natural languages as well as the gains of applying various AI techniques for processing the language-independent entities extracted from the medical text. Using various modules for rule-based text analysis, our IE components in PSIP perform a significant amount of symbolic computations. Future enhancements are planned for extension of the name and dosage recognition rules, to cope with certain specific exceptions and section filtering rules. The preliminary correction of spell errors and other kinds of typos will also increase the IE accuracy.

Acknowledgements

The research leading to these results has received funding from the European Community's Seventh Framework Programme (FP7/2007-2013) under grant agreement n° 216130 – the PSIP project.

References

[1] https://www.i2b2.org/NLP/Medication/, last access on March 2011.
[2] J.G. Mork et al., Extracting Rx Information from Clinical Narrative, *J Am Med Inform Assoc* **17** (2010), 536–39.
[3] S.M. Meystre, G.K. Savova, K.C. Kipper-Schuler, J.F. Hurdle, Extracting Information from Textual Documents in the Electronic Health Record: A Review of Recent Research, *Yearb Med Inform* **1** (2008), 128–44.
[4] D.A. Evans, N.D. Brownlowt, W.R. Hersh, E.M. Campbell. Automating Concept Identification in the Electronic Medical Record: An Experiment in Extracting Dosage Information, *Proc AMIA Annu Fall Symp* (1996), 388–92.
[5] J. Patrick, M. Li. A Cascade Approach to Extracting Medication Events, *In Proc. Australian Language Technology Workshop (ALTA)* (2009), 99–103.
[6] S. Doan, H. Xu, Recognizing Medication related Entities in Hospital Discharge Summaries using Support Vector Machine, *In Proc. of Coling 2010: Poster Volume, Beijing* (2010), 259–66.
[7] S. Halgrim, F. Xia, I. Solti, E. Cadag, Ö. Uzuner, Extracting medication information from discharge summaries, *In Proc. of the NAACL HLT 2010 Second Louhi Workshop on Text and Data Mining of Health Documents* (2010), 61–67.
[8] Y. Miura et al., Adverse-Effect Relations Extraction from Massive Clinical Records, *In Proc. of the 2nd Workshop on NLP Challenges in the Information Explosion Era (NLPIX 2010)*, Coling, Beijing, 75–83.
[9] E. Chazard et al., *Deliverable D2.3 - Results of data & semantic mining, PSIP Project.*
[10] D. Demner-Fushman, W. Chapman, C. McDonald, What can natural language processing do for clinical decision support?, *J Biomed Inform* **42**(5) (2009), 760–72.
[11] S. Boytcheva, I. Nikolova, E. Paskaleva, G. Angelova, D. Tcharaktchiev, N. Dimitrova, Obtaining Status Descriptions via Automatic Analysis of Hospital Patient Records, In: V. Fomichov (Ed.), *Informatica, Int. J. of Computing and Informatics*, *Sp. Issue on Semantic IT* **34** (2010), 269–78.
[12] Bulgarian Drug Agency, *Drug List* at http://www.bda.bg/images/stories/documents/register/Mp.htm
[13] S. Boytcheva, A. Strupchanska, E. Paskaleva, D. Tcharaktchiev, Some Aspects of Negation Processing in Electronic Health Records, *In Proc. of International Workshop Language and Speech Infrastructure for Information Access in the Balkan Countries*, Borovets, Bulgaria, (2005), 1–8.
[14] H. Xu et al., MedEx: a medication information extraction system for clinical narratives, *J Am Med Inform Assoc* **17** (2010), 19–24.
[15] B. Merlin, E. Chazard, S. Pereira, E. Serrot, S. Sakji, R. Beuscart, S. Darmoni, Can F-MTI semantic-mined drug codes be used for Adverse Drug Events detection when no CPOE is available?, *Stud Health Technol Inform* **160**(1) (2010), 1025–29.

Patient Safety Informatics
V. Koutkias et al. (Eds.)
IOS Press, 2011

doi:10.3233/978-1-60750-740-6-129

Health Multi-Terminology Portal: A Semantic Added-value for Patient Safety

Julien GROSJEAN [a], Tayeb MERABTI [a], Badisse DAHAMNA [a], Ivan KERGOURLAY [a], Benoit THIRION [a], Lina F. SOUALMIA [a,b] and Stefan J. DARMONI [a,1]

[a] *CISMeF, Rouen University Hospital and TIBS EA 4108, Rouen University, France*
[b] *LIM&Bio EA 3969, University of Paris 13, Sorbonne Paris Cité, France*

Abstract. Since the mid-90s, several quality-controlled health gateways were developed. In France, CISMeF is the leading health gateway. It indexes Internet resources from the main institutions, using the MeSH thesaurus and the Dublin Core metadata element set. Since 2005, the CISMeF Information System (IS) includes 24 health terminologies, classifications and thesauri for indexing and information retrieval. This work aims at creating a Health Multi-Terminology Portal (HMTP) and connect it to the CISMeF Terminology Database mainly for searching concepts and terms among all the health controlled vocabularies available in French (or in English and translated in French) and browsing it dynamically. To integrate the terminologies in the CISMeF IS, three steps are necessary: (1) designing a meta-model into which each terminology can be integrated, (2) developing a process to include terminologies into the HMTP, (3) building and integrating existing and new inter-terminology mappings into the HMTP. A total of 24 terminologies are included in the HMTP, with 575,300 concepts, 852,000 synonyms, 222,800 definitions and 1,180,000 relations. Height-teen of these terminologies are not included yet in the UMLS among them, some from the World Health Organization. Since January 2010, HMTP is daily used by CISMeF librarians to index in multi-terminology mode. A health multi-terminology portal is a valuable tool helping the indexing and the retrieval of resources from a quality-controlled patient safety gateway. It can also be very useful for teaching or performing audits in terminology management.

Keywords. Abstracting and indexing, cataloguing, controlled vocabulary, information storage and retrieval, subject headings, terminology as subject

Introduction

The Internet is currently the major source of scientific and health information and knowledge. Several Quality-Controlled Health Gateways (QCHG) have now been developed. In [1], Koch defines quality-controlled subject gateways as Internet services that apply a comprehensive set of quality measures to support systematic resource discovery. Most of QCHG are using a thesaurus to index Internet resources, primarily the Medical Subject Heading (MeSH) thesaurus [2] from the US National Library of Medicine. The oldest QCHG is Diseases, Disorders and Related Topics [3] (DDRT),

[1] Corresponding Author: stefan.darmoni@chu-rouen.fr

developed since 1993 by Tor Alhenius, former Medical Librarian of Karolinska Institute in Stockholm, followed by Catalog and Index of Health Resources in French [4] (CISMeF) [5] created in February 1995, then Health on the Net [6] (HON) developed since September 1995, Intute [7], originally Organizing Medical Networked Information [8] (OMNI) created in 1996 [9], and later in 2001 Healthinsite-Au [10-11].

From 1995 to 2005, CISMeF used two standard means to describe and index the most important and quality-controlled sources of institutional health information in French: (1) the MeSH thesaurus and its French translation by the French Medlars Center (French National Institute of Health), and (2) several metadata element sets, in particular the Dublin Core metadata format [12]. In [13] CISMeF have described the various enhancements of the MeSH thesaurus, that the CISMeF team has developed for adapting this terminology to the broader field of health Internet resources (vs. scientific articles in the Medline bibliographic database where the MeSH thesaurus was originally built for).

Since 2005, the CISMeF team has undergone a major strategic shift: switching from a mono-terminological world to a multi-terminology universe for the overall CISMeF Information System (IS), which includes multi-terminology automatic indexing [14], multi-terminology information retrieval [15] and integration of several terminologies (n=24) in the CISMeF terminology database as described in Figure 1.

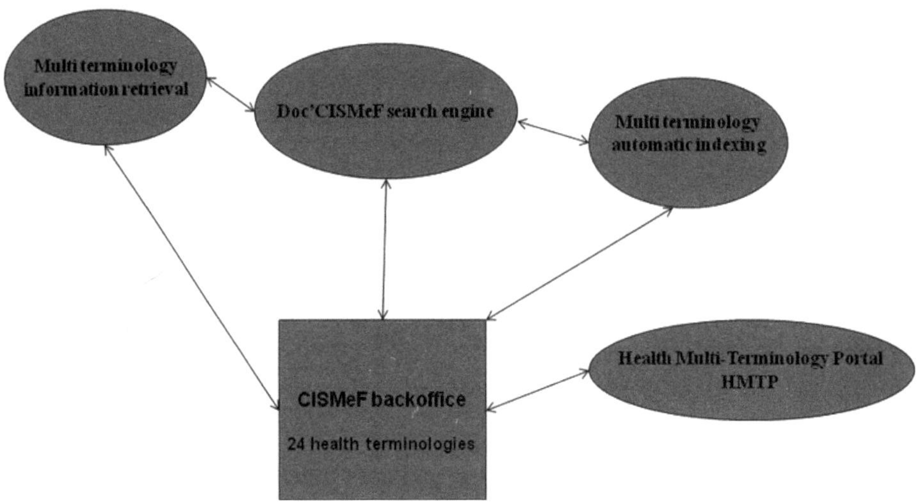

Figure 1. Inter-relationship between CISMeF Terminology Database and the HMTP and interoperability between CISMeF main tools.

There is an increasing amount of interest today not only in developing and maintaining healthcare terminologies but also in making them interoperable within information technology systems delivering services to applications. A "Terminology Server" is a tool that manages and gives access to several terminologies [16]. Many terminology servers have already been developed, mostly in English [16-20].

The principal aim of this work is to (A) create a Health Multi-Terminology Portal (HMTP) largely inspired by the most recent advances [21], to (B) connect it to the CISMeF terminology database for searching concepts and terms among all the health terminologies available in French (or in English and translated in French), in particular for patient safety included in this portal and to (C) browse it dynamically. The ultimate goal is to use the results of this research: (a) to index resources manually or automatically in the quality-controlled health gateway, such as CISMeF or its Drug Information Portal [15]; (b) to permit multi-terminology information retrieval; (c) to evaluate the integrity of terminological data (audit); (d) to provide a new source of education for students.

1. Material and Methods

1.1. List of Terminologies included in the HMTP

The six terminologies of the PSIP project (Patient Safety through Intelligent Procedures in medication) [22] have been integrated in the HMTP:

- WHO-ICD10 (International Classification of Diseases, 10th revision) [23] for diagnoses,
- WHO-ATC (Anatomical Therapeutic Chemical Classification System) [24] for drugs, developed by the Collaborating Centre for Drug Statistics Methodology,
- WHO-ICPS (International Classification for Patient Safety) [25] for patient safety vocabulary,
- C-NPU/IUPAC (International Union of Pure and Applied Chemistry) for chemical sciences and laboratory tests [26],
- NCCMERP (National Coordinating Council for Medication Error Reporting and Prevention) [27] for adverse drug event (ADE) description
- PSIP Taxonomy [28] for the description of potential dangerous situations related to medication.

Overall, twenty four terminologies and classifications have been included in the CISMeF terminology database, and therefore in the HMTP. Some of them are issued from the Unified Medical Language System (UMLS) meta-thesaurus (n=8) but not the most (n=18), and in particular:

- the MeSH thesaurus, including the MeSH Supplementary Concepts (MeSH SC), the translation in French of 8,300 MeSH SC and the add-on of over 10,000 synonyms to MeSH terms,
- the SNOMED International to describe electronic health records [29],
- two other terminologies developed by the World Health Organization (WHO): WHO-ART (Adverse Reactions Terminology) [30], for adverse effects and WHO-ICF [31] (International Classification of Functioning, disability and health) for handicap,
- Various codes used for drugs and chemical compounds: Chemical Abstract Service (CAS) for chemistry, brand names and International Non-proprietary Names (INN) for drugs, CIS, UCD, and CIP for French drugs,
- MedDRA, for adverse effects [32].
- FMA (Foundational Model of Anatomy) for the human anatomy.

Some terminologies and ontologies will be integrated in the coming months, in particular LOINC (Logical Observation Identifiers Names and Codes) for laboratory tests identification, SNOMED CT, US National Cancer Institute Terminology and UMLS Metathesaurus.

1.2. Integration of the Terminologies

To integrate the terminologies in the CISMeF database (Oracle 11.1g database), three steps are necessary: (1) the design of a meta-model into which each terminology can be integrated; (2) the design of a process that integrates the terminologies into the HMTP; (3) the construction and integration of inter-terminology mappings into the HMTP. Two inter-terminology mappings were performed: one exploiting UMLS concepts and one using NLP tools developed by the CISMeF team [33].

The meta-model designed for the database in order to fit all the terminologies into one global structure is described in Figure 2. A model of each terminology was designed as a specialization of the meta-model. The purpose of the meta-model is to factor out the artefacts (i.e. classes, relationships and attributes) that are common to all the terminologies, thus facilitating integration of multiple terminologies within a single platform. Some artefacts, although specific to certain terminologies, must nevertheless be represented in order to avoid losing information. This meta-model is generic enough to be applied to: semantic mediation, hierarchical and graphic navigation, automatic indexing, and information retrieval.

Consequently, a cut-off has to be selected in order to faithfully represent a terminology with no loss of information while removing artefacts shared by terminologies in order, subsequently, to offer independent shared services related to a given terminology. A distinction is therefore made between the unified meta-model (namely UMV2) and the extensions specific to each terminology (namely UMV1 x, where x denotes a particular terminology), as illustrated in Figure 3.

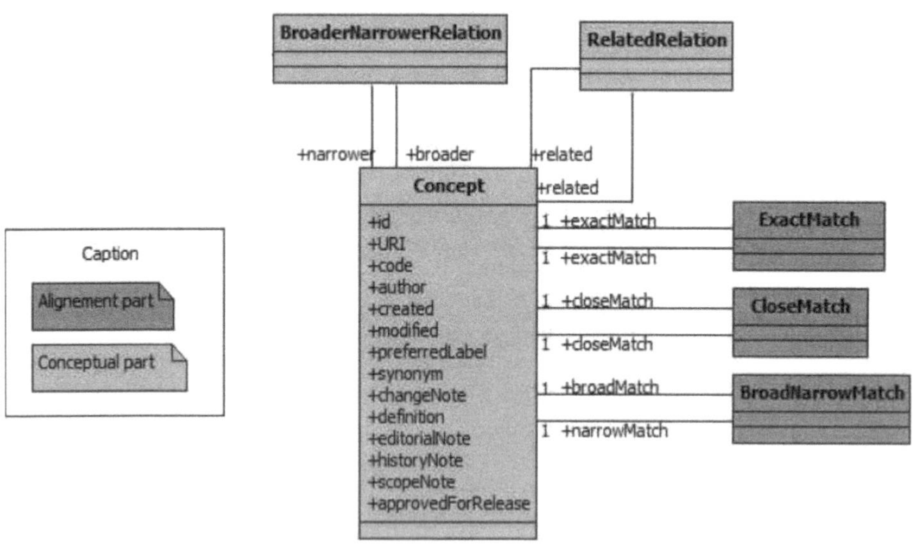

Figure 2. The CISMeF Terminology Database conceptual structure.

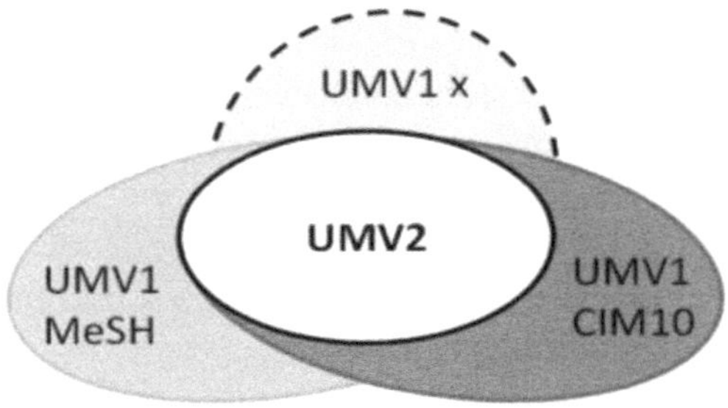

Figure 3. Representation of the unified meta-model (UMV2) and the specific extensions of each terminology (UMV1 x).

1.2.1. The CISMeF Terminology Database

This system was established around the "Descriptor" which is the central concept of the terminologies (or "keyword"). Each descriptor is labelled and may be defined, linked to other descriptors (such as Related-Term relation) and involved in a hierarchy (BT-NT for Broader Term – Narrower Term). A descriptor may also contain specific attributes, synonyms, abbreviations, etc.

It was also necessary to work on the terminologies modelling in order to fit it into the global database structure and to standardize the data in a well known and shared format. That is why the Resource Description Framework (RDF) syntax was chosen with the Ontology Web Language (OWL), standards recommended by the W3C. The workflow of terminology integration is described in Figure 4.

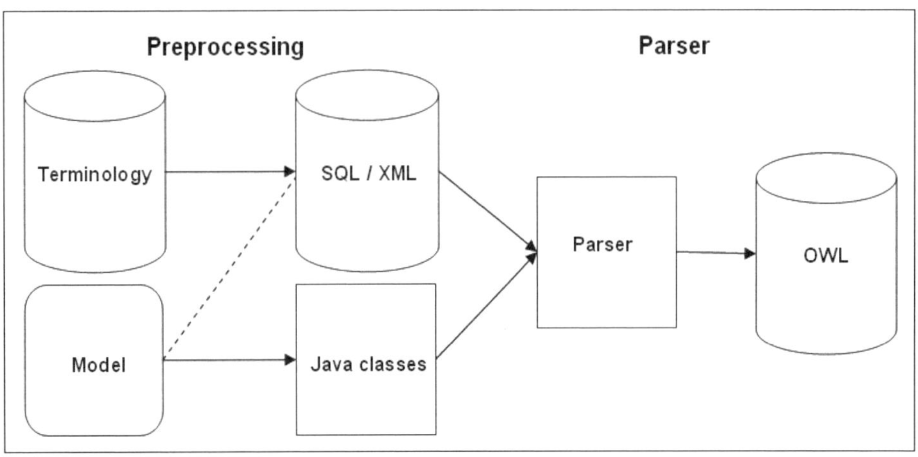

Figure 4. Process for formatting a terminology into OWL.

1.2.2. OWL Models

The first part consists in creating a meta-model in OWL that can include all the terminologies. The Unified Model for Vocabularies has been specified for these requirements. The next stage consists in creating one model for each terminology. Thus, the original data was collected and the native structure of each terminology needed to be well understood.

1.2.3. OWL Data Files

The second part of the work consists in developing a parser for each terminology. The input is the original data (or normalized original data) and the output is a representation of the terminology in OWL. As data could be in different shapes and structures, in some cases additional processes were performed (temporary databases, files in several formats, etc).

1.2.4. Database Integration

The final stage is the integration of the OWL files into the CISMeF Information System (IS). A generic parser was developed to directly insert each terminology into the database. A special model was designed to represent each terminology in a "CISMeF Terminology Database view". The parser can use this model as an input to recognize descriptor classes, definitions, synonyms, relations in order to insert it very easily into the database.

1.3. Creation of the HMTP

The HMTP was designed as a graphic interface of a Web Service, entirely dedicated to information retrieval and semantic relations between terms of several terminologies. Thus, the main objective was to dissociate the substance from the form, in particular the interface.

1.3.1. The HTMP Web Service

This Web Service was the most important part of the task: retrieve information and major schemes to allow the fullest display in the HMTP interface. The HMTP Web Service has been developed to respect Web Services Standards with Simple Object Access Protocol (SOAP) and Web Service Description Language (WSDL) signatures. It presents some methods to search terms by a concept or by a database unique identifier: in all terminologies/ontologies, concepts are unique Ids. A specific assessment of SQL queries on the database has been performed to obtain the best response time. This program queries a special version of the CISMeF IS with extended tables. Another important point of this Web Service is the security management. Axis2 (Apache) is used to deploy Web Services and its module Rampart, which deals with security to authenticate users that want to access the signatures of the HMTP Web Service. Finally, the Jena API was used to generate the final Simple Knowledge Organization System (SKOS) file to be sent by the Web Service as a response. Consequently, this file is well formed and deals with W3C standards.

1.3.2. The HTMP Website

As the HMTP exploits a SKOS file, the graphic interface that renders the final HTML was build based on Java Server Pages (JSP) files including eXtensible Stylesheet Language (XSL) functions. Additional Cascading Style Sheets (CSS) and JavaScript functions are implemented to offer a better Website design. The final HTML rendering is processed by the client navigator. This method is a major positive factor for the Web application because it works with a minimum of effort.

For optimal performance, special Asynchronous JavaScript And XML (AJAX) methods are implemented. Since the whole SKOS file data is not directly displayed on the navigator screen, it is useless to transform the entire document in XHTML with the XSL. Therefore, with JavaScript methods, it is possible to re-transform specific portions of the SKOS file immediately (e.g. semantic relations, hierarchies, results of search by terminology). This technology is a very powerful way to increase load speed and to reduce the XSLT processor load for the client navigator. It is also very interesting because usually AJAX utilisation means a direct server request. With the combination of a Web Service, XSLT and AJAX, this step is not necessary (it also reduces the server load and the transformation speed).

1.3.3. Hardware, Software and Standards

The HMTP Web Service responds in SKOS language and conforms to Web Services Standards such as WSDL and SOAP. It is written in Java (J2EE on JRE 1.6). The HMTP is composed of several servlets that query the different WSDL signatures of the Web Service. The graphic interface is a set of JSP containing XSL functions and templates. Advanced JavaScript methods and CSS are used to finalize characteristics and the client functionalities of the final XHTML Web page. The HMTP has been mainly developed for Firefox 3.x Web browsers but it also works on Internet Explorer 6 and later, Google Chrome and Safari. The final output (XHTML) conforms to the W3C standards.

2. Results

This terminology portal is available online with a restricted access: http://pts.chu-rouen.fr/ (click on "Log in"; id=cismef; password=demo10). To perform mappings between PSIP terminologies (terms alignments), it was necessary to use CISMeF semantic tools because 5 out of 6 PSIP terminologies were not included in the UMLS. Therefore, it was not possible to use concept mappings based on UMLS. Table 1 provides the mapping square matrix between the six PSIP terminologies.

Due to various optimizations, the average response time for one concurrent user takes less than 500 milliseconds. HMTP is daily used by CISMeF librarians to index health resources in multi-terminology mode for the CISMeF catalogue and the Drug Information Portal.

Among the 38,237 CISMeF resources which are manually indexed, 32,970 (86.22%) are indexed with only one thesaurus (the MeSH, which is the CISMeF main terminology since 1995). A total of 3,866 (10.11%) are indexed with two terminologies, 1,397 (3.65%) with three terminologies and 4 with four terminologies.

All the CISMeF resources are manually indexed with at least one MeSH term, even though the perfect term does not yet exist. For example, in the case of a resource where the main subject is the "*Rokitansky syndrome*", there is no MeSH term for this rare disease. The CISMeF indexer used two MeSH terms *vagina/abnormalities* and *uterus/abnormalities,* and have added one SNOMED term *Rokitansky sequence*.

Among the 34,679 CISMeF resources which are automatically indexed, 33,935 (97.85%) are indexed with MeSH and 25,568 (73.72%) with SNOMED. Only 1,051 CISMeF resources are automatically indexed with one terminology (3,137 with two, 5,379 with three, 5,997 with four and 13,514 with more than four terminologies).

Besides MeSH, two terminologies are in constant use: the CCAM is used if possible in the case of technology evaluation of procedures mainly by the French Health Authority (equivalent to the US AHRQ) and the WHO-ATC to index resources about drugs [15, 34].

HMTP is also used by various CISMeF academic partners in different French and European projects (ANR below is a French acronym for National Research Agency):

- InterSTIS [35] project (ANR-07-TECSAN-010);
- ALADIN [36] project (ANR-08-TECS-001);
- L3IM [37] project (ANR-08-TECS-00);
- PlaIR [38] project, funded by FEDER;

Table 1: Numbers of mappings between all the PSIP terminologies.

	ATC	ICD-10	IUPAC	NCCMERP	PSIP Taxonomy	WHO-ICPS	TOTAL
ATC		256	62	24	3	9	**354**
ICD-10	256		27			16	**299**
IUPAC	62	27		4	4	19	**116**
NCCMERP	24		4		123	200	**351**
PSIP taxonomy	3		4	123		43	**173**
WHO-ICPS	9	16	19	200	43		**287**

3. Discussion

The Health Multi-Terminology Portal is daily used by several partners, in particular to maintain the PSIP taxonomy and to access the other ones included in the project. More generally, the main HMTP users are the health students to learn how to manipulate health terminologies (e.g. about rare disease with Orphanet thesaurus or anatomy with the FMA ontology) and to extract knowledge from it, in particular from hierarchies and relations (e.g. various siblings of a rare disease, symptoms of this rare disease or to obtain all the muscles of the forearm in one click). The HMTP has been evaluated by some medical student groups and gave 58% satisfaction for its user interface and 76% for its functionalities and content.

The validation of the HMTP has been performed by the CISMeF librarians and indexing professionals (e.g. pharmacologists, physicians). These days, about 65 people are daily working with the HMTP with a final objective of 10,000 users per month from February 2011 (in fact, the HMTP is going to replace the "Terminologie" tool of CISMeF [39] that allows to access the MeSH thesaurus and which is visited by an average of 9,816 unique users per month in 2010).

Many conceptual and technical issues have been encountered, especially in the model creation for several terminologies (MedDRA model, FMA ontology to terminology). It was necessary to understand the whole structure and the functional purpose of each terminology to propose a good representation for human. Another problem is the space complexity when data is very large (e.g. SNOMED international with more than 80,000 terms and 62,000 relations). We always have to adapt our tools to allow integration in short time while keeping a control on data. For every new terminology integrated in the CISMeF Terminology Database, we learnt more and more about structure and data to be able to integrate all kinds of terminology in our system. Other portals propose to search and navigate through ontologies (e.g. FMA) such as NCBO Bioportal [40] and the EBI Ontology Lookup Service [41-42]. Those tools are also very friendly but do not allow users to navigate through terms or search among synonyms in different languages. They are also not adapted to a daily use to index or to present the FMA to medical students.

Via its Web services, the HMTP may also be used by several interactive applications. The targeted users include the entire range of medical information technology players (e.g. institutions, hospitals, software publishers, information portals) and, through them, all those involved in the healthcare sector, in particular healthcare professionals and patients.

The HMTP presented here has the main functionalities of any terminology server, except the extensive management of terminologies (e.g. adding a new hierarchy). To the best of our knowledge, the HMTP is the first of its kind. The main added value of HMTP when compared to any UMLS browser [43-44] is the possibility to access the main health terminologies or the multi-lingual terminologies and classification coming from WHO, which are not (yet) included in the UMLS (e.g. ATC for drugs or ICPS for patient safety). Currently, the HMTP is a necessary basic tool to index any document in a multi-terminology mode.

Even if the HMTP Web service does not deal with the HL7/CTS specification, it could be an interesting perspective to implement it in order to be compliant with other terminological providers. It would be also convenient to get responses from other similar portals such as NCBO BioPortal, UMLS browser or EBI Ontology Lookup Service to enhance our results and to provide the best possible service to users.

A health multi-terminology portal is a valuable tool to help to index and retrieve resources from a quality-controlled health gateway. It can also be very useful for teaching or performing audits in terminology management.

Acknowledgements

The research leading to these results has received funding from the European Community's Seventh Framework Programme (FP7/2007-2013) under grant agreement n° 216130 – the PSIP project.

The authors thank Richard Medeiros for his advice in the editing of this manuscript and the eight students of the INSA Rouen Engineering School that partially developed the multi-terminology portal.

References

[1] T. Koch. Quality-controlled subject gateways: definitions, typologies, empirical overview, *Subject Gateways, Special issue of "Online Information Review"*, **24** (2000), 24–34.
[2] http://www.nlm.nih.gov/mesh, last access on January 2011.
[3] http://www.mic.stacken.kth.se/Diseases/, last access on January 2011.
[4] http://www.cismef.org, last access on February 2011.
[5] S.J. Darmoni et al., CISMeF: a structured Health resource guide, *Methods Inf Med* **39** (2000), 30–5.
[6] C. Boyer et al., Health On the Net automated database of Health and medical information, *Int J Med Inf* **47** (1997), 27–9.
[7] http://www.intute.ac.uk, last access on January 2011.
[8] http://omni.ac.uk/, last access on January 2011.
[9] F. Norman, Organising Medical Networks' information (OMNI), *Med Inf* **23** (1998), 43–51.

[10] http://www.healthinsite.gov.au/, last access on January 2011.
[11] P. Deacon, J.B. Smith, S. Tow, Using metadata to create navigation paths in the HealthInsite Internet gateway, *Health Info Libr J* **18** (2001), 20–9.
[12] S.L. Weibel, T. Koch, The Dublin Core Metadata Initiative, D-Lib Magazine, 2000 [http://www.dlib.org/dlib/december00/weibel/12weibel.html>]
[13] M. Douyère et al., Enhancing the MeSH thesaurus to retrieve French online health resources in a quality-controlled gateway, *Health Info Libr J* **21** (2004), 253–61.
[14] S. Pereira et al., Using multi-terminology indexing for the assignment of MeSH descriptors to health resources in a French online catalogue, *AMIA Annu Symp Proc* (2008), 586–90.
[15] S. Sakji et al., Drug information portal in Europe: information retrieval with multiple health terminologies, *Stud Health Technol Inform* **150** (2009), 497–501.
[16] A. Burgun et al., A Web terminology server using UMLS for the description of medical procedures, *J Am Med Inform Assoc* **5** (1997), 356–63.
[17] H. Navas et al., Creation and evaluation of a terminology server for the interactive coding of discharge summaries, *Stud Health Technol Inform* **129** (2007), 650–4.
[18] M.L. Gambarte et al., A practical approach to advanced terminology services in health information systems, *Stud Health Technol Inform* **129** (2007), 621–5.
[19] S.H. Brown et al., Using SNOMED CT as a reference terminology to cross map two highly pre-coordinated classification systems, *Stud Health Technol Inform* **129** (2007), 636–9.
[20] G.A. Komatsoulis et al., caCORE version 3: Implementation of a model driven, service-oriented architecture for semantic interoperability, *J Biomed Inform* **41** (2008), 106–23.
[21] S.J. Darmoni, M. Joubert, B. Dahamna, J. Delahousse, M. Fieschi, A French Health Multi-terminology Server, *AMIA Annu Symp Proc* (2009), 808.
[22] R. Beuscart et al., Patient safety: detection and prevention of adverse drug events, *Stud Health Technol Inform* **150** (2009), 968–71.
[23] http://www.who.int/classifications/icd/en/index.html, last access on January 2011.
[24] http://www.whocc.no/atcddd/, last access on January 2011.
[25] http://www.who.int/patientsafety/taxonomy/april_2008-response_technical_expert_comments_nov08.pdf, last access on January 2011.
[26] http://www.iupac.org/, last access on January 2011.
[27] http://www.nccmerp.org/, last access on January 2011.
[28] www.psip-project.eu, last access on January 2011.
[29] Y.A. Lussier, D.J. Rothwell, R.A. Côté, The SNOMED model: a knowledge source for the controlled terminology of the computerized patient record, *Methods Inf Med* **37** (1998), 161–4.
[30] http://www.umc-products.com/DynPage.aspx?id=4918, last access on January 2011.
[31] http://www.who.int/classifications/icf/en/, last access on January 2011.
[32] http://www.meddramsso.com/MSSOWeb/index.htm, last access on January 2011.
[33] T. Merabti et al., An Automated Approach to map a French terminology to UMLS, *Stud Health Technol Inform* **160** (2010), 1040–4.
[34] S. Sakji et al., Automatic indexing in a drug information portal, *Stud Health Technol Inform* **148** (2009), 112–22.
[35] http://www.interstis.org/, last access on January 2011.
[36] http://www.aladin-project.eu/, last access on January 2011.
[37] http://projet4-limbio.smbh.univ-paris13.fr/, last access on January 2011.
[38] http://www.plair.org, last access on January 2011.
[39] http://terminologiecismef.chu-rouen.fr/, last access on February 2011.
[40] N.F. Noy et al., BioPortal: ontologies and integrated data resources at the click of a mouse, *Nucleic Acids Research* Web Server Issue 10 (2009).
[41] R.G. Cote, P. Jones, R. Apweiler, H. Hermjakob, The ontology lookup service, a lightweight cross-platform tool for controlled vocabulary queries, *BMC Bioinformatics* **7** (2006), 97.
[42] R.G. Cote et al., The Ontology Lookup Service: more data and better tools for controlled vocabulary queries, *Nucleic Acids Res* Web Server issue 36 (2008).
[43] K. Zeng, O. Bodenreider, Integrating the UMLS into an RDF-Based Biomedical Knowledge Repository, *AMIA Annu Symp Proc* (2007), 1170.
[44] A.T. McCray, A. Razi, The UMLS Knowledge Source server, *Medinfo* **8** (1995), 144–7.

Patient Safety Informatics
V. Koutkias et al. (Eds.)
IOS Press, 2011

doi:10.3233/978-1-60750-740-6-139

Towards a Standardised Representation of a Knowledge Base for Adverse Drug Event Prevention

Vassilis KOUTKIAS [a,1], Katerina LAZOU [a], Paul DE CLERCQ [b] and Nicos MAGLAVERAS [a]
[a] *Aristotle University, Medical School, Lab of Medical Informatics, Thessaloniki, GREECE*
[b] *Medecs BV, Eindhoven, The Netherlands*

Abstract. Knowledge representation is an important part of knowledge engineering activities that is crucial for enabling knowledge sharing and reuse. In this regard, standardised formalisms and technologies play a significant role. Especially for the medical domain, where knowledge may be tacit, not articulated and highly diverse, the development and adoption of standardised knowledge representations is highly challenging and of outmost importance to achieve knowledge interoperability. To this end, this paper presents a research effort towards the standardised representation of a Knowledge Base (KB) encapsulating rule-based signals and procedures for Adverse Drug Event (ADE) prevention. The KB constitutes an integral part of Clinical Decision Support Systems (CDSSs) to be used at the point of care. The paper highlights the requirements at the domain of discourse with respect to knowledge representation, according to which GELLO (an HL7 and ANSI standard) has been adopted. Results of our prototype implementation are presented along with the advantages and the limitations introduced by the employed approach.

Keywords. Knowledge engineering, knowledge base (KB), medical knowledge representation, knowledge interoperability, standardisation, clinical decision support systems (CDSS), adverse drug events

Introduction

Adverse Drug Events (ADEs) due to medication errors and human factors constitute a major public health issue. They endanger the patients' safety and cause considerable extra healthcare costs. In this regard, in the context of the PSIP (Patient Safety through Intelligent Procedures in medication) project, a knowledge-based approach has been designed and developed for the construction of a framework suitable for the management and effective use of knowledge related to ADE prevention [1]. The framework has as its core part a Knowledge Base (KB) comprising of rule-based knowledge sources, which is accompanied by the necessary inference and query mechanisms to provide healthcare professionals and patients with decision support services in clinical practice, in terms of alerts and recommendations on preventable ADEs [2]. To this end, appropriate knowledge engineering formalisms and

[1] Corresponding Author: bikout@med.auth.gr

methodologies have been investigated, resulting in the adoption of the Computer-Interpretable Guideline (CIG) formalism [3-5]. This choice was primarily due to the fact that the representation of the underlying knowledge required the implementation of procedures, and that ontologies, rules and protocols that constitute the inherent nature of this knowledge are effectively supported and uniformly integrated in CIG. The application of the CIG formalism to construct knowledge-based Clinical Decision Support Systems (CDSSs) has been reported in several studies [5-7].

Towards this aim, among the various knowledge engineering challenges faced, a major one involved elaborating on a standardised knowledge representation, in order to support knowledge interoperability, sharing and reuse. Several approaches have been investigated in this regard, with primary focus on those targeting the medical domain per se, such as Arden syntax [8] and, secondarily, quite general-purpose ones employed in Computer Science such as RuleML and R2ML [9], as well as OWL (Web Ontology Language) combined with SWRL (Semantic Web Rule Language), which are based on Description Logic and semantic rules. From this analysis, it turned out that an appropriate (as it is based on the CIG formalism) and well promising potential is GELLO [10], an HL7 and ANSI standard, providing the benefit of being part of HL7 that is quite dominant for communicating data within the healthcare enterprise. Thus, GELLO was employed to encode the respective KB, in order to further enhance the exploitation of this development.

In this paper, we first present the major initiatives and technologies concerning medical knowledge representation with primary focus on standardised or widely used approaches, we then highlight the application domain, i.e. knowledge representation of ADE signals, and present the effort made towards the standardised representation of a KB for ADE prevention via GELLO, illustrating this development via excerpts of the KB. The paper concludes by referring to the limitations that were identified when employing existing standard means for representing medical knowledge.

1. Medical Knowledge Representation

Medical knowledge representation is a major research area in Medical Informatics and Artificial Intelligence, going through constant development and change due to the particular characteristics of the domain. Medical knowledge relies on the opinions of experts, individual clinical experiences, accepted practices and evidence-based studies [11], while it can be separated into two main types, namely, *declarative knowledge* (e.g. domain-specific knowledge) and *procedural knowledge* (e.g. inference or the method of decision support) [4].

Many different approaches exist for representing medical knowledge. Some of the most well known are Arden syntax, Asbru, EON, Prodigy, GLIF, GUIDE/NewGuide, PROforma and GELLO. More specifically, Arden syntax was initially proposed to address the issue of enabling transfer of medical knowledge among heterogeneous systems [8]. However, it was not designed for representing complex knowledge, such as clinical guidelines [12]. GLIF2 is a model for representing sharable computer-interpretable guidelines [13]. However, the attributes of its constructs were defined as text strings that could not be parsed, preventing the resulting guidelines from being able to make inferences during computerised execution. GLIF3, an extended version of GLIF2, offers several additional constructs and elaborates on a more formal definition of decision criteria, action specifications and patient data. GLIF's expression language

GEL [14] was later evolved into the object-oriented (OO) query and expression language for clinical decision support, GELLO which was approved by HL7 and ANSI in 2005 as a standard. GELLO complies with the guiding principles of the ANSI Healthcare Informatics Standards, as it provides a standard representation and encoding of healthcare knowledge. Another approach, Asbru, enables the definition of the intentions and goals of a guideline, as well as the associated temporal aspects and uncertainties, as an intrinsic part of that guideline [15]. The EON architecture is a component-based suite of models and software for the creation of guideline-based applications [16]. The Prodigy model enables a guideline to be organised as a network of patient scenarios, management decisions and action steps, which produce further scenarios [17]. GUIDE is part of a guideline modelling and execution framework designed to integrate modelled guidelines into organisational workflows [18]. PROforma is a formal knowledge representation language for modelling clinical processes; the language forms the basis of a method and a technology for developing and publishing executable clinical guidelines [19].

From the above-mentioned technologies/approaches, only Arden syntax and GELLO have been approved as standards (both by HL7) for representing medical knowledge. However, both approaches have their limitations. For example, knowledge cannot be easily disseminated from KBs represented in Arden syntax, due to the lack of standard database linkages. Another limitation is that the HL7 Reference Information Model (RIM) is OO and, hence, incompatible with the data model supported by Arden syntax [20]. Due to these constraints, knowledge interoperability is difficult to be sufficiently achieved using Arden syntax. On the other hand, GELLO seems to be a promising alternative, as it is based on the CIG formalism [21], along with an abstract virtual medical record (VMR) [22], so that the same representation can be interpreted and executed in multiple systems accessing data stored in different formats. However, complex knowledge constructs such as meta-rules, i.e. procedures or instructions about how to apply ADE prevention signals that are central in the application domain we are targeting at, cannot be supported in GELLO.

2. A Knowledge Base for ADE Prevention

The developed knowledge framework is designed to support ADE prevention via decision support modules that deliver appropriate alerts and recommendations to the clinical personnel. It incorporates rule-based signals and a context-sensitive, meta-rule level, which is used to address rule ranking and determine the applicability of ADE signals per case, in order to eliminate over-alerting. Its underlying knowledge model is mapped to a data schema specifically designed for querying the KB with actual patient data [23]. The ADE signals elaborated in the knowledge model constitute production rules of the following form [24]: C_1 AND C_2 AND ... AND $C_n \rightarrow R$, where $C_1, C_2, ..., C_n$ are atomic formulae of some accepted language (e.g., propositional logic, attributive logic, first order logic, etc.) and R is the conclusion, action or decision. In the specific case, C_i are pseudo-variables which correspond to groups of (a) *drug codes* expressed in the ATC (Anatomical Therapeutic Chemical) classification system, (b) *laboratory examination results* expressed in C-NPU/IUPAC (Committee on Nomenclature, Properties and Units/International Union of Pure and Applied Chemistry), or (c) *diagnosis codes* expressed in ICD-10 (International Classification of Diseases) classification. The R part constitutes the effect of the rule, i.e. the actual ADE, which typically corresponds to a diagnostic pseudo-variable.

Such rules are statistically inferred by applying data mining techniques to diverse EHRs [25]; thus, the importance and applicability of each rule is determined based on its statistical significance in the local context that is being triggered, i.e. hospital/department. Hence, statistical features such as the confidence (probability of having the effect knowing that the conditions are met), the support (probability of having the effect and matching the conditions at the same time), the Fisher test p-value and so forth constitute rule meta-data that may be particularly used to address over-alerting. It is interesting to note that besides data mining originated rules, a commercial knowledge source (provided by the partner VIDAL - http://www.vidal.fr/) capturing drug to drug interactions, drug contraindications, drug to allergy class associations, as well as drug to laboratory examination values or medical parameter associations, is also embodied in the knowledge framework via an appropriate interface. This knowledge is also expressed via a rule-based formalism and based on the abovementioned standard terminologies.

Overall, the knowledge employed in PSIP belongs in three categories: a) *domain knowledge*, defining types and facts, which are generally static and structured via concepts (i.e., classes), relations-associations, attributes, and rule types (expressions); b) *task knowledge*, in terms of functional decomposition, and control; in this regard, knowledge is elaborated with respect to combination of tasks to reach a goal/workflow, or oppositely, decomposition of complex tasks into separate processes; c) *inference knowledge*, corresponding to the basic reasoning steps that can be followed in the domain and are applied by tasks.

According to the above, the KB comprises of a set of ontology-based structures, either application-specific or standard classifications. In addition, a rule-based component is included that is defined via a set of classes and populated with ADE rules. The ontology-based structures and the rule-based component constitute the fundamental elements to define complex procedural logic in terms of protocols and guidelines, according to the CIG formalism. Being the core knowledge engineering methodology for KB design and development in this work, CIG enables the unification of the former knowledge components, so as to provide a common knowledge framework.

3. Standard Representation of the Knowledge Base

In the current implementation, the KB is represented as Protégé CLIPS files (frame-based ontology) and as a single RDF/XML file (both supported by the adopted development framework, GASTON – http://www.medecs.nl/). Aiming to address the requirement of knowledge interoperability and reuse, an effort has been made to encode the KB in GELLO, which was recently established for expressing CDSS-driven knowledge in healthcare information systems. GELLO was initially conceived as a standard expression language for decision support, and quite recently it evolved as an HL7 and ANSI standard decision support language. GELLO has its roots in the Object Constraint Language (OCL), though optimised and extended for decision support. Its primary role is to serve as a query language for obtaining clinical information from an EHR system in a standard way. Based on the abstract VMR, i.e. a simplified view of

HL7 RIM V3, the same GELLO code can be executed on multiple systems accessing data stored in different formats. In summary, the GELLO language can be used to:

- build-up expressions to extract and manipulate data from medical records;
- construct decision criteria by building up expressions to reason about particular data features/values; these criteria can be used in decision-support KBs, and
- create expressions, formulae etc., for other applications.

In order to facilitate the encoding and evaluation of expressions, and more importantly to maximise the ability to share such expressions, GELLO includes basic built-in data types (such as primitive types, model types, collection types, tuple types and enumeration types), while providing the necessary syntactic mechanisms to manipulate an OO data model compatible with the HL7 RIM, and access all the data-model associated classes and methods. This is especially important in enabling decision rules and guidelines to successfully support different data models. In this regard, GELLO has been proposed as a platform-independent standard expression language for sharing and manipulating knowledge in a medical context as it is vendor and platform independent, while offering modularity, encapsulation and extensibility, due to its OO nature.

At the current stage, GELLO was used to encode part of the KB, i.e. the intermediate and main ADE rules [2]. The KB also incorporates a number of meta-rules, i.e. procedures or instructions about how to apply the main ADE rules. One type of meta-rules controls the appropriate application of rules and in particular the correct evaluation of condition variables as regards the timing by filtering out lab measurements and drug admissions that were older than a specified threshold, defined in number of days. A second type of meta-rules employed aims at contextualisation and reducing over-alerting. This is done by using rules' meta-data to filter out rules that should not be applicable in specific circumstances. GELLO has the potential to depict a "static" structure very well, but it is difficult to represent dynamic behaviour, such as data manipulation, meta-data and meta-rules. In this case, intermediate rules and ADE rules are properly represented. On the other hand, meta-rules that require the use of data that are derived upon execution of the main rules, cannot be described. Additionally, limitations of the current VMR model, upon which GELLO is based, do not allow the encoding of meta-rules. For example, it is not possible to check whether previous alerts for the same condition and patient had been generated, since the current VMR specification does not contain concrete classes for representing alerts [26].

Besides the above limitations, GELLO has been employed in this work, since it constitutes the only relevant standard for targeted application.

4. Results

The KB consists of rules, intermediate rules, meta-data and meta-rules, as explained in the following. From these elements only the core knowledge was represented in GELLO, namely the rules and the intermediate rules.

Figure 1 illustrates an example rule for ADE prevention represented in GELLO. The rule is given as: "high blood pressure **&** aminoglycoside **&** NO potassium lowering diuretic **&** age less than 70 → renal failure (creat.>135 micromol/L or urea>16.6 mmol/L)". In order for this rule to be represented in the KB, it is split in the "Conditions" part, which contains the conditions that are linked together with the

"AND" operator and the "Result", which is the predicted effect, if all conditions are met. The conditions of the rule are denoted by pseudo-variables as explained in section 2. The result constitutes the effect of the rule, i.e. the actual ADE. These pseudo-variables are implemented in the KB in the form of intermediate rules. Each "Condition" is composed by the following elements:

- a variable name,
- an operator (<, >, <=, >=, ==), and
- a reference value.

Each rule contains only one effect, which is expressed also as a pseudo-variable. The pseudo-variables in turn are expressed in the form of binary variables. Such a variable is defined by using mappings to standard coding systems. For example, the expression "*renal failure (creat.>135 micromol/L or urea>16.6 mmol/L)*" is mapped to the variable `bi.kidney_i`, which is defined as a binary variable that takes the value 1, if the lab result with C-NPU/IUPAC code equal to NPU01459 is more than 16.6, else it equals to 0. This variable indicates that urea is higher than the normal bound. The variable `dr1.antithrombotic_aminoglycoside` is assigned the value 1, if the administered drug has ATC code within the set `{J01GA01, J01GB01, J01GB03, J01GB06, ..., J01XX04}`, else it equals to 0. The physical meaning of this variable is the existence of any drug from a group of aminoglycoside type of drugs.

In this regard, the aforementioned example rule can be expressed in the following form:

```
IF di1.cardiovasc_hbloodpressure = 1 AND
dr1.antibiotic_aminoglycoside = 1 AND
dr1.diuretics_potassiumLowering =0 AND mi1.age.quanti < 70
THEN bi.kidney_i
```

The rule consists of four conditions, with the first one referring to diagnoses, the next two referring to drugs and the last one referring to patient specific information, while the effect of the rule refers to a lab result. All the conditions, apart from the condition that describes the age, correspond to intermediate rules which are mapped to groups of either drug codes in ATC, or lab results in C-NPU/IUPAC, or diagnosis codes in ICD-10 classification.

The representation of the above sample rule in GELLO involves initially the description of the individual conditions of the rule, thus the intermediate rules are defined first. A Boolean variable is defined, since it represents a binary variable denoting the presence or absence of a drug, named *ATC_DRUG_A01AD11*. This variable takes the value 1, if the drug having SNOMEDCD code equal to 'A01AD11' is present; otherwise the variable is equal to 0. This is defined using the following expression:

```
Let   ATC_DRUG_A01AD11:Boolean   =   Medications   ->   select(code.
implies(Factory.SNOMEDCD('A01AD11||')).value).size() > 0
```

Similarly, a variable that represents the presence of a diagnosis code is defined as shown below:

```
Let ICD10_E10:Boolean = ProblemList ->
select(code.implies(Factory.SNOMEDCD('E10||')).value).size() > 0
```

An additional variable of type real, named Patientage is also defined to depict the age given in the patient record. The definition is as follows:

```
Context SinglePatient
--Declarations
Let ATC_DRUG_A01AD11:Boolean = Medications ->
    select(code.implies(Factory.SNOMEDCD('A01AD11||')).value).size() > 0
Let ATC_DRUG_A07AB03:Boolean = Medications ->
    select(code.implies(Factory.SNOMEDCD('A07AB03||')).value).size() > 0
...
Let ICD10_E10:Boolean = ProblemList ->
    select(code.implies(Factory.SNOMEDCD('E10||')).value).size() > 0
Let ICD10_E102:Boolean = ProblemList ->
    select(code.implies(Factory.SNOMEDCD('E102||')).value).size() > 0
...
Let Patientage:Real = Observation ->
    select(code.implies(Factory.SNOMEDCD('Patientage||')).value)->
    last().value.oclAsType(PQ).value

Let PSIP_Guidelines_13888:Boolean=
(ICD10_I10 or ICD10_I11 or ICD10_I110 or ICD10_I119 or ICD10_I13 or ICD10_I130
or ICD10_I131 or ICD10_I132 or ICD10_I139 or ICD10_I15 or ICD10_I150 or
ICD10_I151 or ICD10_I152 or ICD10_I158 or ICD10_I159 or ICD10_O101 or ICD10_O103)

Let PSIP_Guidelines_01013:Boolean=
(ATC_DRUG_J01GA01 or ATC_DRUG_J01GB01 or ATC_DRUG_J01GB03 or ATC_DRUG_J01GB06
or ATC_DRUG_J01GB07 or ATC_DRUG_J01XX04)

Let PSIP_Guidelines_04281:Boolean=
(ATC_DRUG_C02LA01 or ATC_DRUG_C03AA03 or ATC_DRUG_C03BA11 or ATC_DRUG_C03BX03
or ATC_DRUG_C03CA01 or ATC_DRUG_C03CA02 or ATC_DRUG_C03CA03 or ATC_DRUG_C03EA01
or ATC_DRUG_C03EA04 or ATC_DRUG_C03EB01 or ATC_DRUG_C09BA01 or ATC_DRUG_C09BA02
or ATC_DRUG_C09BA03 or ATC_DRUG_C09BA04 or ATC_DRUG_C09BA05 or ATC_DRUG_C09BA06
or ATC_DRUG_C09BA07 or ATC_DRUG_C09BA09 or ATC_DRUG_C09BA15 or ATC_DRUG_C09DA01
or ATC_DRUG_C09DA02 or ATC_DRUG_C09DA03 or ATC_DRUG_C09DA04 or ATC_DRUG_C09DA06
or ATC_DRUG_C09DA07 or ATC_DRUG_C09DA08)


--Rule: b217_0
Let b217_0: String =
If
(PSIP_Guidelines_13888)
 and
(PSIP_Guidelines_01013)
 and
((Patientage<70))
 and
not(PSIP_Guidelines_04281)
then
'ALERT: Aminoglycosides can cause acute renal failure'
else
''
endif
```

Figure 1. Representation of an example ADE prevention rule in GELLO.

```
Let Patientage:Real = Observation ->
select(code.implies(Factory.SNOMEDCD('Patientage||')).value)->
last().value.oclAsType(PQ).value
```

The intermediate rules that are used in the actual implementation of the rule are defined by grouping together the Boolean variables that correspond to the drug codes that are present in the given drug group. For example, the definition of the intermediate rule *dr1.aminoglycoside* is the following:

```
Let PSIP_Guidelines_01013:Boolean= (ATC_DRUG_J01GA01 or
ATC_DRUG_J01GB01 or ATC_DRUG_J01GB03 or ATC_DRUG_J01GB06 or
ATC_DRUG_J01GB07 or ATC_DRUG_J01XX04)
```

The rule is implemented by joining the individual conditions, as shown below:

```
Let b217_0: String =
If (PSIP_Guidelines_13888) and (PSIP_Guidelines_01013) and
((Patientage<70)) and not(PSIP_Guidelines_04281)
then
'ALERT: Aminoglycosides can cause acute renal failure'
endif
```

5. Conclusion

Standardised formalisms and technologies play a significant role in confronting knowledge interoperability. Especially in the medical domain, where knowledge may be tacit, not articulated and highly diverse, the development and adoption of standardised knowledge representations is highly challenging and of outmost importance to facilitate knowledge sharing and reuse. In this paper, we presented our research effort towards a standardised represenattion of a KB encapsulating rule-based signals and procedures for ADE prevention. The paper highlighted the requirements at the domain of discourse with respect to knowledge representation, according to which the CIG formalism was adopted, as well as our effort to represent the KB in GELLO. Although this knowledge representation approach has several advantages, our prototype implementation revealed that it was not possible to encode the entire KB, as more complex knowledge contracts, such as meta-rules that are central in the targeted application, could not be supported.

Evidently, the medical domain lacks a generic knowledge representation standard capable of addressing the various and complex requirements typically met in knowledge engineering tasks. Further research needs to be conducted towards finding an appropriate technique that will support the representation of static along with dynamic information that is part of the KB. An available approach that can be a suitable candidate for the representation of the procedural logic incorporated in such a KB is Business Process Execution Language (BPEL), a standard executable language for specifying actions within business processes with Web services.

Acknowledgments

The research leading to these results has received funding from the European Community's Seventh Framework Programme (FP7/2007-2013) under grant agreement n° 216130 – the PSIP project.

References

[1] V. Koutkias et al., A knowledge engineering framework towards clinical support for adverse drug event prevention: the PSIP approach, *Stud Health Technol Inform* **148** (2009), 131–41.

[2] V. Koutkias et al., Constructing clinical decision support systems for adverse drug event prevention: a knowledge-based approach, *AMIA Annu Symp Proc* (2010), 402–6.
[3] M. Peleg et al., Comparing computer-interpretable guideline models: a case-study approach, *J Am Med Inform Assoc* **10** (2003), 52–68.
[4] P. de Clercq, K. Kaiser, A. Hasman, Computer-interpretable guideline formalisms, *Stud Health Technol Inform* **139** (2008), 22–43.
[5] M.A. Musen, Y. Shahar, E.H. Shortliffe, Clinical Decision-Support Systems, In: E.H. Shortliffe (Ed.). *Biomedical Informatics: Computer Applications in Health Care and Biomedicine*, Springer-Verlag, 2006.
[6] E.M.W. van Oosterhout et al., Three-layer model for the design of a protocol support system, *Int J Med Inf* **74** (2005) 101–10.
[7] A. Latoszek-Berendsen, J. Talmon, P. de Clercq, A. Hasman, With good intentions, *Int J Med Inf* **76S** (2007), S440–6.
[8] P.D. Clayton, T.A. Pryor, O.B. Wigertz, G. Hripcsak, Issues and structures for sharing knowledge among decision-making systems: The 1989 Arden Homestead Retreat", In: Proc. of the 13th IEEE Annual Symp. on Computer Applications in Medical Care (1989), 116–21.
[9] H. Boley et al., "Rule interchange on the Web", *Lecture Notes in Computer Science* **4636** (2007), 269–309.
[10] ANSI/HL7 V3, GELLO: A Common Expression Language, Release 2, May 2010.
[11] M. Peleg, Guideline and workflow models. In: R.A. Greenes (Ed.). *Clinical Decision Support: The Road Ahead*, Elsevier, 2007.
[12] M. Peleg, A.A. Boxwala, E. Bernstam, S. Tu, R.A. Greenes, E.H. Shortliffe, Sharable representation of clinical guidelines in GLIF: relationship to the Arden Syntax, *J Biomed Inform* **34** (2001), 170–81.
[13] A.A. Boxwala et al., GLIF3: a representation format for sharable computer-interpretable clinical practice guidelines, *J Biomed Inform* **37** (2004), 147–61.
[14] S. Quaglini, L. Dazzi, L. Gatti, M. Stefanelli, C. Fassino, C. Tondini, Supporting tools for guideline development and dissemination, *Artif Intell Med* **14** (1998),119–37.
[15] Y. Shahar, S. Miksch, P. Johnson, The Asgaard project: A task-specific framework for the application and critiquing of time-oriented clinical guidelines, *Artif Intell Med* **14** (1998), 29–51.
[16] S.W. Tu, M.A. Musen, Modeling data and knowledge in the EON guideline architecture, *Stud Health Technol Inform* **84** (2001), 280–4.
[17] P. Johnson, S. Tu, N. Jones, Achieving reuse of computable guideline systems, *Stud Health Technol Inform* **84** (2001), 99–103.
[18] M. Peleg et al., Using features of Arden Syntax with object-oriented medical data models for guideline modeling, *Proc AMIA Symp* (2001), 523–7.
[19] J. Fox, N. Johns, A. Rahmanzadeh, Disseminating medical knowledge: the PROforma approach, *Artif Intell Med* **14** (1998), 157–81.
[20] R.A. Jenders, R. Corman, B. Dasgupta, Making the standard more standard: a data and query model for knowledge representation in the Arden syntax, *AMIA Annu Symp Proc* (2003), 323–30.
[21] M. Sordo, O. Ogunyemi, A.A. Boxwala, R.A. Greenes, GELLO: an object-oriented query and expression language for clinical decision support, Decision Systems Group, Bringham & Women's Hospital, Harvard Medical School, Boston, MA, DSG-TR-2003-02, 2003.
[22] C. Huang, L.A. Noirot, K.M. Heard, R.M. Reichley, W.C. Dunagan, T.C. Bailey, Implementation of virtual medical record object model for a standards-based clinical decision support rule engine, *AMIA Annu Symp Proc* (2006), 958.
[23] E. Chazard et al., Detection of adverse drug events: proposal of a data model, *Stud Health Technol Inform* **148** (2009), 63–74.
[24] A. Ligêza, Logical foundations for rule-based systems, Springer-Verlag Berlin Heidelberg, 2006.
[25] E. Chazard et al., Data-mining-based detection of adverse drug events, *Stud Health Technol Inform* **150** (2009), 552–6.
[26] Y. Denekamp, O. Ogunyemi, A.A. Boxwala, R.A. Greenes, Using new object oriented expression language (GELLO) to encode Arden Syntax's Medical Logic Modules, *Proc AMIA Symp* (2002), 1006.

Patient Safety Informatics
V. Koutkias et al. (Eds.)
IOS Press, 2011

doi:10.3233/978-1-60750-740-6-148

Analysis of the Medication-use Process in North American Hospital Systems: Underlining Key Points for Adoption to Improve Patient Safety in French Hospitals

Agnes BROUARD [a,1], Jean Yves FAGON [a] and Charles E. DANIELS [b]
[a] *Assistance Publique-Hôpitaux de Paris (AP-HP), France*
[b] *University of California San Diego Medical Center, UCSD Skaggs School of Pharmacy and Pharmaceutical Sciences*

Abstract. This project was designed to underline any actions relative to medication error prevention and patient safety improvement setting up in North American hospitals which could be implemented in French Parisian hospitals. A literature research and analysis of medication-use process in the North American hospitals and a validation survey of hospital pharmacist managers in the San Diego area was performed to assess main points of hospital medication-use process. Literature analysis, survey analysis of respondents highlighted main differences between the two countries at three levels: nationwide, hospital level and pharmaceutical service level. According to this, proposal development to optimize medication-use process in the French system includes the following topics: implementation of an expanded use of information technology and robotics; increase pharmaceutical human resources allowing expansion of clinical pharmacy activities; focus on high-risk medications and high-risk patient populations; develop a collective sense of responsibility for medication error prevention in hospital settings, involving medical, pharmaceutical and administrative teams. Along with a strong emphasis that should be put on the identified topics to improve the quality and safety of hospital care in France, consideration of patient safety as a priority at a nationwide level needs to be reinforced.

Keywords. Medication-use process, patient safety, medication error prevention

Introduction

The Assistance Publique-Hôpitaux de Paris (AP-HP) is a large French academic Institution, including 38 hospitals, 20,000 physicians, 23,000 beds, 1 million inpatients and 4 millions outpatients per year; seven Universities are associated with AP-HP, including 7 medical schools, 2 pharmaceutical schools and 2 odontology schools.

In 2009, the Institution had to work on its new strategic plan for the following four years (2010-2014). The pharmaceutical part of the strategic plan needed new proposals for medication-use process improvement.

[1] Corresponding Author: agnesbrou@me.com

In the U.S., major actions dedicated to preventing medication errors took place in the early 1990s. The United States Pharmacopeia (USP) and the Institute for Safe Medication Practices (ISMP) jointly set up the Medication Error Reporting Program (MERP) in 1991 [1]. The action of the National Coordinating Council for Medication Error Reduction and Prevention (NCC MERP) needs also to be noticed [2].The Institute of Medicine (IOM) played an undeniable role in launching the debate on human errors, medication error prevention and patient safety with the release of three major publications in the early 21st century [3-5].The model of the North American hospital medication-use process could thus leverage the evolution of the French model.

The main goal of the study was to underline any actions relative to medication error prevention and patient safety improvement that could be implemented in French Parisian hospitals.

The work considered the various factors leveraging the process to improve patient safety in both countries: stakeholders acting all along the process -politics, health-care professionals, professional associations, patients, third party agencies, regulations, informatics and technology industry, hospital pharmacy staffing.

1. Methods

The methods consisted of a two-step analysis:

The first step included a manual literature research and review to encompass the challenges of the North American system -especially in California- to improve patient safety and medication error prevention; and to get a better understanding of regulation surrounding hospital medication-use process.

Different websites were consulted: Federal agencies and bodies (Federal and Drug Administration (FDA), Agency for Healthcare Research and quality (AHRQ) from the US Department of Health and Human Services); the Joint Commission; the American Society of Health-System Pharmacists (ASHP); and third party agencies: Institute of Safe Medication Practices (ISMP), United States Pharmacopeia (USP), Institute of Medicine (IOM), the National Coordinating Council for Medication Error Reduction and Prevention (NCCMERP).

The second step consisted of a visit of the San Diego area hospital pharmacist managers to discuss the main points of their own medication-use process, to get a better approach of their practices and to understand the issues faced to improve medication safety in hospital settings. The discussion was conducted with the support of a questionnaire listing the main medication-use process topics highlighted after the literature review:

- general data on drug and medical device expenses, committees and pharmacy team type setting of their hospital,
- the medication-use process organization set up in their hospital: prescription, dispensation, administration, patient education (including the contribution of informatics and technology (IT) and robotics),
- any strategic initiatives developed in their hospital relative to patient safety: cooperation with medical teams to enhance organization, IT program development, medication-use adherence policies evaluation,
- impact of financial aspects underlying any step of the decision process with regard to patient safety.

2. Results

The results are presented in three different parts: the main documents published on medication error prevention and medication-use process; a comparison between North American and French hospital system regulation and context; a list of proposals developed to improve patient safety and medication-use process for the French hospitals.

2.1. Literature Review

The literature review highlighted several main documents, all of them pointing out expanded and disseminated actions or requirements geared towards professional to prevent medication errors and improve patient safety:

- the Institute of Medicine (IOM) reports, especially the one released in 2007 on medication error prevention [5];
- the National Patient Safety Goals (NPSG) [6] and the Joint Core Measures [7], two essential actions taken over by the Joint Commission;
- the four last ASHP national surveys (U.S. national data) on medication-use process: Prescription and Transcription in 2007 [8], Dispensation and Administration in 2008 [9], Monitoring and Patient Education in 2009 [10], Informatics in 2007 [11] and the last issue on Hospital Best Practices [12];
- the ISMP reports (i.e. Look-alike-Sound-alike medication, error-prone abbreviations etc.) [13].

The Code of Federal Regulations (CFR) [14] and the Californian Code of Regulations (CCR) [15] were analyzed in depth in their respective parts dedicated to hospital and pharmaceutical services (part 482-25 of the CFR and 70261 to 70269 of the CCR) to point out specific requirements mentioned to prevent medication errors.

2.2. Comparison between U.S. Hospitals and the French System

The literature analysis, along with the discussion with the hospital pharmacist managers in the San Diego area, helped us to highlight major points of organization in the two countries.

Table 1 shows a comparison between hospital healthcare systems in the U.S. and France, allowing to design the context of patient safety and medication error prevention in both countries, at three different levels: nationwide level, hospital level and pharmaceutical service level.

2.3. List of Proposals Pointed out for Hospitals

The first proposal concerns the fact that patient safety needs to be considered as a priority for public health at the nation level. The patient needs to become a real actor of the success of its treatment thanks to an enhanced therapeutic education. The role and actions of independent and third party organizations dedicated to patient safety should be envisioned.

Table 1. Comparison between U.S. hospitals and the French system.

United States of America	France
Nationwide level	
Healthcare funding: mainly private (public: Medicare, Medicaid)	Healthcare funding: universal social security; equal access to cares
Prevention of medication errors: large influence of IOM reports ; large and constant communication [3-5]	Prevention of medication errors: large national survey (ENEIS 2004) [16, 17] on medication errors; very limited communication (compared to the U.S.)
Dedicated supportive resources for patient safety and medication error prevention: -Third Party organizations as a support for healthcare professionals -ASHP: 30,000 members (critical mass of human resources to produce work)	Minimum resources dedicated to patient safety and medication error prevention: -Regulation and accreditation Bodies -No organization specifically dedicated to patient safety -French Society of Clinical Pharmacy (SFPC): 200 members; European Society of Clinical Pharmacy (ESCP): 1,000 members
Healthcare costs are a real concern: 16% GDP (2007) [18]	Healthcare costs are a real concern: 11% GDP (2007) [18]
Informatics, technologies and robotics: large industry; diversity of commercially available products…	Informatics, technologies and robotics: access on European market increases slowly
Hospital level	
Hospital regulation codes: a tremendous emphasis in the FCR and CCR on medication error prevention in addition to the quality and security of care [14, 15]	Hospital regulation codes: Main objectives: quality and security of care; a minor emphasis on medication error prevention
The individual motivation for safety improvement is due to professional accountability in addition to the competition driven by the healthcare industry market Possible impact of private and competitive system organizations to increase the quality of care (impact of benchmarking requirements, impact of patient lawsuits) [5]	The individual motivation for safety improvement is mainly due to professional accountability No official benchmarking in France
Hospital funding: strong impact of incentives and regulatory requirements	Hospital funding: penalties started in France in 2005 for high-risk and high-cost medications: off-label use has to be justified by a strong level of Evidence-Based Medicine
Large and repetitive communication on costs of medication errors (IOM report [5])	Minor communication on costs of medication errors
Pharmaceutical services	
Areas of pharmaceutical service responsibilities: medications and some medical devices (used for drug administration)	Areas of pharmaceutical service responsibilities: medications and all medical devices used for inpatients
Pharmacy Human Resources:	Pharmacy Human Resources:

1 FTE for 10 occupied beds (average) [10]	1FTE for 185 occupied beds (average) [19]
Clinical Pharmacy: value-added clinical pharmacy activities are recognized; the collaborative role of a Clinical Pharmacist is expected and recognized by medical team	Clinical Pharmacy: Pharmaceutical service staffing doesn't allow to involve a lot of pharmacists in clinical pharmacy activities
Continuing education is a requirement for pharmacist license renewal	Continuing education just started to be required (not mandatory for license renewal)

The second proposal outlines the necessity to establish a large policy and a culture of patient safety in the hospital. Medication error reporting to specific agencies or "Patient Safety organizations" should become a requirement. A specific pharmaceutical human resources dedicated to prevent medication error prevention in the hospital (i.e. Medication Safety Officer-MSO) could help to coordinate this action.

The third proposal deals with a collective and shared accountability within healthcare professionals to secure the medication-use process in the hospitals. This accountability, traditionally devoted to institutional committees (Executive committee and medical staff committee) and to the Pharmaceutical and Therapeutics Committee (P&T Committee) should be reinforced and disseminated to all the staff in the hospital.

The fourth proposal includes incentives to stimulate actions for quality and security of care improvement. French hospital policy already includes these goals. Health professionals need to be motivated to increase professional practices assessments, morbidity and mortality conferences. Financial incentives (collective or individual) as well as external communication on the results of quality and safety of care and benchmarking actions have to be routinely managed.

The fifth proposal asks for a large implementation of informatics and technology tools necessary at all the steps of the medication-use process (Prescribing, Dispensing, Administration, Therapeutic monitoring, Patient education). Main examples are: Electronic Medical Record (EMR), Computer Prescriber Order Entry (CPOE) plus Clinical Decision Support System (CDSS), Medication Administration Record (MAR), Bar-coding for dispensation, administration and patients identity checking.

The sixth proposal concerns a large promotion of equipments for pharmaceutical services: automated dispensing systems to optimize drug inventory and to secure the dispensation: robots (centralized distribution) and Automated Dispensing Cabinets-ADC- (decentralized distribution); robotic tools to automate pharmaceutical repackaging and compounding: robotic systems for preparation compounding (parenteral nutrition, pediatric oral preparations...) and robotic systems for unit-dose repackaging and bar-coding.

The seventh proposal brings up specific points of the medication-use process. In addition to the benefits carried by informatics and technology to improve the process, some key points can contribute to the quality and safety of care and medication error prevention: limitation of oral process prescription (if necessary, asking for a prescriber validation and signature); increasing the number of analyzed and validated prescriptions by the pharmacist (which is actually a requirement); check the patient's identity in the absence of bar code system, double-check for high-risk medications and drugs taken by the patient.

The eighth proposal intends to promote incentives in terms of resource allocation and action (with the support of independent agencies; see first proposal), so that institutions particularly focus on: high-risk clinical areas (oncology, anesthesiology, intensive care, etc.), high-risk populations (pediatrics, elderly), high-risk medications (anticoagulants, chemotherapy, drugs administered by injection including hypertonic concentrations); and use and communicate the list of "look-alike and sound-alike medications" and the list of "error-prone abbreviations".

The ninth proposal asks to: strongly consider the need of increasing pharmaceutical human resources especially dedicated to clinical pharmacy activities; and to pursue strategic organization of pharmaceutical services (and of clinical services in the area of medication-use process) to allow the increase of clinical pharmacy activities.

The tenth proposal suggests: a recognition of the cost of preventable adverse drug effects and of the economic impact of clinical pharmacy services when return on investment are calculated; and a consideration for expanded economic assessment of non formulary drug policy (including cost of human resources and medication errors).

3. Discussion

Patient safety and medication error prevention are real political issue in both countries. Results published by the IOM [5] concluded that there are at least 1.5 million preventable adverse drug events occurring in the U.S. each year. Assuming that 400,000 of those adverse drug events took place in a hospital, the estimated total annual cost would be $3.5 billion. In France, the ENEIS survey on severe adverse events published in 2004, concluded that 350,000 to 450,000 serious adverse events occurred annually in hospitalized patients, 35% being preventable and 26.7% due to health products [16].

The difference between the two countries mainly concerns the methods of communication towards health stakeholders after the release of the national surveys; they were modest in France and huge in the U.S. Likewise, specific resources dedicated at both national and health facility levels are not as intense in France as in the U.S. [5]. However, the recent law entitled Hospital Patient Health County Law (Loi HPST; Hôpital Patients Santé Territoires) enacted in France in 2009 [20], keeps reinforcing the needs for safety and quality of care.

The model of "Patient Safety" organization has not been reproduced in France. Independent associations, responsible for the dissemination of tools to support healthcare professionals are essential [13].

Like the Medication Error Reduction Plan (MERP) set up in California in 2007 [21], the 2005 French hospital regulation, asked for a large involvement of the hospital in "Good Practices" by signing a contract of good use, CBU (Contrat de Bon Usage) [22]. The contract, signed between French hospitals and their own Health Regional Agency, ARS (Agences Régionales de Santé) aims to improve and secure within the health facility the medication-use process. The request for improvement insists on: a higher level of computerization at all steps of the medication-use process, a comprehensive and individual prescription and dispensation, the development of a quality assurance system. In return for compliance with their commitments, French hospitals get financial incentives; they are be reimbursed for 100% of their expanses of innovative drugs. In the framework of the Californian MERP, noncompliant hospitals can be strongly sanctioned with an extensive suspension of funding.

Like in the U.S., the role of a strong politics of the P&T committee (with the endorsement of the Medical staff committee) in enforcing drug and medical devices policies, medication-use process procedures and application of policies by hospital healthcare professionals, is essential. Recently, the manual for hospital certification developed by the High Health Authority (HAS; Haute Autorité de Santé) required in its last version (2010) that medication regimen management is a priority [23].

The difference between French and North American system is based on two major differences: a private system of organization in the US encouraging a strong competition between health-care facilities; the motivation of health professionals for a higher performance is stimulated by both factors- accountability and competition where in France accountability is the major driver for performance improvement [5]; the request for improvement from the payers is based in France on the process set up for quality assurance more than the final results.

Although medication error reporting is widely encouraged, this action is not mandatory in the French hospitals. Health professionals are not enough stimulated to report medication errors and the fear of punishment is still predominant. A responsible culture of safety with staff training, positive attitude sharing and horizontal approach of risk management facilitating has to be promoted [24].

Finally, human resources dedicated to pharmaceutical services and essential for patient safety and medication error prevention are dramatically low in France, twenty times less in terms of hospitals pharmacists and ten times less in terms of technicians [19], [10]. On the other hand, the area of responsibility for the French hospital pharmaceutical services includes the drugs and the medical devices while it includes drugs only for the North Americans. Moreover, various studies conducted in the U.S. shows that the impact of hospital-based clinical pharmacy services and pharmacy staffing continue to be associated with lower mortality rates [25]; and that clinical pharmacy services keep up providing a significant return on investment in the hospitals [26].

4. Conclusion

The work clearly underlines that the U.S. and France have two different hospital healthcare organization systems.

Political, economical and cultural backgrounds of the respective healthcare systems are different and have not been compared. Economic efficiency of the U.S. system is still uncertain: in the U.S., 16% of the Gross Domestic Product is dedicated to Health, where this part reaches 11% in France [20].

However, a strong emphasis should be put on specific topics which should help to improve the quality and security of hospital cares in France: a large informatics, technology and robotics deployment; an increase of pharmaceutical human resources allowing clinical pharmacy activities; a specific concern for high-risk medications, high-risk population; a collective sense of responsibility for medication error prevention in the hospital settings, involving medical, pharmaceutical and administrative teams.

References

[1] https://www.ismp.org/orderforms/reporterrortoISMP.asp, last access on February 2011.

[2] NCC MERP, Available at: http://www.nccmerp.org/, last access on February 2011.

[3] Institute of Medicine, *To Err Is Human: Building a Safer Health System*, National Academy Press, Washington DC, 2000.

[4] Institute of Medicine, *Crossing the Quality Chasm: A new Health System for the 21st Century*, National Academy Press, Washington DC, 2001.

[5] Institute of Medicine, *Preventing medication errors*, National Academy Press, Washington DC, 2007.

[6] The Joint Commission, National Patient Safety Goals, Available at: http://www.jointcommission.org/PatientSafety/NationalPatientSafetyGoals/, last access on February 2011.

[7] http://www.jointcommission.org/PerformanceMeasurement/PerformanceMeasurement/, last access on February 2011.

[8] C.A.Pedersen, P.J. Schneider, D.J. Scheckelhoff, ASHP national survey of pharmacy practice in hospital settings: Prescribing and transcribing—2007, *Am J Health Syst Pharm* **65** (2008), 827–43.

[9] C.A.Pedersen, P.J. Schneider, D.J. Scheckelhoff, ASHP national survey of pharmacy practice in hospital settings: dispensing and administration—2008, *Am J Health Syst Pharm* **66** (2009), 926–46.

[10] C.A.Pedersen, P.J. Schneider, D.J. Scheckelhoff, ASHP national survey of pharmacy practice in hospital settings: Monitoring and patient education—2009, *Am J Health Syst Pharm* **67** (2010), 542–58.

[11] C.A.Pedersen, K.F.Gumpper, ASHP national survey on informatics: assessment of the adoption and use of pharmacy informatics in U.S. hospitals—2007, *Am J Health Syst Pharm* **65** (2008), 2244–64.

[12] Best Practices for Hospital and Health-System Pharmacy 2009-10. Bethesda, MA: ASHP.

[13] ISMP's List of Confused Drug Names, Available at: http://www.ismp.org/tools/confuseddrugnames.pdf, last access on February 2011.

[14] Code of Federal Regulations. Title 42- Appendix A- State Operations Manual Part 482-11 to 482-27, Available at: https://www.cms.gov/manuals/downloads/som107ap_a_hospitals.pdf, last access on February 2011.

[15] Californian Code of Regulations. Title 22- Pharmaceutical services, Available at: http://www.cshp.org/uploads/file/Shared Resources/2008/title_22_pharmacy.xls, last access on February 2011.

[16] Etude Nationale sur les Evènements Indésirables Graves lies aux soins (ENEIS) 2004. Direction de la Recherche, des Études, de l'Evaluation et des Statistiques, Available at: http://www.fhpr2a.fr/portail/IMG/pdf/10.05._infections_nosocomiales.pdf, last access on February 2011.

[17] Etude Nationale sur les Evènements Indésirables Graves lies aux soins (ENEIS) 2010, Available at: http://www.sante.gouv.fr/l-enquete-nationale-sur-les-evenements-indesirables-lies-aux-soins-eneis.html, last access on February 2011.

[18] Les dépenses de santé aux Etats-Unis. M. Pearson. Communication. Septembre 2009, Available at: http://www.observateurocde.org/news/fullstory.php/aid/2611/Les_d_E9penses_de_sant_E9_aux__C9tats-Unis.html, last access on February 2011.

[19] Étude d'impact organisationnel et financier de la sécurisation du circuit du médicament dans les établissements de santé. Ministère de la Santé. DHOS. Octobre 2009, Available at: http://www.sante-jeunesse-sports.gouv.fr/IMG/pdf/RAPPORT_NATIONAL_SECURIMED.pdf, last access on February 2011.

[20] Loi n°2009-879 du 21 juillet 2009 portant réforme de l'hôpital et relative aux patients, à la santé et aux territories.

[21] Justia US Laws, Available at: http://law.justia.com/california/codes/hsc/1339.63.html, last access on February 2011.

[22] Décret n° 2005-1023 du 24 août 2005 relatif au contrat de bon usage des médicaments et des produits et prestations mentionné à l'article L. 162-22-7 du code de la sécurité sociale.

[23] Manuel V2010 certification des établissements de santé. Haute Autorité de santé, Available at: http://www.has-sante.fr/portail/jcms/c_714928/manuel-v2010-de-certification-des-etablissements-de-sante-version-juin-2009, last access on February 2011.

[24] Patient Safety and the "Just Culture": A Primer for Health Care Executives. Marx D. New York, NY: Columbia University; 2001. Available at: http://www.mers-tm.org/support/Marx_Primer.pdf, last access on February 2011.

[25] C.A. Bond, C.L. Raehl, Clinical pharmacy services, pharmacy staffing, and hospital mortality rates, *Pharmacotherapy* **27** (2007), 481–93.

[26] A. Perez et al., Economic evaluation of Clinical Pharmacy Services: 2001-2005, *Pharmacotherapy* **28** (2008), 285–323.

Patient Safety Informatics
V. Koutkias et al. (Eds.)
IOS Press, 2011

doi:10.3233/978-1-60750-740-6-156

An Approach to 'Dynamic - DDD (Defined Daily Dose) Monitoring' to Reduce Adverse Clinical Outcomes and Increase Patient Safety: Information Repositories and Event Triggers in Clinical Practice

Esat N. ERYILMAZ [1]
Independent HCICT Consultant, Educator, Knowledge Management Mentor

Abstract. The goal of every effort and actions/interventions in almost all healthcare settings throughout the world's health systems -primary care, inpatient, outpatient encounters, diagnostic and therapeutic interventions, peri-operative settings- is and has been to achieve a well defined outcome (a kind of improvement in health status of the patient under consideration, an observable and significant change(s) in selected set(s) of clinical parameters confirmed by laboratory results and pathology findings, improvements in clinical outcomes). Clinical inefficiencies, in this context, should be addressed very systematically and scientifically. This is achieved through a continuously monitoring approach to adverse drug events based on information repositories and evidence-based rule sets. For monitoring drug-related outcomes and clinical outcomes in general, the concept of DDD (Defined Daily Dose) compliance is explained in this article to eliminate and avoid adverse clinical outcomes.

Keywords. Medication-related irrelevancies, adverse clinical outcomes, adverse drug events, clinical interventions, nursing classifications, triggers in healthcare, evidence-based medicine, evidence-based nursing

Introduction

The goal of every effort and actions/interventions in almost all healthcare settings throughout the world's health systems -primary care, inpatient, outpatient encounters, diagnostic and therapeutic interventions, peri-operative settings- is and has been to achieve a well defined outcome (a kind of improvement in health status of the patient under consideration, an observable and significant change in selected set(s) of clinical parameters confirmed by laboratory results and pathology findings, improvements in clinical outcomes). This goal remained unchanged for centuries; but clinical process management approaches have not reached a mature state and as a result of this, clinical processes are far from being managed scientifically, especially care coordination competencies at individual and team levels.

---

[1] Corresponding Author: esatnadir@gmail.com

This immature status of clinical process management hinders care related teamwork to be managed properly. Majority of adverse outcomes are medication related in most cases. Saboor et al. [1] points out the need for supporting the systematic assessment of clinical processes. They claim that: '*...Healthcare is characterized by complex cooperation between highly specialized healthcare departments. This often leads to inefficient clinical processes. In order to improve these processes, a systematic assessment method is needed.*' Saboor et al.'s positioning of the Complexity of clinical processes can be deemed to be valid to some extent. However, this approach does not explain all the inefficiencies encountered in clinical process management in clinical settings.

Addressing this critical issue of clinical process inefficiencies should be considered as the most urgent item in healthcare domain. In this respect, it will be attempted first to give a short account of underlying causes of those inefficiencies in the following section.

The intent throughout the paper is to introduce a conceptual layout for dynamically monitoring of DDD (Defined Daily Dose) in clinical applications to reduce and even eliminate by means of appropriate methodologies and software applications developed in compliance with state-of-the-art frameworks. In particular, CMMI (Capability Maturity Model Integrated) is a powerful framework for business excellence owing to its highly effective and integrated approach to process management, product-service management and project management. For this purpose, the concept of medication errors has been limited to individual drug administration processes. Software development aspects are out of the scope of this paper. Another study as to the optimum management of multi-drug application is under consideration for chemotherapy protocols[2].

1. Major Reasons for Clinical Inefficiencies

In this section, I would like to first give short descriptions of World Healthcare Organization's ATC and DDD to make the situation clearer. Views and proposal about ATC-DDD monitoring to reduce medication related errors and increase patient safety will be based on these short descriptions.

ATC classification system divides drugs into different groups according to the organ or system on which they act and/or their therapeutic and chemical characteristics. Each bottom-level ATC code stands for a pharmaceutically used substance in a single indication (or use). This means that one drug can have more than one code: acetylsalicylic acid (aspirin), for example, has A01AD05 as a drug for local oral treatment, B01AC06 as a platelet inhibitor, and N02BA01 as an analgesic and antipyretic. On the other hand, several different brands share the same code if they have the same active substance and indications.

Defined Daily Dose(s) (DDDs) is a WHO (World Health Organization) statistical measure of drug consumption. DDDs are used to standardize the comparative usage of various drugs between themselves or between different health care environments.

The DDD is the assumed average maintenance dose per day for a drug used for its main indication in adults. A common problem when comparing drugs is that different

---

[2] Esat N. ERYILMAZ and Senem Özgür SARI: Investigation of full control possibilities and related methodologies in Medication Process Improvement – Ongoing Investigation.

medication can be of different strengths and different potency. Simply comparing 1g of one, with 1 mg of another can be confusing, particularly if different countries use different doses. DDDs aim to solve this by relating all drug use to a standardized unit which is analogous to one day's worth.

The DDD system is most frequently used in academic articles and reports, as well as a tool for comparison and control over nationwide total drug consumption. For example the overall drug consumption of e.g. opioids, can be measured in DDDs and compared between different countries and nations.

The formula for calculating DDDs is as follows:

$$Drug\ Usage(DDDs) = \left(\frac{Items\ issued \times Amount\ of\ Drug\ per\ item}{WHO\ DDD\ Measure}\right)$$

For example, paracetamol has a DDD of 3g, which means that an average patient who takes paracetamol for pain relief (Paracetamol main indication) uses 3 gram per day. This is equivalent to six standard (500 mg) tablets. If a patient consumes twenty four (500 mg) tablets (i.e. 12 g of paracetamol in total) over the space of six days, he can have said to have consumed four DDDs of this drug.

12g (total amount of drug) / 3g (amount of drug in a DDD) = Number of DDDs

1.1. Lack of a Robust and Adoptable Clinical Practice Model

Although the Evidence Based Clinical Practice (EBCP) discourse seems to provide a strong potential for improving clinical process efficiency, there has not been a sign for rapid deployment of EBCP in clinical specialties in clinical settings. The issue of a generic model of clinical practice is elaborated by Tange et al [2], though this kind of elaborations are not common in various healthcare domains.

Tange et al writes: '*...Shared medical care involves different professionals from different organizations who need to communicate their findings and decisions effectively. To support this communication, an EPR system must be more than just a technical integration of the systems of the different parties involved. It has to support different professions with different information needs and connect different organizations with different information systems.*' This point is of critical importance to the healthcare professionals and hospital managements and will be on the top of healthcare agenda, considering the urgent need for sustainable systems. Achieving this requires semantic interoperability in all respects: clinical process efficiencies, effective clinical outcomes management, compliance monitoring and management, high quality and safe healthcare services, etc.

1.2. Lack of a Simplified Definition of Healthcare Quality

In author's opinion, healthcare quality has two dimensions: [A] Providing relevant, required healthcare services in time according to scientific knowledge management framework(s). The detailed account of this issue is outside the scope of this manuscript. [B] No harm to the patient during the delivery of healthcare services. This outline definition will be adopted through all the studies related to medication safety and investigations.

1.3. Lack of a Common Linguistic/Semantic Framework for 'Clinical Data Standards'

This corrupts and fragments the clinical data for the improvement of clinical processes in terms of better clinical outcomes [3-5]. For the classification of diseases and medical procedures there are some hierarchically-structured classification systems such as ICD (International Classification of Diseases and Procedures family of classification) systems, ICPC (International Classification of Primary Care), NIC (Nursing Intervention Classifications), NOC (Nursing Outcomes Classifications), ICD-X CM (ICD 9-10 Clinical Modification), etc.. The semantic structure of ICNP (International Classification of Nursing Practice), ICD-10 PCS (ICD-10 Procedure Coding System) differ in some respects, compared to hierarchically-structured terminology systems. A comprehensive evaluation and elaboration of healthcare terminology systems, taxonomies and ontologies should be considered for another tutorial in the context of healthcare quality and patient safety. However, with the exception of some limited efforts, there are not mature semantically-oriented terminology systems and taxonomies in use for clinical outcomes, complications and adverse outcomes. One important reason for this situation is well stipulated in [6]. Senge writes *'From a very early age, we are taught to break apart problems, to fragment the world. This apparently makes complex tasks and subjects more manageable, but we pay a hidden, enormous price. We can no longer see the consequences of our actions; we lose our intrinsic sense of connection to a larger whole. When we then try to "see the big picture," we try to reassemble the fragments in our minds, to list and organize all the pieces. But, as physicist David Bohm says, the task is futile -similar to trying to reassemble the fragments of a broken mirror to see a true reflection. Thus, after a while we give up trying to see the whole altogether'.*

This makes the preventing adverse outcomes nearly impossible especially within a rather broad scope of medication management contexts, because ICT (ICT: Information and Communication Technologies) does not provide easy-to-use rule based and case based reasoning platforms to detect adverse events/outcomes prior to their occurrence(s).

1.4. Lack of Multidisciplinary/Inter-professional Clinical Pathways

In clinical practice: healthcare professionals' perceptions of algorithms, guidelines, consensus frameworks in medical specialties and clinical maps are not still well-appreciated and the level of penetration of those concepts into clinical practice is not at a significant level. In this context, availability of clinical maps/pathways is a critical issue and requires a comprehensive approach in all respects. An example of such infrastructure is the Map of Medicine (http://www.mapofmedicine.com/), developed and put into service with appropriate updates by NHS-Institute for Innovation and Improvement. This information infrastructure seems to be a strategic framework for controlled scientific content. On the other hand, according to the author's opinion, Map of Medicine content does not contain a comprehensive SEMANTIC terminology framework to be implemented in different cultural and clinical contexts, for the time being. Map of Medicine infrastructure can be used in integration with BNF (British National Formulary). This portal should be inserted in healthcare education through relevant modifications and enrichments for innovative healthcare delivery approaches with special emphasis on inter-professional medical team formation and clinical outcomes monitoring.

1.5. Lack of Consensus on Health/Medical and Patient Records in Various Clinical and Cultural Contexts

Electronic patient-record (EPR) systems based on a theoretical model of clinical practice have never been successful [3]. Existing approaches to those systems EHR (Electronic Health Records), EPR (Electronic Patient Records), CPR (Computerized Patient Records), CMR (Computerized Medical Records), PHR (Personal Healthcare Records etc. do not provide acceptable functionalities for healthcare professionals and care record functionalities for nurses in critical care and peri-operative settings among others. As a result of all the factors listed above preventing adverse outcomes and complications become nearly impossible, worsening the patient safety indicators, increasing expenditures and extending LOS (Length of Stay).

2. Addressing Medication Irrelevancies in Clinical Settings and Adverse Outcomes

This section should not be understood as an elaboration of clinical pathways/maps or care plans. Both pathways and care plans are considered to be tools for relevant clinical practice and must support the approach explained. This is a very large complex domain requiring inter-professional attention and collaborative work.

2.1 The Issues of Clinical Interventions and Outcomes

For patient safety and back-traceability of clinical interventions and achieved outcomes accurate, valid and accessible 'INFORMATION' is an ingredient of vital role. The most prominent barriers for this type of 'INFORMATION' cover existence, availability, usability and accessibility when needed by a healthcare professional (or a team) in a given context in a clinical setting (Point of Care). The situation may be explained through the cultural variations in addition to the differences in professional practice and legislative regulations as to the sharing of personal medical records. McClanahan writes '*...Electronic information is a vital but complex component in the modern healthcare system, fueling ongoing efforts to develop a universal electronic health record infrastructure. This innovation creates a substantial tension between two desirable values: the increased quality and utility of patient medical records and the protection of the privacy of the information they contain.*' [7].

However, our focus, today, is oriented towards the impact of CPOE (Computerized Provider Order Entry Systems) medication systems on medication orders [8]. On the other hand, scholars question the potential of whether CPOEs support the inter-professional medication process or not [9]. There are other more detailed elaborations on the inter-professional nature of clinical processes from diagnosis to patient care [10].

This article does not intend to elaborate the HCICT (Healthcare Information and Communication Technologies) - related infrastructure issues. Instead, the knowledge management dynamics of medication processes will be attempted to be explained to enable healthcare teams to avoid irrelevant medication-related actions in clinical care processes. Beyond this, most important classification systems for care - related interventions and outcomes achieved. Diagnostic aspects are out of the scope of this article, since it requires a more comprehensive approach for achieving diagnosis by consensus [11]. The core concept for diagnosis involves MDTs (Multi-disciplinary Medical Teams).

One important point to be emphasized here is that in 1999, the promotion of ordering compliance and appropriate test utilization was among the core functionalities of CPOE systems [12]. Integrity of gathered data and semantic interoperability were far from established methodologies and software development efforts. This was mainly due to weaknesses in requirements elicitation effectiveness [13-14].

2.2 Causal Structure of Healthcare Interventions and Patient Outcomes

Whatever the diagnosis (diagnoses) of a patient - whether pathologically confirmed or not- be many events take place during her/his clinical care , some of them being interventions and some being patient outcomes. All the interventions and outcomes can be expressed by means of causal propositions (statements). The most comprehensive general statement is of the form sketched in Figure 1. Specifically, the right hand side of the conceptual equation depicted is the result of the left-hand side, namely, '*Outcomes*' are the result(s) of *'Interventions'*. '*Interventions'* and '*Outcomes'* could be of the following sub-categories, no matter which ontological framework and classification systems are being utilized:

- PATIENT STATUS-RELATED
- DIAGNOSTIC
- MEDICAL
- SURGICAL
- NURSING
- MEDICATION RELATED
- FINANCIAL

Any *'Intervention'* or a set of them cause(s) a set of *'Outcomes'*. In this respect, any *'Outcome'* or a set of them may have been caused by an *'Intervention'* or a set of them with a given probability after a time period [ΔT]. All the statements (propositions) represent an *'Information Element'* or an *'Information Set'*. *'All Information Elements'* and *'Information Sets'* manifest themselves within the context of healthcare processes of different natures (Diagnostic, Medical, Clinical Care, Nursing Care, Surgical, Medication Related). Some informative statements (one or more) could be utilized for preventing and/or controlling a substantial amount of adverse outcomes; ADEs (Adverse Drug Events) and ADRs (Adverse Drug Reactions) from our point of interest. *'Information'* categories and *'Information'* repositories needed at the 'Point of Care' are sketched in Figure 2 [15] (with the permission of Editors).

Within the framework of the causality relationship sketched in Figure 1, whenever the left hand side of the equation comes into the picture (workflow, ordering, etc.) the outcome on the right hand side can be expected to occur with the highest probability. In this case, through alerting functionalities and information repository queries the unexpected/unwanted outcomes could be avoided. Based on the availability and full functionality of those *'Information'* repositories some rule sets are obtained in the outpatient and inpatient settings, namely in real clinical settings. Once these rule sets are obtained, those sets enable clinical practitioners apply RBR and CBR (Rule-Based Reasoning, Case-Based Reasoning). The above mentioned '*Information Repositories'* form the foundations of *'Diagnostic, Medical, Surgical, Nursing, Medication-Related*

Evidence'. The extent to which this type of evidence and existing/accessible evidence-based literature converges is an indication of the success for EBM (Evidence Based Medicine), EBN (Evidence Based Nursing), EBHC (Evidence Based Healthcare) [16-19].

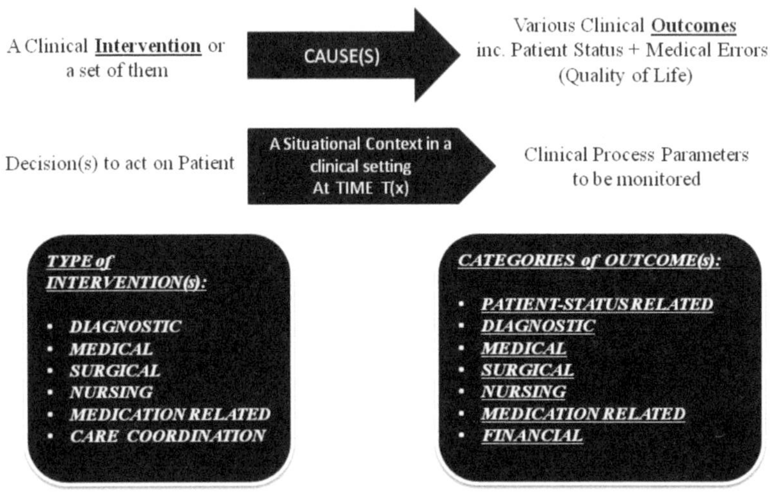

Figure 1. Causal relationship between clinical interventions and outcomes.

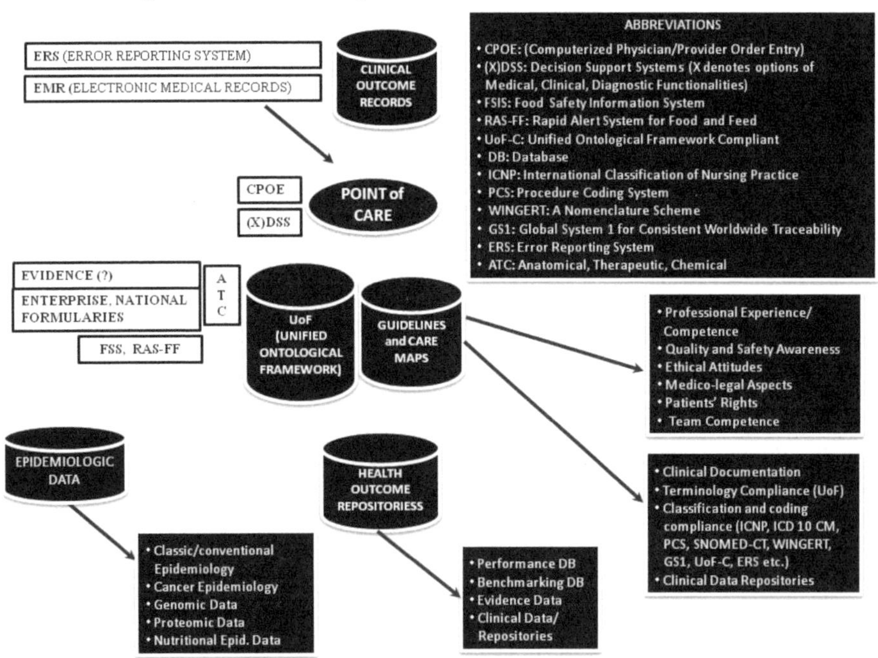

Figure 2. Information Categories at the Point-of-Care.

At this point, it should be emphasized that the critical success factor for ADE/ADR (Adverse Drug Events/Adverse Drug Reactions) reduction is the causal statements (propositions) in clinical contexts in addition to the systematic classification of *'All Outcomes'* and *'All Interventions'*. If the unwanted and/or unexpected outcomes take place within the framework of any kind of *'Intervention'* there are some measures to be taken to reduce or eliminate adverse outcomes (ADEs, ADRs) and increase patient safety especially in medication processes-related contexts. All clinical actions and interventions likely to cause adverse outcomes (through gathered data/information according to relevant data standards such as ICNP (International Classification for Nursing Practice), SNOMED CT (Systematized Nomenclature of Medicine-Clinical Terms), ATC-DDD etc.) are triggers of clinical nature.

Putting this patient safety increasing and adverse outcome(s) reducing team competencies into practice in a given clinical context requires rule-based applications according to clinical requirements by different healthcare professionals and team members (See Figures 2 and 3).

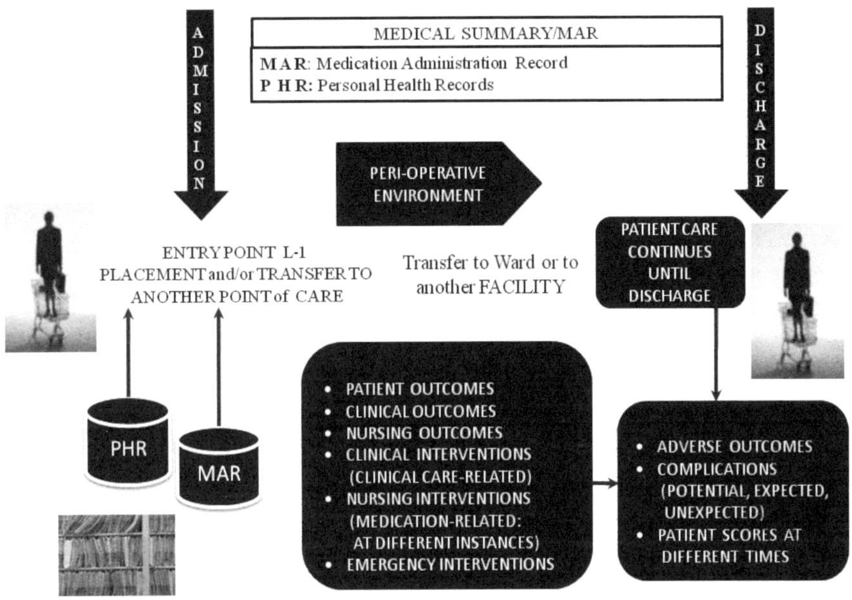

Figure 3. Causal relationship between clinical interventions and outcomes through care processes.

3. Discussion and Conclusion

As has been the case for medical processes in general, medication is a very complex process in interacting with all clinical processes and workflows. This complexity well-defines the most fundamental functionality requirements of clinical record systems. The author of this paper proposes a DDD-based backward traceability approach for every individual drug ordered in clinical settings. This approach imposes each drug-administration decision to be evaluated thoroughly in compliance with available DDD information repositories. Evaluations and control decisions are effected according to time periods of 24 hours, starting from a new drug administration time; but not to calendar days, shifts and different timeframes. A tentative framework for achieving this control approach is sketched in Figure 4.

Important points to be remembered are: (1) Ordering a medication is a complex, highly information intensive, knowledge based inter-professional process. (2) The most fundamental functional requirement of a software application is the capability of dynamically monitoring of DDD of each individual drug. (3) Any multi-drug clinical application should be based on the dynamic DDD control data for reducing and eliminating Adverse Clinical Outcomes including Adverse Drug Reactions. (4) All drug-related interactions should be standardized based on a UoF (Unified Ontological Framework) covering all available state-of-the-art terminology systems.

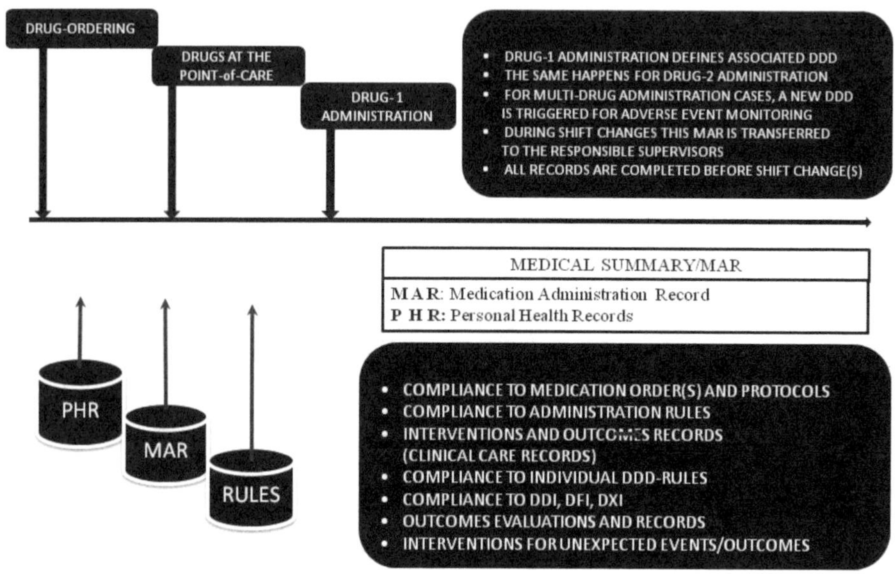

Figure 4. Definition of DDDs according to a multi-drug application in an appropriate time-axis frame.

In high risk patients with co-morbidities patient safety is a critical issue for patient herself/himself for healthcare providers, healthcare professionals, researchers and payers. For the common benefit of all stakeholders, healthcare processes should be monitored very systematically through scientific approaches and relevant tools. Most of the patient related life threatening risks are caused by medication related adverse events throughout the world.

To reduce and eliminate medication related risks and overcome adverse clinical outcomes for every drug -used for a specific indication and targeted clinical goal- a very strict DDD-compliance is a must in all clinical settings. This compliance requires MARs (Medication Administration Records) to be prepared in compliance with state-of-the-art standard-terminologies. MARs arranged according to state-of-the-art standard terminologies is a fundamental requirement for assuring continuity of care in all clinical settings. Another approach for achieving increased patient safety is utilizing 'Triggers' based on proven information repositories formed by strong and reliable medical/clinical evidence.

Finally, it must be emphasized that without a Unified Ontological Framework [15] it is unlikely to achieve high-level patient safety and reduce medication related irrelevancies caused by medication errors. Clinical outcome classification systems and nursing outcome classifications should be addressed and utilized more intensely, requiring inter-professionally coordinated, collaborative efforts. Otherwise, using our limited resources for reporting medical errors and building expensive systems, mostly medication-related ones would be inevitable.

References

[1] S. Saboor, J. Chimiak-Opoka, E. Ammenwerth, Supporting the systematic assessment of clinical processes: the MedFlow method, *Methods Inf Med* **46** (2007), 586–94.

[2] H.J. Tange et al., A generic model of clinical practice: a common view of individual and collaborative care, *Methods Inf Med* **42** (2003), 203–11.

[3] Clinical Data Standards in Healthcare: Five Case Studies. iHealth Reports, July California Healthcare Foundation, California, 2005.

[4] Introduction of a Clinical Terminology in NETHERLANDS – Needs, Constraints, Opportunities NICTIZ, Amsterdam, 2003.

[5] P.J. Brown, P. Sönksen, Evaluation of the quality of information retrieval of clinical findings from a computerized patient database using a semantic terminological model, *J Am Med Inform Assoc* **7** (2000), 392–403.

[6] P.M. Senge, The Fifth Discipline – The Art & Practice of The Learning Organization, Currency Doubleday, New York, 1994.

[7] K. McClanahan, Balancing good intentions: protecting the privacy of electronic health information, *Bulletin of Science, Technology and Society* **28** (2008), 69–79.

[8] R. Khajouei, M.W. Jaspers, The impact of CPOE medication systems' design aspects on usability, workflow and medication orders: a systematic review, *Methods Inf Med* **49** (2010), 3–19.

[9] Z. Niazkhani, H. Pirnejad, H. van der Sijs, A.de Bont, Jos Aarts, Computerized provider order entry system--does it support the inter-professional medication process? Lessons from a Dutch academic hospital, *Methods Inf Med* **49** (2010), 20–7.

[10] B. Kane, S. Luz, Achieving Diagnosis by Consensus, *Computer Supported Cooperative Work* **18** (2009), 357–92.

[11] J.E. Bardram, T.R. Hansen, Context-based workplace awareness, *Computer Supported Cooperative Work* **19** (2010) 105–38.

[12] H.H. Hawkins, R.W. Hankins, E. Johnson, A computerized physician order entry system for the promotion of ordering compliance and appropriate test utilization, *J Healthc Inf Manag* **13** (1999), 63–72.

[13] M.F. Collen, General requirements for a medical information system (MIS), *Computers and Biomedical Research* **3** (1970), 393–406.

[14] A. Hoerbst, E. Ammenwerth, Electronic Health Records. A systematic review on quality requirements, *Methods Inf Med* **49** (2010), 320–36.

[15] E.N. Eryilmaz, Gül Dündar, S.O. Sari, Inevitable components of and steps for ADE management systems: the need for a Unified Ontological Framework (UOF) and a more effective collaboration in medication safety, *Stud Health Technol Inform* **148** (2009), 149–58.

[16] A.K. Kakkar, S. Rushton-Smith, Venous thromboembolism pharmacologic prophylaxis after major surgery-are we doing well or not well enough?, *Ann Surg* **253** (2011), 221–2.

[17] S. Halimi, Acute consequences of hypoglycaemia in diabetic patients, *Diabetes Metab* **36** (2010), S75–S83.

[18] F. Nobels et al., Tight glycaemic control: clinical implementation of protocols, *Best Pract Res Clin Anaesthesiol* **23** (2009), 461–72.

[19] K.A. Caddell et al., Patient-specific insulin-resistance–guided infusion improves glycemic control in cardiac surgery, *Ann Thorac Surg* **90** (2010), 1818–23.

Part E

Novel Applications of Patient Safety Informatics

Patient Safety Informatics
V. Koutkias et al. (Eds.)
IOS Press, 2011

doi:10.3233/978-1-60750-740-6-169

The ADE Scorecards: A Tool for Adverse Drug Event Detection in Electronic Health Records

Emmanuel CHAZARD[a,1] Adrian BĂCEANU[b] Laurie FERRET[c,d] and Grégoire FICHEUR[a]

[a] *Department of Medical Information and Archives, CHU Lille; UDSL EA 2694; Univ Lille Nord de France; F-59000 Lille, France*
[b] *IDEEA Advertising, Romania*
[c] *Central dispensary, CH Denain, France*
[d] *CERIM, UDSL EA 2694; Univ Lille Nord de France;F-59000 Lille, France*

Abstract. Although several methods exist for Adverse Drug events (ADE) detection due to past hospitalizations, a tool that could display those ADEs to the physicians does not exist yet. This article presents the ADE Scorecards, a Web tool that enables to screen past hospitalizations extracted from Electronic Health Records (EHR), using a set of ADE detection rules, presently rules discovered by data mining. The tool enables the physicians to (1) get contextualized statistics about the ADEs that happen in their medical department, (2) see the rules that are useful in their department, i.e. the rules that could have enabled to prevent those ADEs and (3) review in detail the ADE cases, through a comprehensive interface displaying the diagnoses, procedures, lab results, administered drugs and anonymized records. The article shows a demonstration of the tool through a use case.

Keywords. Adverse drug events, adverse drug reactions, data mining, electronic health records

Introduction

The Institute Of Medicine defines ADEs as "injuries due to medication management rather than the underlying condition of the patient" [1]. That definition emphasizes that ADEs are due to a combination of causes, including drugs (drug administration, dose variations, and drug discontinuations) and characteristics of the patient (such as the age, diseases, renal and hepatic functions) [2].

When computerized provider order entries (CPOEs) are used to prescribe drugs, it is possible to detect situations at risk of ADE via prevention rules, such as *"Heparin & age>70 → increased bleeding risk"*. Those rules enable to detect risky situations and to prevent from an ADE by alerting the prescriber. The ADE is still not observed when the alert fires: that can be called *prospective ADE prevention*.

Another subject of research is *retrospective ADE detection*. It aims at analyzing past hospital stays to discover cases where ADEs really occurred. An ADE case is a hospital stay where an outcome occurred, and where that outcome is explained by a set of causes related to drug administration or discontinuation, possibly combined with

[1] Corresponding Author: emmanuel.chazard@univ-lille2.fr

characteristics of the patient. Several approaches have been developed in the field of retrospective ADE detection [3-4]. They can be classified into expert-operated methods, or automated methods. The expert-operated methods suppose that an expert explicitly identifies the ADE cases. Those methods consist of retrospective medical chart reviews and reporting systems. The development of automated methods is more recent. Those methods include natural language processing of discharge summaries [5-8], and data mining of electronic health records [9].

Whatever the method used for ADE retrospective detection, a tool that could display the detected ADE cases and related statistics to the physicians of medical units does not exist yet. As a consequence, the physicians are not aware of how many ADEs occur in their medical unit, and they cannot improve their medication management.

The objective of the present work is to develop and deploy a tool that can be installed in any hospital to automatically detect past ADE cases and to display those cases to the physicians. The tool must take as input records of past hospitalizations extracted from the Electronic Health Records (EHR) of the hospital, and a set of ADE detection rules. The tool must run the rules, and provide the physicians of the hospital with comprehensive statistics about ADEs in the current department, the ADE detection rules that are interesting in the current department, and the ability to review the ADE cases that are detected by the system.

1. Material

The material consists of data that correspond to past hospital stays, and a set of ADE detection rules obtained by means of data mining.

1.1. Records of Past Hospital Stays

As the objective is to mine past hospital stays to discover ADE cases, the Scorecards must be provided with structured description of the stays extracted from the EHR of the hospital where it is installed. This description fits a data model that has been designed previously within the PSIP Project [10]. It only uses routinely-collected data: no data have to be specifically recorded or computed for the Scorecards. The data model includes:

- medical and administrative information (e.g., age, gender, admission date);
- diagnoses encoded using the International Classification of Diseases (ICD10);
- medical procedures;
- drugs administered daily to the patient, encoded using the Anatomical Therapeutic Chemical classification (ATC);
- laboratory results encoded using the International Union of Pure and Applied Chemistry classification (IUPAC) or local terminologies, and
- anonymized free-text records, such as discharge letters.

The Scorecards are installed in four hospitals (in Denmark, France and Bulgaria) and provided with about 90,000 records over 3 years (2007-2010). In some of those hospitals, the data are updated monthly.

1.2. Adverse Drug Events Detection Rules

The knowledge about ADEs can be summarized by means of ADE detection rules. An ADE detection rule is made of one or several Boolean conditions that lead to an outcome, with a given probability, such as $Cause_1$ & $Cause_2$ & $Cause_3$ → *Outcome*. That representation is widely used either for prospective ADE prevention or retrospective ADE detection [11]. Generally, the conditions are simple: two drugs, a drug and a lab result, a drug alone, a drug and a patient's characteristic, or a drug and a drug allergy [4, 12-23]. In this work we use a set of 236 rules that have been discovered in a previous work by data mining of EHRs [9]. Those rules involve 1 to 4 conditions that lead to an outcome. The conditions can be of demographic characteristics of the patients, drug administrations or discontinuations, laboratory results, or diagnoses. The number and the kind of the conditions were not constrained by the methods but were optimized by the use of statistical procedures. The rules enable to discover 56 kinds of outcomes, displayed in Table 1.

Table 1. Number of ADE detection rules per outcome

Outcome	**Rules**
Coagulation disorders	
Hemorrhage (detected by the administration of haemostatic)	7
Heparin overdose (activated partial thromboplastin time>1.23)	5
VKA overdose (INR>4.9 or administration of vitamin K)	59
Thrombopenia (count<75,000)	24
Other coagulation disorders	23
Ionic and renal disorders	
Hyperkalemia (K^+>5.3 mmol/l)	63
Renal failure (creatinine>135 µmol/l or urea>8 mmol/l)	8
Other ionic disorders	4
Miscellaneous	
Anemia (Hb<10g/dl)	2
Bacterial infection (detected by the administration of antibiotic)	4
Diarrhea (detected by the administration of an anti-diarrheal)	2
Fungal infection (detected by the administration of an antifungal)	10
Hepatic cholestasis (alk. Phos.>240 UI/l or bilirubins>22 µmol/l)	3
Hepatic cytolysis (ala. trans.>110 UI/l or asp. trans.>110 UI/l)	4
Hypereosinophilia (eosinophilocytes>10^9/l)	4
High level of pancreatic enzymes (amylase>90 UI/l or lipase>90 UI/l)	7
Neutropenia (count<1,500/mm^3)	2
Others	5
Total	*236*

The rules are described as a set of structured XML files [24]. Those files include:

- Mappings, that enable to transform the raw data into Boolean variables, e.g. *potassium≥5.3 → hyperkalemia=1*.
- The set of rules, identified as set of conditions linked to outcomes.
- A lexicon that enables to automatically replace the names of the variables by understandable English, French or Danish labels.
- A set of free-text explanations that describe each rule and provide with bibliographic references. Those explanations are available in three languages for several uses (short label, long label, "what to do" label) and for several users (physicians, nurses and patients).

2. Methods

The display of statistics on ADEs and ADE cases relies on two steps (Figure 1). The first step, *computation step*, consists in applying the ADE detection rules to the hospital stays in order to detect ADE cases and to compute statistics about ADEs. The second step, *Web-based display tool*, consists in displaying the statistics and the ADE cases.

The Method section mainly deals with the computation step. The conception of the display tool is briefly explained in this section, and then the Web-based interface is illustrated in the Results section.

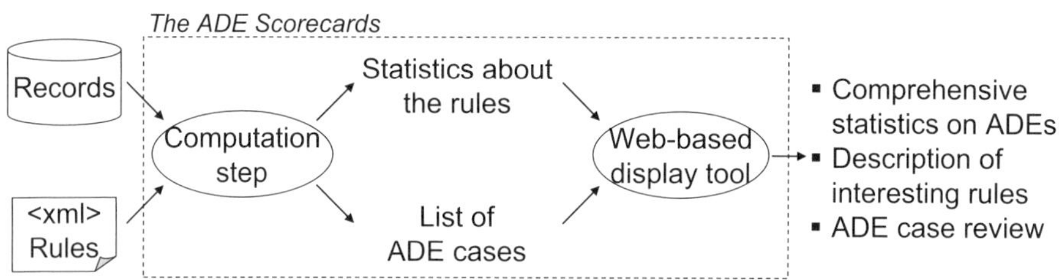

Figure 1. The ADE Scorecards rely on a computation step and a Web-based display tool.

2.1. Computation Step

The computation step consists in applying the rules on the hospital stays that are extracted from the EHR. A rule is a set of conditions leading to an outcome, such as C_1 & ... & $C_k \rightarrow O$. A stay that "matches the conditions of the rule" is a stay that belongs to the set $C_1 \cap \ldots \cap C_k$, if in addition the conditions are compatible regarding time: $max(startTimeC_1, \ldots, startTimeC_k) \leq min(stopTimeC_1, \ldots, stopTimeC_k)$. A stay that "matches the rule" is a stay that belongs to the set $C_1 \cap \ldots \cap C_k \cap O$, if in addition the conditions and the outcome are compatible regarding time: $max(startTimeC_1, \ldots, startTimeC_k) \leq startTimeO \leq min(stopTimeC_1, \ldots, stopTimeC_k)$. This enables to compute several statistics for each rule in the hospital. The same statistics are also computed separately in each medical department, we call them "contextualized statistics". The statistics are:

- Support = $P(O \cap C_1 \cap \ldots \cap C_k)$.
- Confidence = $P(O \mid C_1 \cap \ldots \cap C_k)$.
- Relative risk $RR = \dfrac{P(O / C_1 \cap \ldots \cap C_k)}{P(O / \overline{(C_1 \cap \ldots \cap C_k)})}$.
- P value of the Fisher's exact test for independency between the outcome (O) and the set of conditions($C_1 \cap \ldots \cap C_k$).
- Median delay between t_1 (the conditions are met) and t_2 (the outcome occurs).
- Description of the background of the patients: average age, sex ratio, prevalence of renal insufficiency, hepatic insufficiency, and alcoholism.
- Description of what happens to the patients thereafter: average length of stay, death rate, etc.

2.2. Conception of the Web-based Display Tool

A Web-based tool is developed to display the statistics described above, the rules that are interesting, and the ADE cases. The following constraints are taken into account.

The Scorecards must be easily accessible: they are developed in PHP as a Web-based application and made available through an Apache HTTP server connected to a MySQL relational database. Any member of the staff equipped with a Web browser can use the Scorecards, assuming he has valid credentials.

The Scorecards must preserve the anonymity of the patients: the data used in the Scorecards concern patients who have already been discharged. The knowledge brought by the Scorecards is generic and there is no need to connect the data to the original records by name. The free-text records (e.g. discharge summaries) are automatically anonymized. The structured data do not contain any directly or indirectly nominative data (identifiers, names, birth date, dates of the stay, precise age, ZIP code…). Finally, the Scorecards are deployed in the intranet of each hospital.

The Scorecards must be easy to use: the users must be able to quickly and simply find the relevant information, and not to be flooded by too much useless information. The scorecards have been developed using a Human-centered design process [25].

The Scorecards must provide the users with contextualized information: the information displayed to the user must depend on the user's characteristics and requirements. The statistics that are displayed are computed especially in the medical department of the user, and the cases that are displayed really occurred in his department. In addition, the Scorecards are fully multilingual. For the moment, the following languages are supported: English, French and Danish.

The Scorecards must be easy to deploy: the Scorecards are developed as a bootable ISO image, so that it requires a few time to deploy them into a new hospital, assuming that the data extraction are available in the form of tabulated text tables.

3. Results

This section describes the ADE Scorecards. The main features are described in the first section, and the second part consists of a use-case that demonstrates the tool.

3.1. Main Features

The ADE Scorecards are a Web tool for ADE detection and ADE-related knowledge visualization. The basic course of events consists of 3 steps (Figure 2). Once logged in, the user can visualize global statistics about ADEs in his department. On a comprehensive page, it is possible to know how many ADEs occurred with respect to their kind. Then, by choosing a type of ADE, the user accesses the list of rules that are interesting in his department, i.e. the rules that would have enabled to prevent some ADEs in the department. Those rules are complemented by contextualized statistics. There is a hypertext link to the ADE cases, which allows the user to visualize all the anonymized data, including demographics, diagnoses, procedures, lab results (in tabular or graphical form), drugs administered to the patient (in tabular or graphical form), and anonymized free-text reports. This helps the user making his opinion about the case.

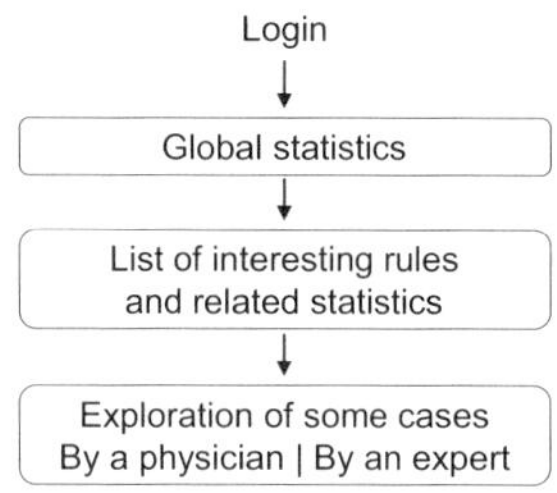

Figure 2. Basic course of events.

From a technical viewpoint, the Scorecards are distributed as a bootable ISO image that contains a Web server and a set of PHP scripts. It is to be installed onto the intranet of a hospital; the installation is immediate. The hospital records have to be extracted in tabulated text according to the data model, and are automatically loaded into the database. If they are available, the free-text reports have to be anonymized first. The rules are stored as a set of XML files that can be easily updated or replaced by a customized rule set. The users have to be registered into a specific table. Then, the tool is available from the intranet through a HTTP connection.

3.2. Use Case

The features of the Scorecards are presented through a sequence of commented screenshots that correspond to the following possible scenarios: "A physician working in a hospital, from which the ADE Scorecards are available, uses the Scorecards for various purposes. (Scenario 1) He wants to have a comprehensive overview of the ADEs that have been detected in his medical department during the last 6 months. (Scenario 2) Among those kinds of ADEs, he wants to explore the rules that lead to hyperkalemia (Scenario 3). Then he wants to explore one of the probable ADE cases to form his own opinion."

3.2.1. Scenario 1: Comprehensive Overview about ADEs in a Department

The user has to use a computer connected to the intranet and equipped with a Web browser. Once logged in, he has access to the synthesis page (Figure 3). The language select box allows for choosing the language: French, English or Danish. The synthesis page (Figure 3) consists of 3 zones. The table (part 1 of Figure 3) displays the number of ADEs detected month per month. Each line of the table is a kind of ADE; each column is a month of the current year. The line chart displays the same information using a chart (part 2 of Figure 3). In the third zone (part 3 of Figure 3), the user can chose a period of the analysis, from 2007 to 2010. He is also able to choose some kinds of ADEs and validate the form in order to generate the scorecards per kind of ADE.

3.2.2. Scenario 2: Exploring Interesting Rules in a Department

Once the user has chosen one or several types of ADEs and validated the form, he is displayed one page per kind of outcome chosen in the previous list. In this use case, the user focuses on the cases of hyperkalemia. The potassium is an electrolyte; its level in the plasma is regulated by the kidneys and might be influenced by some drugs and diseases. In case the potassium level raises up to 5.3 mmol/l, there is a hyperkalemia: this kind of anomaly could lead to lethal cardiac rhythm troubles.

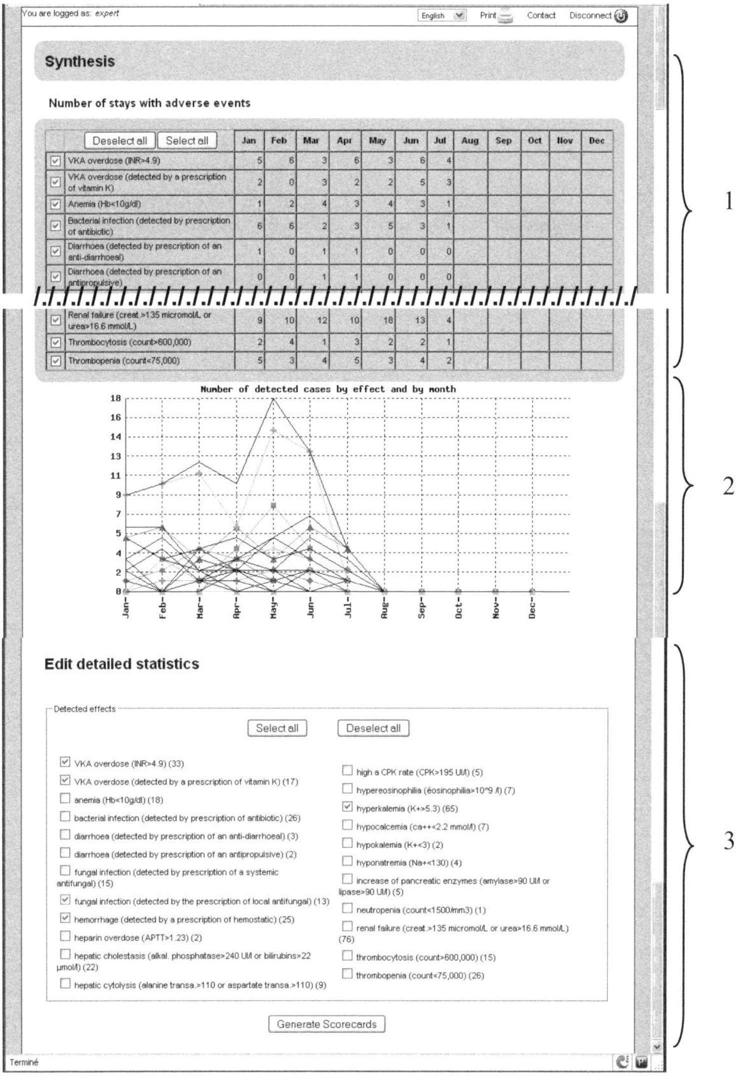

Figure 3. Synthesis page of the Scorecards.

The complete scorecard is displayed (Figure 4). The page contains 4 zones, and is conceived to be either explored on the screen or printed on paper. At the top of the page, the user can read the period, the place, and the outcome that is traced (part 1 of Figure 4). In the second area, descriptive statistics are computed (part 2 of Figure 4); they describe the stays that have been detected within all the rules. In the third area, all (and only) the rules that enable to detect potential ADE cases in the current department are displayed (part 3 of Figure 4). For instance, the user can read that Low Molecular Weight Heparins (LMWH) can induce hyperkalemia especially for patients suffering from renal insufficiency (rule N°1). In the current department, 17% of patients with

LMWH and renal failure encountered a hyperkalemia in a median delay of 4.5 days. At the bottom of the page (part 4 of Figure 4), more detailed explanations are provided for each rule. They can be reached by clicking on the internal hypertext links placed on the number of each rule. If the user wants to check one of those stays, he just has to click on the number of stays beside a given rule, on the right. Doing this, a popup displays the different cases that match the rule. The user can reach the corresponding stay by clicking on its identifier.

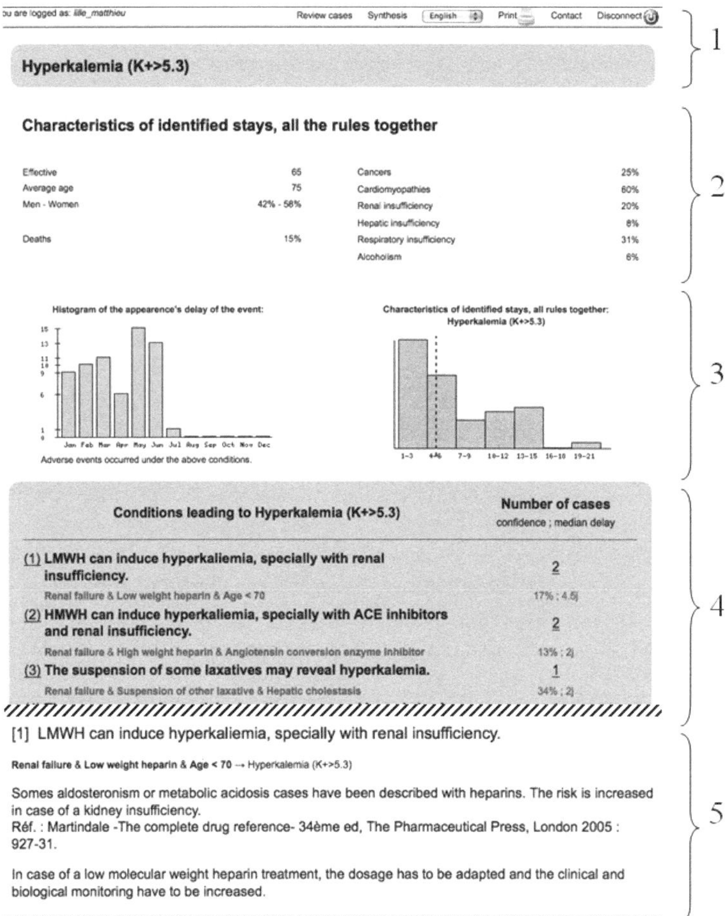

Figure 4. Scorecard of hyperkalemia (K^{+}>5.3).

3.2.3. Scenario 3: Review of an ADE Case

By clicking on its identifier, it is possible to review a potential ADE case. The user can reach several pages that display all the available information according to the data model. A page also provides comprehensive information about the stay; we present here only this screen (Figure 5). This screen is made up of 3 main parts. The top frame contains several buttons that will be described later. The left panel enables to review all the drugs that have been administered to the patient. The right panel enables to review all the laboratory results.

In the lab panel (right), by clicking on the "Potassium" checkbox (label 1 on Figure 5), the user makes the Potassium chart appear on the screen. The Potassium checkbox has a colored background because it is identified as the outcome within the rules that fire on the present stay. Several charts can appear on the same page if necessary. In this case the Potassium ion reaches a value of 5.7 on the seventh day (label 2 on Figure 5).

If the user wants to see the rules that fire for that stay, he just has to click on the button "Rule info" in the head panel. A popup appears as displayed in Figure 6.

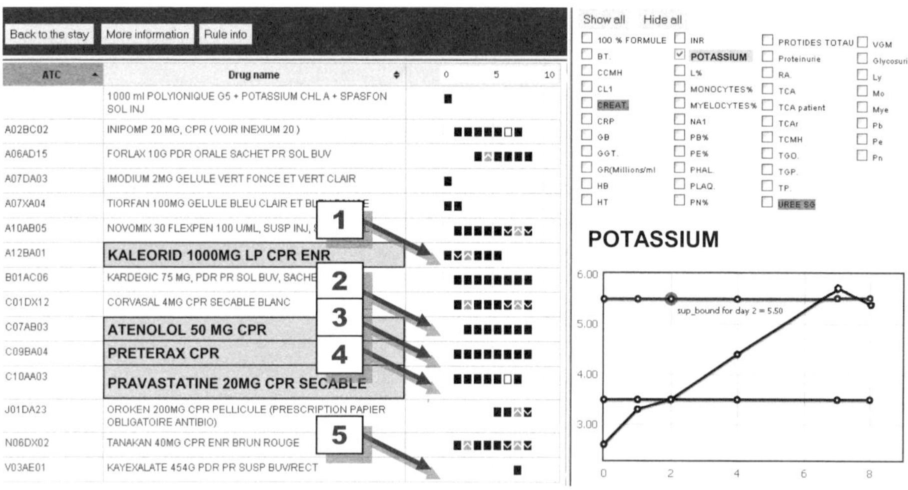

Figure 5. Main screen of the stay review facility.

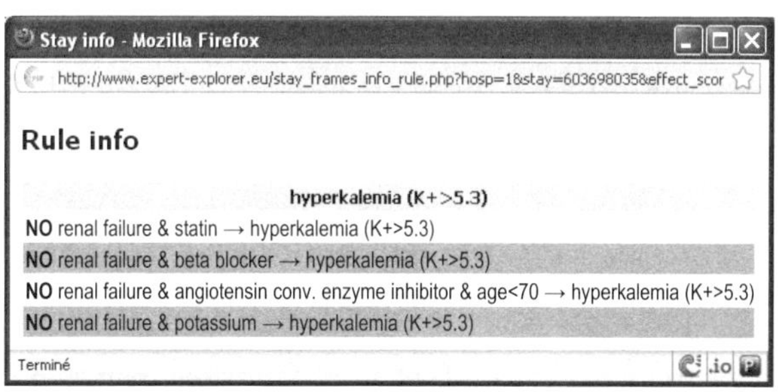

Figure 6. Popup displaying information about the rules of the current stay.

In the present case, according to the rules, the drugs involved are statins, beta blockers, angiotensin conversion enzyme inhibitor, and potassium. On the drug panel (left part of Figure 5), the user can review the drugs. The drugs that correspond to the various rules appear on a colored background (labels 3-6). The user can check that the potassium (label 3), the beta blocker (label 4), the association of the angiotensin conversion enzyme inhibitor and potassium sparing diuretic (label 5) and the statin (label 6) have been administered before day 7, the date of the outcome. All those drugs are known to increase the potassium blood level. In the present example, the user can also notice the reactions of the physicians. Hopefully the potassium is suspended before the hyperkalemia occurs (label 3). But as the potassium level reaches a very high level, a potassium lowering drug is administered during the seventh day (label 7).

The user can also access additional information by clicking on the "more information" button of the head panel. A popup appears and displays the age, the gender, the length of stay, the exit mode, and the diagnoses. In the present case, the hypokalemia is encoded (it was probably the admission ground), but the hyperkalemia is not. Finally, the Scorecards also enable the user to read the anonymized letters and reports that are previously anonymized. In that precise case, the hypokalemia is mentioned in the report but not the hyperkalemia. The physician concludes "woman admitted for a hypokalemia in relation to a gastro-enteritis (...) after correction, the potassium level is normal (...)".

4. Discussion & Conclusion

The ADE Scorecards are an innovative tool that enables to automatically detect occurred ADE cases, by screening anonymized data extracted from an EHR with a set of rules. The detection is automated and doesn't need any expert review, contrary to chart reviews or voluntary declarations. The rules used here have been obtained by data mining of EHRs but, as the rules consist of a set of XML files, it is simply possible to use a custom set of rules instead. Occurred ADE cases are detected, and several statistics are automatically computed, allowing the physicians to get quantitative knowledge about ADEs. The physicians are also provided with contextualized knowledge about ADEs, in the form of the set of rules that are interesting for them in their own department. This feature is important, as the knowledge about ADEs is very profuse, and not sorted by probability. Using the Scorecards, the physician can get a reasonable amount of qualitative knowledge: that knowledge is contextualized and describes their own medical unit. Moreover, the users are more responsive to that knowledge because it concerns ADEs that really occurred in their own medical unit, and they are able to review the cases in detail.

The ADE Scorecards can very easily be deployed in any hospital, as they consist of a Web server that is distributed as a bootable ISO image. The hospital has to be able to provide the Scorecards with structured extraction of data from the EHR, including administrative data, diagnoses, lab results and drug administration. If the hospital is able to provide the Scorecards with anonymized reports, then the users will benefit from them.

The Scorecards are currently being evaluated through three aspects. (1) The accuracy and the reliability of the set of rules are evaluated by medical experts who are reviewing the ADE cases detected by the tool. (2) A team of ergonomists and psychologists is evaluating the usability of the tool. (3) A prospective impact assessment is performed, to assess if the tool could help reducing the incidence of ADEs in a French hospital.

Acknowledgements

The research leading to these results has received funding from the European Community's Seventh Framework Programme (FP7/2007-2013) under Grant Agreement n°216130 – the PSIP project.

The authors would like to acknowledge every healthcare

professionals (physicians, nurses, head nurses and pharmacists) and technicians whose involvement made completion of this study possible.

References

[1] Institute of Medicine, *Preventing medication errors: Quality Chasm Series*, National Academies Press, 2007.

[2] J.R. Nebeker, P. Barach, M.H. Samore, Clarifying adverse drug events: a clinician's guide to terminology, documentation, and reporting, *Ann Intern Med* **140** (2004), 795–801.

[3] D.W. Bates, R.S. Evans, H. Murff, P.D. Stetson, L. Pizziferri, G. Hripcsak, Detecting adverse events using information technology, *J Am Med Inform Assoc* **10** (2003), 115–28.

[4] T. Morimoto, T.K. Gandhi, A.C. Seger, T.C. Hsieh, D.W. Bates, Adverse drug events and medication errors: detection and classification methods, *Qual Saf Health Care* **13** (2004), 306–14.

[5] M.N. Cantor, H.J. Feldman, M.M. Triola, Using trigger phrases to detect adverse drug reactions in ambulatory care notes, *Qual Saf Health Care* **16** (2007), 132–4.

[6] M. Gysbers et al., Natural language processing to identify adverse drug events, *AMIA Annu Symp Proc* (2008), 961.

[7] G.B. Melton, G. Hripcsak, Automated detection of adverse events using natural language processing of discharge summaries, *J Am Med Inform Assoc* **12** (2005), 448–57.

[8] E. Aramaki et al, Extraction of adverse drug effects from clinical records, *Stud Health Technol Inform* **160** (2010), 739–43.

[9] E. Chazard et al., Detection of adverse drug events detection: data agregation and data mining, *Stud Health Technol Inform* **148** (2009), 75–84.

[10] E. Chazard, B. Merlin, G. Ficheur, J.C. Sarfati, R. Beuscart, Detection of adverse drug events: proposal of a data model, *Stud Health Technol Inform* **148** (2009), 63–74.

[11] V. Koutkias et al., Constructing clinical decision support systems for adverse drug event prevention: a knowledge-based approach, *AMIA Annu Symp Proc* (2010), 402–6.

[12] D.W. Bates et al., Potential identifiability and preventability of adverse events using information systems, *J Am Med Inform Assoc* **1** (1994), 404–11.

[13] A.K. Jha, G.J. Kuperman, E. Rittenberg, J.M. Teich, D.W. Bates, Identifying hospital admissions due to adverse drug events using a computer-based monitor, *Pharmacoepidemiol Drug Saf* **10** (2001), 113–9.

[14] G. Del Fiol, B.H. Rocha, G.J. Kuperman, D.W. Bates, P. Nohama, Comparison of two knowledge bases on the detection of drug-drug interactions, *Proc AMIA Symp* (2000), 171–5.

[15] T.K. Gandhi et al., Outpatient prescribing errors and the impact of computerized prescribing, *J Gen Intern Med* **20** (2005), 837–41.

[16] J. Judge et al., Prescribers' responses to alerts during medication ordering in the long term care setting, *J Am Med Inform Assoc* **13** (2006), 385–90.

[17] M.D. Paterno al., Tiering drug–drug interaction alerts by severity increases compliance rates, *J Am Med Inform Assoc* **16** (2009), 40–46.

[18] A. Schedlbauer et al., What evidence supports the use of computerized alerts and prompts to improve clinicians' prescribing behavior?, *J Am Med Inform Assoc* **16** (2009), 531–8.

[19] J.M. Teich et al., The Brigham integrated computing system (BICS): advanced clinical systems in an academic hospital environment, *Int J of Med Inform* **54** (1999), 197–208.

[20] G.J. Kuperman et al., Detecting alerts, notifying the physician, and offering action items: a comprehensive alerting system, *Proc AMIA Annu Fall Symp* (1996), 704–8.

[21] B. Honigman et al., Using computerized data to identify adverse drug events in outpatients, *J Am Med Inform Assoc* **8** (2001), 254–66.

[22] T.S. Field et al., Strategies for detecting adverse drug events among older persons in the ambulatory setting, *J Am Med Inform Assoc* **11** (2004) 492–8.

[23] S.M. Handler et al., A systematic review of the performance characteristics of clinical event monitor signals used to detect adverse drug events in the hospital setting, *J Am Med Inform Assoc* **14** (2007) 451–8.

[24] E. Chazard, G. Ficheur, B. Merlin, E. Serrot, R. Beuscart, Adverse drug events prevention rules: multi-site evaluation of rules from various sources, *Stud Health Technol Inform* **148** (2009), 102–11.

[25] ISO 13407:1999, Human-centered design processes for interactive systems, 1999.

Patient Safety Informatics
V. Koutkias et al. (Eds.)
IOS Press, 2011

doi:10.3233/978-1-60750-740-6-180

Three Different Cases of Exploiting Decision Support Services for Adverse Drug Event Prevention

Stéphanie BERNONVILLE [a,1], Julie NIES [b], Henrik Gliese PEDERSEN [c], Bertrand GUILLOT [b], Mostafa MAAZI [a], Anna-Lis BERG [c], Jean-Charles SARFATI [d] and Vassilis KOUTKIAS [e]

[a] *CHU Lille, UDSL EA2694, Univ Lille Nord de France F-59000 Lille, France*

[b] *MEDASYS, Gif-Sur-Yvette, France*

[c] *IBM Global Business Services, Healthcare, Denmark*

[d] *ORACLE FRANCE, Colombes, France*

[e] *Aristotle University, Medical School, Lab of Medical Informatics, Thessaloniki, Greece*

Abstract. Clinical Decision Support Systems (CDSSs) are implemented in clinical settings in order to improve patient outcomes and/or clinical practices. However, they are still not widely accepted by healthcare professionals due to over-alerting. The aim of the "Patient Safety through Intelligent Procedures in medication" (PSIP) project is to develop and demonstrate innovative tools so as to generate and provide relevant knowledge to healthcare professionals and patients for Adverse Drug Event (ADE) prevention by means of Information and Communication Technologies (ICT). PSIP employs a Knowledge Base (KB) as the core of its CDSS. This KB encapsulates signals capable of automatically detecting potential ADEs and contextualizing the CDSS output to the patient and healthcare professionals. To exploit the KB, a Global Knowledge Platform (GKP) has been created comprising of a KB system, a Connectivity Platform and appropriate user interface modules. The GKP has been tested to demonstrate integration of the KB in different work situations and it has been deployed in three different medical applications. The first is a Web application; the second involves a commercial French EHR (Electronic Health Record) and the third is a Danish CPOE (Computerised Physician Order Entry) system. This paper presents recent progress as regards the exploitation of the PSIP KB and the results obtained in the three different medical applications.

Keywords. Adverse drug event (ADE), clinical decision support system (CDSS), computerised phycisian order entry (CPOE), electronic health record (HER), knowledge base (KB), usability driven design

[1] Corresponding author: stephanie.bernonville@univ-lille2.fr

Introduction

Clinical Decision Support Systems (CDSS) are increasingly implemented in clinical settings with significant expectations as regards improving patient outcomes, clinical practices and especially prescription reliability [1-2]. Despite many years of research and development, CDSSs are still not in mainstream use by Healthcare Professionals (HCPs). Many feel that they do not meet the needs of clinical care. Current CDSSs generate multiple alerts, which often inappropriately interrupt a clinician's workflow. Consequently, HCPs ignore alerts or become habituated to them. As a result, events with potentially serious consequences may be disregarded or not recognized [3].

The work presented in this paper takes place in the European project: Patient Safety through Intelligent Procedures in medication (PSIP) [4]. One of the project sub-objectives is to develop innovative and contextualized knowledge resources for HCPs and patients derived by extracting and aggregating data from large numbers of clinical records. In this regard, a Knowledge Base (KB) has been elaborated, contaning ADE detection rules [5], which can be contextualized per hospital and medical unit thanks to specific computed statistical features. It aims at providing contextualized knowledge usable to prevent ADE in a prospective way through a decision support service, as well as in a retrospective fashion through a scorecards tool [6].

In this paper, we focus on the exploitation of the PSIP KB to prevent ADE through the decision support service, in three different medical applications and show its use in different work situations.

1. Methods for Exploiting the Knowledge Base

To exploit the PSIP KB for decision support services, the PSIP Global Knowledge Platform (GKP) has been elaborated. This platform consists of three components: (1) The KB system allowing managing and representing rules derived from data-mining techniques [7]; (2) A Connectivity Platform (CP) providing transformation and routing services between any medical application and the KB system; (3) A user interface module allowing the incorporation of PSIP knowledge into medical applications. Instantiating the GKP allows for deploying a CDSS tailored to the targeted environment.

1.1. The Knowledge Base System

The PSIP KB system enables to systematically represent and manage the ADE detection rule base derived from data-mining techniques (236 rules constitute currently the PSIP rule base). The KB system is based on the conceptual model depicted in Figure 1 [8]. *Rule* constitutes the primary concept corresponding to the main rules on predicting ADE and is linked with *Conditions* and *Effect*. The condition consists of the value of one variable, a comparison operator and one reference value, while a TRUE/FALSE value is returned according to the result of the comparison. The variable checked by each condition may be a prescribed or suppressed *Drug*, a *Diagnosis* and a patient characteristic or a *Lab* examination value. Pseudo-variable expressions have been used to define diagnoses and medication. These pseudo-variables express groups of conditions or drugs that (may) have the same effect. The *Patient* concept is associated with patient data that participate in *Conditions*. The mechanism that controls the applicability of rules to a particular *Context* and the subset of alerts to be displayed as decision support output is handled via *Meta-rules*.

This knowledge model has been implemented using GASTON [9], a framework supporting the design, the development and the validation of CDSS.

Finally, ADE PSIP detection rules can be contextualized by hospital and by medical unit thanks to specific computed statistical features. To take into account this aspect, contextualized PSIP KB systems are created for each hospital and contain the corresponding rule statistics. Thus, medical applications can be connected to the corresponding KB system and display relevant information for each specific hospital.

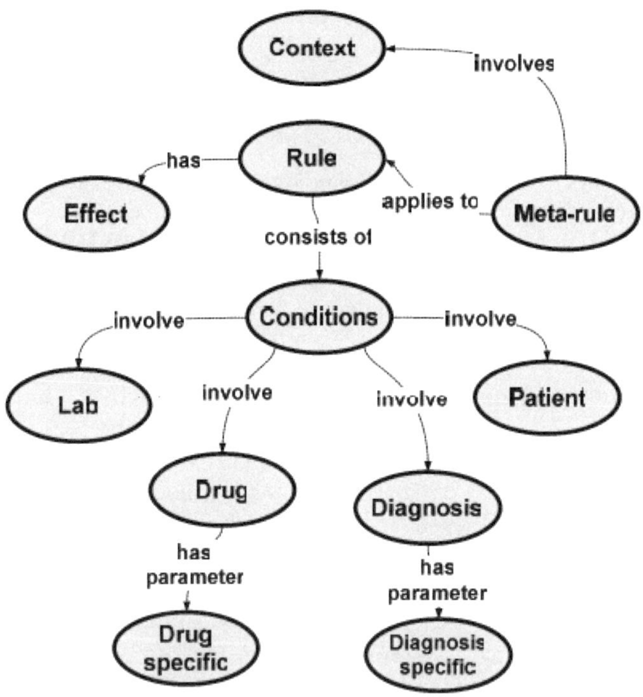

Figure 1. Conceptual model of PSIP knowledge for ADE prevention.

1.2. The Connectivity Platform

The CP provides the interoperability service between medical applications and the KB system. The development of the CP is based on Oracle© products. It enables to minimize the effort needed to achieve system integration regardless of system structure and language. The main characteristics of the CP are: (1) capacity to be generic, (2) openness, (3) adoption of standards (XML, Web services, SOAP), and (4) usage of industrial tools and techniques (Oracle SOA suite) for its development and deployment. This architecture was fully tested in a real integration environment, using the KB system and diverse medical applications

(Results section). Figure 2 illustrates an instantiation of the GKP, especially highlighting the messages exchanged among its components.

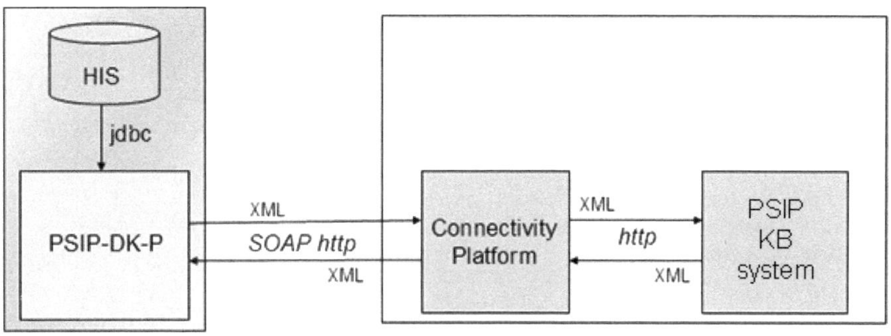

Figure 2. Example of instantiation of the PSIP GKP.

1.3. The User Interface Module

To display the ADE information derived from the KB system, appropriate user interface modules have to be developed. Those modules depend on the structure and nature of the targeted medical applications. Thus, ADE information is displayed in different way and consequently for different work situations. In the PSIP project, three user interface modules have been developed. The design of those prototypes has been driven by usability approaches. For example, to face the complexity of ADE prevention activity, a Human Factor (HF) based analysis of the existing work systems has been performed. This analysis provided a set of design recommendations. As each partner has their own development strategy, recommendations were taken into account but followed when it was feasible (due to technical and time constraints). Usability inspections have also been used [10]. This is an informal method where ergonomists judge whether each dialogue element of user interface follows established usability principles. To improve the usability of the user interface modules, ergonomists involved in the project applied this method to detect ergonomic problems and to propose recommendations. An example ergonomic problem detected and the relevant recommendation for addressing it is presented in Figure 3.

2. Three Different Decision Support Services Exploiting the PSIP Knowledge

To test the exploitation of the KB and the use of the GKP, three decision support services have been deployed. The first decision support service exploits the KB in a Web application and allows providing ADE information at anytime via Web access. The second decision support service exploits the KB in a commercial EHR and allows providing ADE information on different places of the system. The third decision support service exploits the KB in a CPOE system and allows providing ADE information during the prescription activity of the physician.

Critère	Description du problème	Conséquences	Recommandations	Degré de gravité
Compatibility	Only 10 drugs can be displayed for the drug selection module. nevertheless, sometime, for the same drug there are more than 10 type of dose / packaging. As a consequence, the user won't be able to display all the existing drugs.	Time lost Risk of error	Do not limit the list at 10 drugs. For example, a vertical scroll bar could be used.	✹✹✹

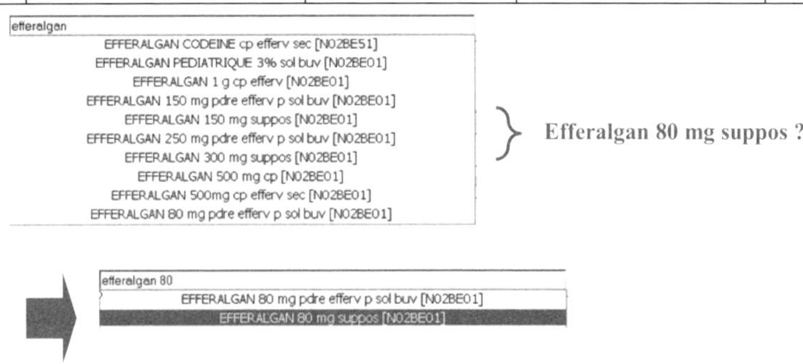

Figure 3. Example of ergonomic problem detected during the usability inspection.

2.1. Access to ADE Information via a Web Application

The Web prototype was built to support the prevention of ADE through an access to the PSIP KB independently of any CPOE. It enables (1) the display of anonymous clinical data for a specific patient, i.e. a patient hospitalization summary, the step of the patient hospitalization, the diagnoses of the patient, the lab results of the patient obtained during his/her hospitalization, the document associated with the patient hospitalization; (2) the simulation of patient prescription, i.e. addition and deletion of drugs; (3) the display of potential risk(s) of ADEs, i.e. PSIP ADE information. Figure 4 shows the display of PSIP ADE information in the Web prototype.

The display of ADE information is categorized by effect. Then each rule triggering this effect is displayed. For each rule, the conditions, a textual explanation and the confidence computed for the specific clinical department are displayed. Some tooltips guide the users and help them to understand particular items (e.g. a tooltip has been added to explain the confidence term). Finally, the user can modify alerts display parameters, as the confidence, by setting a new threshold value (for example, the user can display all the alerts of his/her medical unit by setting a confidence value equal to 0). It is possible also to display alerts from other existing knowledge sources (for example, complementary information derived from an external KB provided by the partner Vidal© KB can be displayed by activating an interface implemented). Currently, the Web prototype has been realized as a standalone application that operates with a local database that contains clinical patient data previously extracted from an existing Hospital Information System. Progressive versions of the Web prototype are released. The most recent version has been developed according to the results of a heuristic inspection.

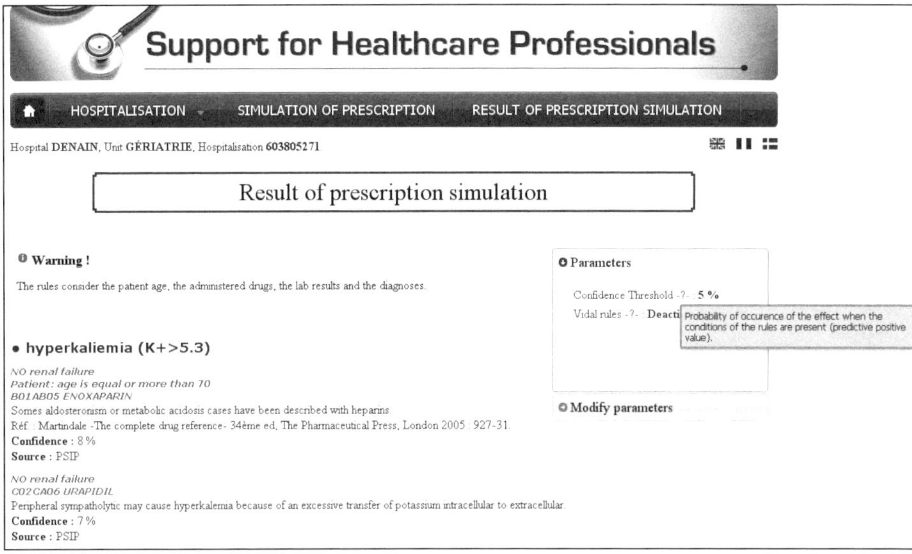

Figure 4. Sample page of the Web prototype displaying PSIP ADE information.

2.2. Access to ADE Information via an Electronic Health Record System

Medasys is a company delivering a French EHR system (DxCare®) with a CPOE function that covers the prescription, administration and dispensation processes. Following the HF recommendation, the Medasys prototype was integrated into the system as a "team player", in order to display PSIP information as suggested actions rather than as intrusive alerts. PSIP ADE information is available from multiple modules in the system.

When opening DxCare®, the first display is the list of the patients under the user's responsibility. A PSIP icon indicates patients with identified risks. Functions of DxCare® are available, depending on the access rights of the connected user.

This prototype is based on an existing passive Alert module, which manages all the alerts for each patient available in the EHR about lab results, imaging results, PSIP information, etc. The Alert module is composed of an area where search criteria can be defined (Figure 5 – 1) and an area where alerts are displayed (Figure 5 – 2). In the second version of the prototype, the PSIP alert details are displayed in the same way as all the alerts managed by DxCare® (Figure 5 – 3).

The display of ADE information is categorized by effect. Each rule triggering this effect is displayed. For each rule, the conditions, a textual explanation and the confidence computed for the concerned clinical department are displayed. DxCare® displays EHR retrieved information along tab sections. It enables the HCP to consult the ADE information while working with another EHR module.

A third version of the prototype is envisaged from mock-ups derived from collaborative meetings between ergonomists, potential users and designers/developers. These mock-ups aim to take into account recommendations issued from the work situation analysis and focus group.

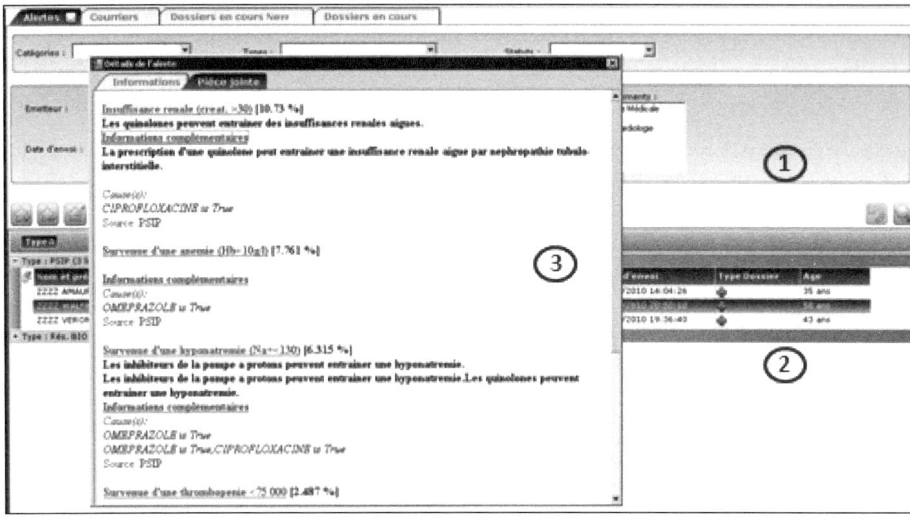

Figure 5. Second version of the Medasys prototype; details are displayed in the same way as all the alerts managed by DxCare®.

2.3. Access to ADE Information via a Computerized Physician Order Entry system

The IBM prototype is an independent graphical component communicating within an existing Danish CPOE. It presents lab results and patient clinical data, providing also PSIP ADE information during the prescription task. This prototype was designed with HCP input during design games sessions. Two mockups were made before the prototype development. The first mockup was based on the principle of placing features and functionality according to the frequency of use. The second mock-up is based on the evaluation of the first one. Users' feedback required placing features and functionality according to importance:

- Patient information at the top;
- Information that is driven by action (selection of drugs or of patient values) in the middle of the screen;
- Patient values, diagnosis and cave information at the left side of the screen;
- Medication selection list and the list of current medication at the right;
- Go forward action button is placed in the lower right corner.

Finally, this second mock-up was implemented in a prototype (Figure 6). The design of the application enables the physician to establish an overview of the conditions and status of the patient. The physician can see diagnosis, drugs administered, lab results. When the physician inputs orders with the "Vælg lægemiddel" (Select drug) part of the application, the information are sent to the PSIP KB system. Potential ADEs are triggering and displayed in the "Effekt" (Effect) part.

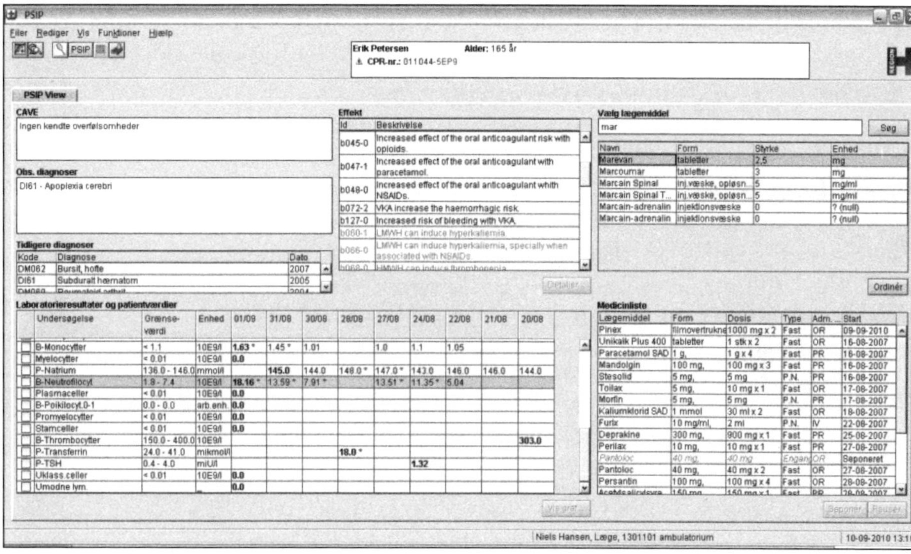

Figure 6. IBM prototype derived from the second mock-up.

3. Discussion and Conclusion

To generate and provide relevant information to HCP for ADE prevention, the PSIP project firstly created a PSIP KB containing ADE detection rules, which can be contextualized by hospital and by medical unit thanks to specific computed statistical features. This paper described a method for the exploitation of this KB in decision support system (i.e. the PSIP GKP) as well as the results obtained concerning the design of three different cases of deploying decision support services. The GKP consists of three components: a KB system allowing managing and representing the KB, a CP providing interoperability service between medical applications and the PSIP KB system, and a user interface module allowing the display of PSIP ADE information. To test the PSIP GKP, three PSIP decision support prototypes have been developed. The first prototype provides ADE information via Web access. The second prototype (the Medasys prototype) integrates the KB in an existing EHR (in a French context). The third prototype (the IBM prototype) integrates the KB in an existing CPOE system (in a Danish context).

Through this work, we show that the PSIP KB can be interoperable, i.e. it can work with other systems and makes easier the sharing of knowledge. Indeed, the majority of CDSSs have their own and specific KB which can be not shared for other projects.

To address the "over-alerting" issue, the PSIP project considers the contextualization of information to display relevant elements to the HCP. Currently, the "environment" parameter is taken into account in the KB system through the computation of statistics allowing screening relevant ADE information by hospital and medical unit. Other work on contextualization of information is progressing [11]. This ongoing work deals with the work situation analysis of the medication ordering activity allowing the identification of contexual elements which could facilitate adapting the display of alerts in the right moment during the activity and in the right form, taking into account “time” and “task” parameters. This new information could reinforce the development of more mature versions of the presented prototypes.

Acknowledgements

The research leading to these results has received funding from the European Community’s Seventh Framework Program (FP7/2007-2013) under Grant Agreement n°216130 – the PSIP project.

References

[1] A.X. Garg, N.K. Adhikari, H. McDonald, M.P. Rosas-Arellano, P.J. Devereaux, J. Beyene, J. Sam, R.B. Haynes, Effects of computerized clinical decision support systems on practitioner performance and patient outcomes: a systematic review, *JAMA* **293** (2005), 1223–38.
[2] K. Kawamoto, C.A. Houlihan, E.A. Balas, D.F. Lobach, Improving clinical practice using clinical decision support systems: a systematic review of trials to identify features critical to success, *BMJ* **330** (2005), 765–68.
[3] H. Van der Sijs, J. Aarts, A. Vulto, M. Berg, Overriding of drug safety alerts in computerized physician order entry, *JAMIA* **13** (2006), 138–47.
[4] R. Beuscart, P. McNair, J. Brender, Patient safety through intelligent procedures in medication: the PSIP project, *Stud Health Technol Inform* **148** (2009), 6–13.
[5] E. Chazard, B. Merlin, PSIP Consortium, R. Beuscart, Detection of adverse drug events: proposal of a data model, *Stud Health Technol Inform* **148** (2009), 63–74.
[6] R. Marcilly, E. Chazard, M.C. Beuscart-Zéphir, W. Hackl, A. Băceanu, A. Kushniruk, E.M. Borycki, Design of Adverse Drug Events-Scorecards, *Stud Health Technol Inform* **164** (2011), 377–81.
[7] V. Koutkias, G. Stalidis, I. Chouvarda, K. Lazou, V. Kilintzis, N. Maglaveras, A Knowledge Engineering Framework towards Clinical Support for Adverse Drug Event Prevention: The PSIP Approach , *Stud Health Technol Inform* **148** (2009), 134–44.
[8] V. Koutkias et al., Constructing clinical decision support systems for adverse drug event prevention: a knowledge-based approach, *AMIA Annu Symp Proc* (2010), 402–06.
[9] P.A. de Clercq, J.A. Blom, A. Hasman, H.H.M. Korsten, Design and implementation of a framework to support the development of clinical guidelines, *IJMI* **64** (2001), 285–318.
[10] J. Nielsen, R.L. Mack (Eds.), Usability inspection methods, John Wiley & Sons, New York, 1994.
[11] R. Marcilly, S. Pelayo, S. Bernonville, N. Leroy, J. Forrierre, Prise en Compte du Contexte pour la Conception d'un Système d'Aide à la Décision Médicamenteuse, Proc. of SELF Conf., Liège, 2010.

Patient Safety Informatics
V. Koutkias et al. (Eds.)
IOS Press, 2011

doi:10.3233/978-1-60750-740-6-189

Patient Summary and Medicines Reconciliation: Application of the ISO/CEN EN 13606 Standard in Clinical Practice

Francisco J. FARFÁN SEDANO [a,1], Marta TERRÓN CUADRADO [a], Yolanda CASTELLANOS CLEMENTE [a], Pablo SERRANO BALAZOTE [b], David MONER CANO [c] and Montserrat ROBLES VIEJO [c]

[a] *Pharmacy Department, Hospital Universitario de Fuenlabrada, Madrid, Spain*
[b] *Medical Director, Hospital Universitario de Fuenlabrada, Madrid, Spain*
[c] *Grupo IBIME, Instituto ITACA, Universidad Politécnica de Valencia, Spain*

Abstract. The comparison of the patient's current medication list with the medication being ordered when admitted to Hospital, identifying omissions, duplications, dosing errors, and potential interactions, constitutes the core process of medicines reconciliation. Access to the medication the patient is taking at home could be unfeasible as this information is frequently stored in various locations and in diverse proprietary formats. The lack of interoperability between those information systems, namely the Primary Care and the Specialized Electronic Health Records (EHRs), facilitates medication errors and endangers patient safety. Thus, the development of a Patient Summary that includes clinical data from different electronic systems will allow doctors access to relevant information enabling a safer and more efficient assistance. Such a collection of data from heterogeneous and distributed systems has been achieved in this Project through the construction of a federated view based on the ISO/CEN EN13606 Standard for architecture and communication of EHRs.

Keywords. Medicines reconciliation, patient safety, semantic interoperability, patient summary, archetypes

Introduction

Medicines reconciliation, or in other words, assuring medication accuracy at the transitions in care, is considered a vital tool to improve patient safety. In fact, it is one of the "Nine Patient Safety Solutions" [1] described by the World Health Organization to help reduce the toll of healthcare-related harm affecting millions of patients worldwide.

Medication errors have a significant impact; it has been estimated that only in the United States medication errors harm 1.5 million people and kill several thousand each year [2]. Medication was found to be the leading cause of injury during medical care, followed by healthcare associated infections and surgical

[1] Corresponding Author: ffarfan.hflr@salud.madrid.org

errors [3].

Some studies report discrepancies varying from 30-70% between the medications patients were taking before admission and the prescriptions ordered in hospitals [4-5] [6]. Omissions were repeatedly found as the most frequent of these discrepancies [7]. In a recent retrospective cohort study [8] medication discrepancies were analyzed to describe their incidence, drug classes, and probable importance. A random sample of adult patients admitted to the general medicine, cardiology or general surgery was examined. Potentially high-risk discrepancies and differences were identified by determining if the medications were included on either the Institute for Safe Medication Practice high-alert list or the North Carolina Narrow Therapeutics Index list. The authors found that of the 178 patients who did have medication listed on admission, 41 had at least 1 discrepancy identified by the reconciliation process on admission (23%; 95% CI, 17-29), 19% (95% CI, 11-31) of these medications were considered to be potentially high risk. Cardiovascular drugs were the most frequent class involved at both admissions (31%) and discharge (27%) in medication discrepancies or differences.

The medicines reconciliation process is therefore designed to prevent those medication errors that take place at patient transitions by identifying the most accurate list of all medication a patient is taking and using this list to provide correct medications for patients anywhere within the health care system.

Many factors may contribute to medicines reconciliation errors [9-10]:

- Lack of access to the patient's prescriptions list from Primary Care: as information is not usually collected in a standardized way, the systems fail to transfer information from Primary Care to Hospital.
- Difficulties in obtaining an accurate account of a patient's medication due to an acute condition, sensory or cognitive impairment, lack of access to family or caregiver, or due to language barriers.
- Errors in transcribing medication details to the hospital clinical record: in the case of hand-written prescriptions, that may contribute to errors if they are illegible, incomplete, or use inappropriate abbreviations.State of the Art

1. Medicines Reconciliation Program Implemented at Hospital Universitario de Fuenlabrada: Use Case of the Patient Summary Project

The Hospital Universitario de Fuenlabrada is a public general hospital located in the Madrid region which started its activity in 2004. It provides assistance to a population of 217.000 inhabitants. The Hospital implemented at its inception a global EHR system that integrates all the specific software applications from different providers installed in the Pharmacy and other Departments (Diagnostic Imaging, Critical Care Unit, Surgery, Pathology and Laboratory).

The Patient Summary Project was developed to provide doctors at both settings, the Hospital and the Primary Care, access to the most complete and updated clinical information about patients collected from all the systems where this information was stored. Actually, we followed the approach of the European Project epSOS [11] in considering a Patient Summary the concise clinical document that provides an electronic patient health data set applicable both for unexpected as well as expected, healthcare contact, and hence, it contains the essential information needed for healthcare coordination and, in case of an unexpected need, for the continuity of care, or when a patient consults a healthcare professional other than his regular general practitioner, for example.

The final aim of the Project was in fact, patient safety as we seek to ensure that the medicines prescribed on admission to hospital correspond to those that the patient was taking at home, unless they need to be modified due to clinical conditions.

The practical implementation of the overall Project was then structured in two main objectives:

- The development of a **Patient Summary** that includes clinical data from three different and distributed systems: the Primary Care Electronic Health Record (EHR), the Hospital EHR, and the Hospital Pharmacy software application.
- The establishment of a clinical **Standard Operating Protocol (SOP)** to prevent medication errors through a medicines reconciliation program.

The SOP for medicines reconciliation contains the complete set of instructions for implementing the process by multiple users, the healthcare professionals, in a consistent and measurable manner. This SOP includes as a first step collecting information on medication history, using the most recent and accurate sources of information to create a full and current list of medicines. This list is completed with the information from the patient or his family or caregiver. Then, the information collected about current medication is checked against the hospital prescriptions, ensuring any discrepancies are accounted for and communicated, if necessary, to the doctor. Such discrepancies are defined as unexplained differences among documented regimens across different sites of care; in our project, prescriptions prior to admission were compared with hospital orders.

The information contained in the home medication list should include:

- Prescription medications
- Sample medications
- Vitamins
- Nutraceuticals
- Other over-the-counter (OTC) medicines
- Herbal medicines

And the specific data to be collected should consider: drug name, strength, pharmaceutical form and route of administration, frequency, indication, timing of last dose, and source of the patient's medications.

2. The Patient Summary based on the ISO 13606 Standard

The electronic information about a person's health, his EHR, consists of data about observations, pathologies, laboratory tests, diagnostic imaging reports, treatments, patient identifying details, alerts, etc. Unfortunately, this information is frequently stored in various locations and in diverse proprietary formats, making access to it a real challenge. The consequent lack of interoperability between EHRs or ability "to talk to each other" causes problems while fully interoperable EHRs would make access to patient's information easier as well as enhance the quality and safety of healthcare by providing professionals with relevant and up-to-date information.

In this context, semantic interoperability designates that the precise meaning of exchanges information is understandable by another system or application not initially developed for this purpose.

The Patient Summary developed in this Project is constructed following the CEN EN13606 Standard for the Electronic Health Record Communication. This Standard specifies the information architecture required for interoperable exchange between EHRs and a centralized repository.

The CEN EN13606 Standard was developed by the European Committee for Standardization (CEN) and applies the dual model approach based on the separation between information (the data) and knowledge (which may change over time). Knowledge is therefore represented in this project as archetypes or formal descriptions of the concepts of the specific domain. Obviously, there is a need for an expert's agreement on the specific data sets; this can be accomplished using archetypes developed by those experts, mainly doctors, pharmacists and nurses.

The core part of the Standard, the Reference Model, represents the global characteristics of healthcare record data, the way these data are aggregated, and the context information expected to addressing ethical, legal and provenance requirements. The model defines the set of classes that constitute the generic building blocks and stable characteristics of any EHR.

The other important feature of the Standard is the incorporation of archetypes for sharing semantic structures defined in the second part, the Archetype Model. Archetypes are formal definitions of domain-level concepts in the form of structured and constraint combinations of classes contained in the Reference Model. Their main purpose is to provide a powerful, reusable and interoperable mechanism for managing the creation, description, validation and query of EHRs. Archetypes provide semantics to data instances that conform to some reference model by assuring that the data obey a particular structure and satisfy a set of semantic constraints.

In this Project three archetypes were developed reusing ("specialized archetypes") the repository of archetypes of the openEHR organization:

- Alerts (including allergies)
- Problem list
- Medication

We "specialized" the current openEHR archetypes for those three sections of the Patient Summary in order to include local particularities. openEHR is an international not-for-profit Foundation, whose aim is making interoperable, life-long EHR a reality, improving healthcare in the information society by creating specifications, open source software and tools. Specially, openEHR maintains a repository of archetypes.

The final federated view of the patient vital information was accomplished through a standardization platform which allows the edition of archetypes, the specification of mappings between archetypes and data sources and the semi-automated generation of data conversion scripts that translate not normalized data into XML documents conforming to the selected reference model and at the same time satisfy all the data constraints imposed by archetypes. Hence, the use of archetypes provides a means to standardization and semantic interoperability. In fact, archetypes convert existing information into standardized EHR extracts. Figure 1 shows an overview of the edition process of an integration archetype with four different stages.

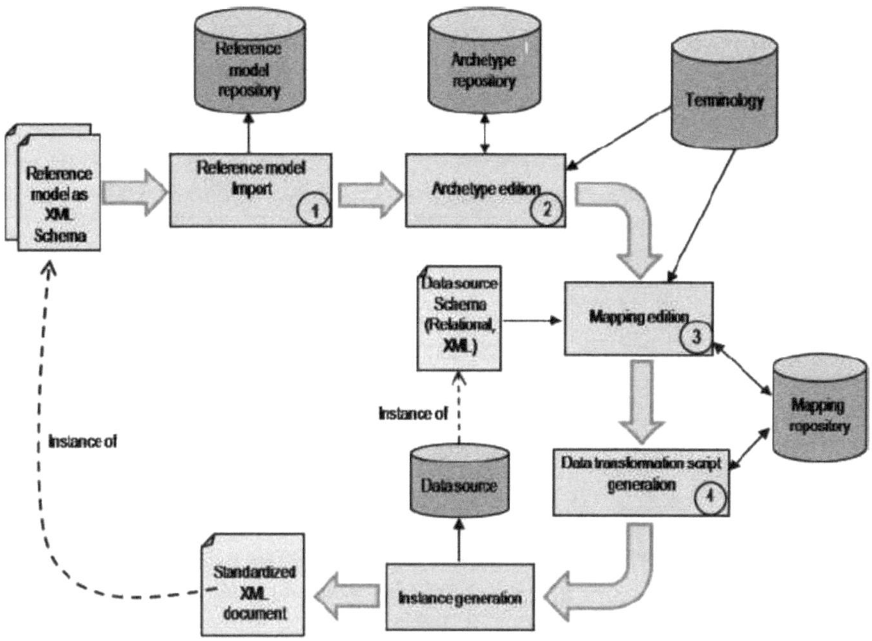

Figure 1. Overall integration of archetype edition process in the standardization platform.

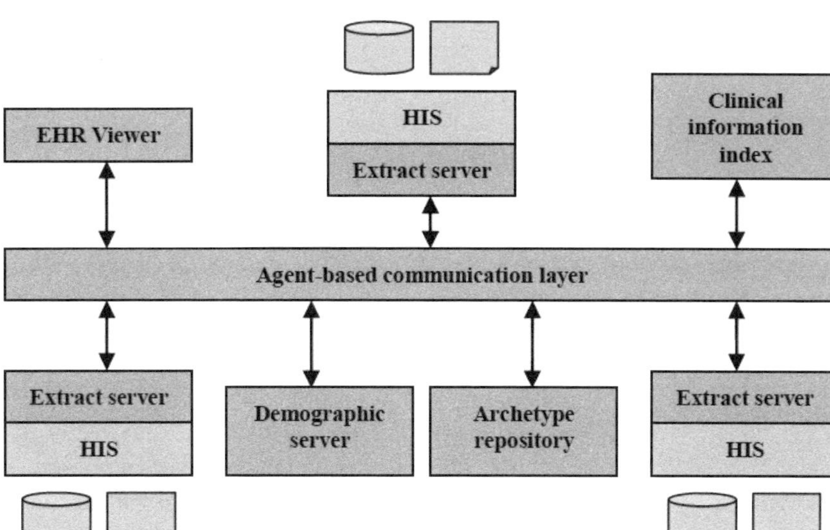

Figure 2. Standardization platform architecture.

After the integration archetype has been defined an XQuery program is automatically generated to extract and normalize data; the next step is building an infrastructure for the global EHR. The standardization platform creates the virtual or federated view of the patient EHR the data of which are stored among heterogeneous systems. Figure 2 shows the standardization platform architecture.

3. The Medicines Reconciliation Program

To implement the medicines reconciliation program a SOP was developed involving doctors, nurses and pharmacists. Each healthcare professional role and responsibilities were specified. Figure 3 shows the flowchart designed to diagram the process.

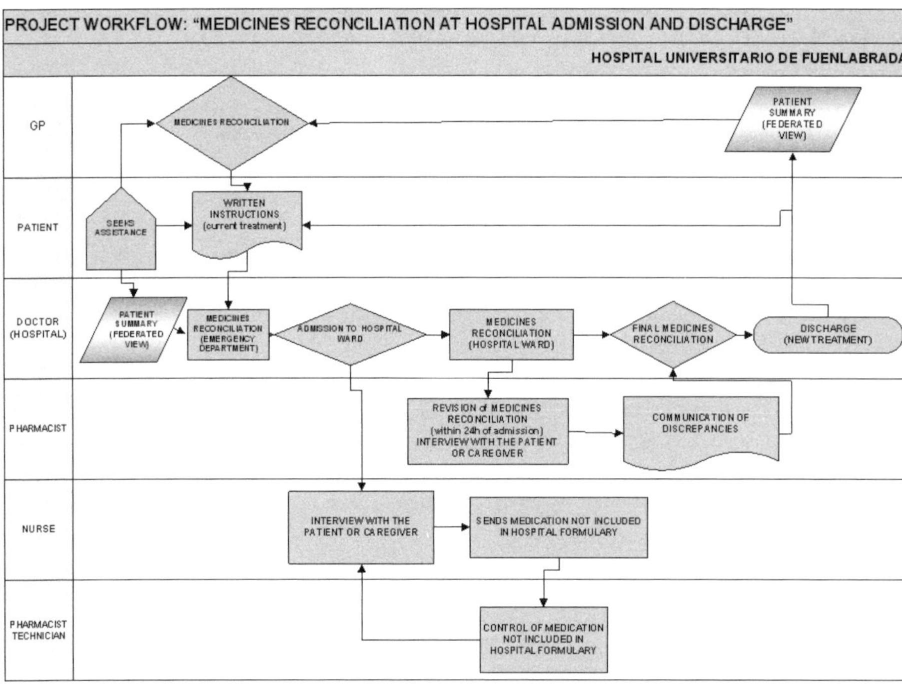

Figure 3. Flowchart for the Medicines Reconciliation Program.

Patients who fulfilled the following criteria were eligible to enter the program:

- Admitted to Internal Medicinal Department
- Age ≥ 65 years
- Chronic treatment including more than 4-5 medicines

Pharmacists play a central role in the program: after collecting information on the patient's home medications, problems and alerts, an interview with the patient or caregiver is conducted. We consider patient involvement of the greatest importance, as they are in the best position to be aware of all the medications they are prescribed by multiple healthcare professionals. Precisely, one valuable source of information is, in fact, the medication brought by patients to hospital.

Asking patients about compliance can also clarify the possible lack of effect of a specific medicine.

A template for collecting information prior the interview was used as a tool to guide the pharmacist when analyzing the information provided by the patient as well as when comparing the treatment prescribed at Hospital. Finally, a template collecting discrepancies between both list (current treatment and hospital orders) was designed to notify physicians the discrepancies encountered.

The Patient Summary was considered the first source of information to obtain the patient's current medication (Figure 4).

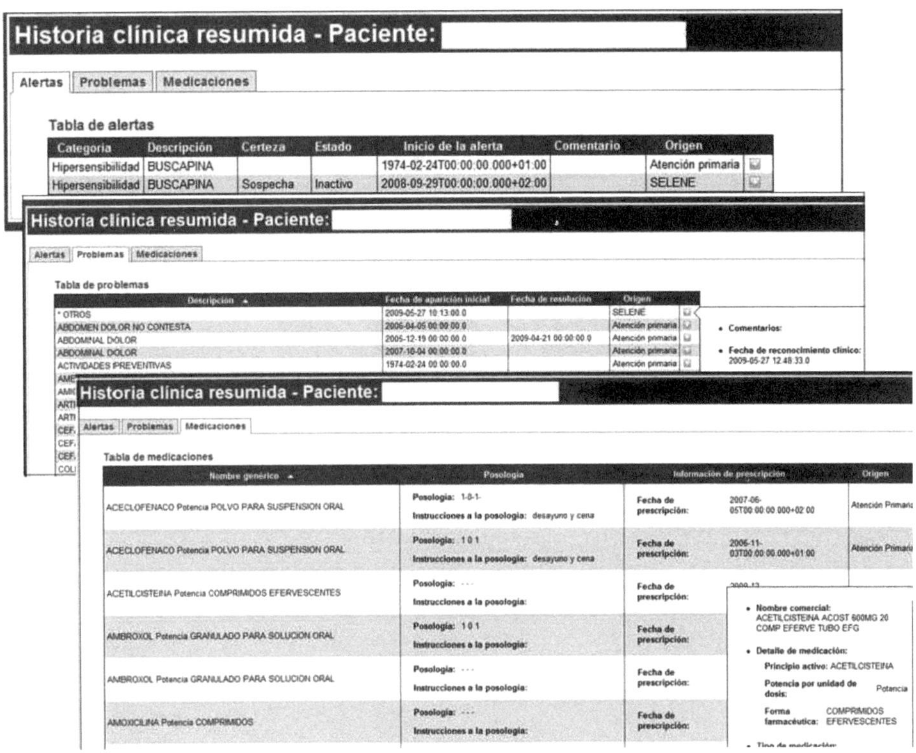

Figure 4. Sections of the Patient Summary: alerts, problem list and medication.

4. Conclusions

The development of a Patient Summary that includes clinical data from different electronic systems (the Primary Care EHR, the Hospital EHR and the Pharmacy Department software application) was achieved through the construction of a virtual federated view of those systems using the ISO/CEN EN13606 standard. The first use case of this Project has been a Medicines Reconciliation Program at patient admission to Hospital that allows doctors access to the information about which medicines the patient is taking at home. Pharmacist participate in the program verifying that the orders prescribed at hospital correspond to the current treatment unless there are reasons for discontinuation, changes in dose, frequency or route.

Acknowledgements

This Project has been funded by the Spanish Health Ministry (*Convenio de colaboración para el impulso de prácticas seguras en Centros Sanitarios 2008)* and has been awarded with one of the Quality within the Spanish National Health System Prizes 2009.

References

[1] http://www.who.int/patientsafety/solutions/patientsafety/PS-Solution6.pdf, last access on January 2011.
[2] Institute of Medicine, *Preventing Medication Errors*, Washington DC, 2006.
[3] Institute of Medicine, *To err is human: Building a Safer Health System*, Washington DC, 1999.
[4] P.L. Cornish, S.R. Knowles, Medication safety: one organization's approach to the challenge, *Qual Manag Health Care* **8** (2001), 27–34.
[5] K.M. Gleason J.M. Groszek, C. Sullivan, D. Rooney, C. Barnard, G.A. Noskin, Reconciliation of discrepancies in medication histories and admission orders of newly hospitalized patients, *Am J Health Syst Pharm* **61** (2004), 1689–95.
[6] S. Lessard, J. DeYoung, N. Vazzana, Medication discrepancies affecting senior patients at hospital admission, *Am J Health Syst Pharm* **63** (2006), 740–3.
[7] P.L. Cornish et al., Unintended medication discrepancies at the time of hospital admission, *Arch Int Med* **165** (2005), 424–9.
[8] K.T. Unroe, T. Pfeiffenberger, S. Riegelhaupt, J. Jastrzembski, Y. Lokhnygina, C. Colón-Emeric, Inpatient medication reconciliation at admission and discharge: a retrospective cohort study of age and other risk factors for medication discrepancies, *Am J Geriatr Pharmacother* **8** (2010), 115–26.
[9] Institute for Healthcare Improvement, Medication Reconciliation Review, http://www.ihi.org/IHI/Topics/PatientSafety/MedicationSystems/Tools/Medication+Reconciliation+Review.htm, last access on January 2011.
[10] http://www.nice.org.uk/nicemedia/pdf/PSG001GuidanceWord.doc, last access on January 2011.
[11] http://www.epsos.eu/, last access on January 2011.

Patient Safety Informatics
V. Koutkias et al. (Eds.)
IOS Press, 2011

doi:10.3233/978-1-60750-740-6-197

Engineering the Electronic Health Record for Safety: A Multi-Level Video-Based Approach to Diagnosing and Preventing Technology-Induced Error Arising from Usability Problems

Elizabeth M. BORYCKI [a,1], Andre W. KUSHNIRUK [a],
Shigeki KUWATA [b] and Joseph KANNRY [c]
[a] *School of Health Information Science,*
University of Victoria, Victoria, British Columbia Canada
[b] *Tottori University Hospital, Tottori, Japan*
[c] *Mt. Sinai Medical Center, New York, New York, United States of America*

Abstract. Electronic health records (EHRs) promise to improve and streamline healthcare through electronic entry and retrieval of patient data. Furthermore, based on a number of studies showing their positive benefits, they promise to reduce medical error and make healthcare safer. However, a growing body of literature has clearly documented that if EHRS are not designed properly and with usability as an important goal in their design, rather than reducing error, EHR deployment has the potential to actually increase medical error. In this paper we describe our approach to engineering (and reengineering) EHRs in order to increase their beneficial potential while at the same time improving their safety. The approach described in this paper involves an integration of the methods of usability analysis with video analysis of end users interacting with EHR systems and extends the evaluation of the usability of EHRs to include the assessment of the impact of these systems on work practices. Using clinical simulations, we analyze human-computer interaction in real healthcare settings (in a portable, low-cost and high fidelity manner) and include both artificial and naturalistic data collection to identify potential usability problems and sources of technology-induced error prior to widespread system release. Two case studies where the methods we have developed and refined have been applied at different levels of user-computer interaction are described.

Keywords. Electronic health records, usability testing, clinical simulations, technology induced error, system testing, video analysis, human-computer interaction, patient safety, software engineering

Introduction

Electronic health record systems (EHRs) promise to streamline and modernize healthcare by allowing not only for electronic entry of patient data but also value-added features such as automated clinical decision support (e.g. by providing physicians with

[1] Corresponding Author: emb@uvic.ca

alerts and reminders), public health surveillance capabilities, as well as potential for interconnecting health records across regions and even nations. Despite their potential, in North America the majority of primary care physicians are still using paper-based records for entering and accessing their patients' data [1]. Although in parts of Europe and Asia the rate of EHR use in primary care is higher, there are problems associated with the adoption of these systems that continue to delay large national EHR projects and slow the dissemination of this important technology worldwide. Some of the underlying reasons for this situation arise from the difficulty experienced by implementers in moving health care organizations and health professionals from the use of paper to EHRs. These difficulties arise from organizational issues, technical difficulties in integrating patient data (across systems, institutions and regions) as well as cognitive-socio-technical issues (e.g. issues related to usability problems and potentially negative impacts on workflow and healthcare work activities) [2, 3]. In this paper we report on work we have carried out in developing methods for identifying or detecting technology-induced errors arising from usability and workflow problems. In addition, extensions of the approach can be used to assess if the introduction of a new system will adversely impact on work practices and create safety issues around health professional workflow. Our work is based on the premise that usability problems are highly related to "technology-induced error" – i.e. error introduced by interaction with a system under real conditions that are unlikely to be caught by traditional software testing methods but that may lead to potentially lethal medical errors (i.e. leading to death and disability in patients). In this paper we therefore describe a set of methods we have employed for the engineering of safer and more effective healthcare information systems, in particular EHRs.

1. Background: Technology-Induced Error and Electronic Health Records

Medical errors are a significant cause of death and disability worldwide. Current estimates suggest that in Canada alone approximately 185,000 hospital admissions are associated with an adverse event each year – an event that occurs for which medical error is the cause (e.g. overdose of a medication, or giving a patient a medication they are allergic to) [4, p. 1678]. The numbers are much greater in the United States and worldwide [2]. The EHR, by providing electronic entry and retrieval of data has been shown to reduce error due to illegible handwriting. Furthermore, by interconnecting electronic records throughout an institution, region or even nation, a number of value-added benefits can be obtained directly related to improving safety. These include the ability to obtain information about a patient (e.g. about their drug allergies) across entire regions or a country, allowing for timely and up-to-date information to be used in patient decision making at point of care. In addition, electronic decision support systems that provide healthcare providers with automated alerts or reminders about a patient's condition depend on electronically available information. Finally, large-scale systems with new functionalities, such as regional or national public health surveillance systems, will depend on data ultimately entered at point of care through the EHR. These considerations, coupled with many published studies that have examined the impact of the EHR provide evidence for the argument that EHRs will greatly increase the safety of healthcare and streamline healthcare processes [5].

Despite the incredible potential for EHRs to streamline healthcare processes and improve patient safety, involving recent years, particularly after 2005, a growing body of evidence has accumulated indicating that healthcare information systems (including EHRs) are not unlike systems in many other domains, whereby poorly designed or implemented systems have actually been implicated in causing user errors - resulting in or "inducing" medical error. In our work first published in 2004 we have shown that usability problems associated with a user interface design are highly associated with physician medication order entry errors [6]. In 2005, Koppel and colleagues [7] published a paper about a commercial EHR system and classified over 20 serious "technology-facilitated" errors associated with its use in a hospital setting. In addition, Han et al. [8] have published work indicating that deaths in a neonatal unit rose after the introduction of an EHR.

The findings of our work and of others has lead us to define and delineate a category of "technology-induced errors" in healthcare information technology [6-8]. As noted above, there are now documented examples of tested systems ("proven" to be safe) using traditional software engineering testing approaches (including both white and black box testing) [7], when released in real healthcare settings these systems have resulted in health professionals making errors that lead to mistakes and may have even lead to patient harm (e.g. death and disability) [8]. Technology-induced errors may be complex and may have their sources in user-system interaction at multiple levels, from the individual user interacting with a system in isolation, to the use of the system by a healthcare team in providing care to patients with a given disease process.

In this paper we consider the issue of ensuring the design and deployment of safe and efficient EHRs in terms of the following: (a) levels of user interaction with EHRs - from the perspective of individual users interacting with an individual EHR system in isolation in consideration of workflow level problems and issues, (b) the application of video-based usability testing for analyzing individual EHR-user interactions and, (c) the application of what we refer to as "clinical simulations", which involve detailed video analysis of user interactions with EHR technology in simulated and real-world clinical settings [2, 3].

2. Levels of EHR-User Interaction and Their Relation to Technology-Induced Error

One way to consider user-system interaction, when analyzing technology-induced error in healthcare IT, is to consider user interaction in a series of levels. We have adapted an approach from Eason [9], whereby we examine system-user interaction at different levels (see Figure 1). Level 1 refers to the most basic level of user interaction – namely that of an individual user interacting with a health information system individually, in isolation. For example, this could involve a usability test of a single user interacting with an EHR to assess the relationship between user interface design and technology-induced errors.

At Level 2, we move up to the level of a user (or users) interacting with a health information system such as an EHR in the context of carrying out complex work tasks; for example, a physician interacting with an EHR to record and retrieve patient information during a doctor-patient interview (forming a three way "doctor-patient-computer" interaction).

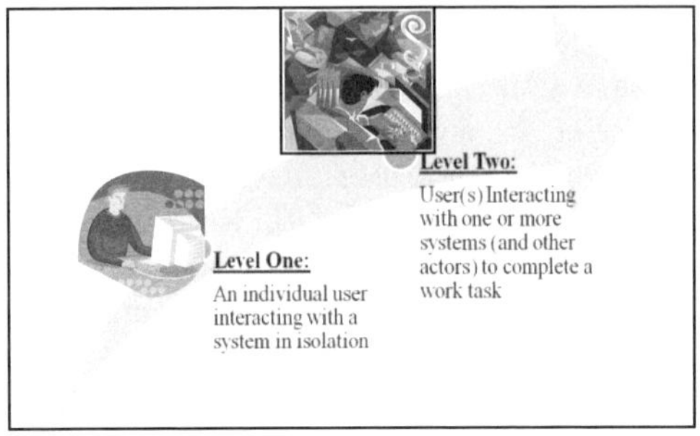

Figure 1. Levels of user-system interaction.

In our work in assessing where technology-induced error may arise from, we have adopted an approach where we provide a step-wise method that isolates the level(s) at which problems and technology-induced errors arise during system-user interaction. To do so, we typically begin by examining a system at the lower level first (e.g. Level 1). For example, if difficulties are encountered in implementing an EHR (with reports of user dissatisfaction with a new system) we might begin by considering Level 1 ergonomic aspects of the user interface in order to isolate any specific features that might need optimizing (e.g. screen design or menu layout). It should be noted this is an important level to analyze in that many technology-induced errors may have their origins here and furthermore, testing of individual users with systems may reveal such errors (we will provide an example of work we have conducted at this level in a subsequent section). In many cases, we have found that by doing such analyses we may isolate a specific usability or interaction problem that may be causing technology-induced errors. However, we have also found that a system shown to be adequate at the level of the individual user, when subjected to the real-world expectations and stresses of real practice, the system may still not be deemed usable by health professionals and may still pose a safety hazard. In this case we then move up to the Level 2 of system-user interaction in Figure 2, and we begin to test the system under more realistic conditions involving multiple participants in real clinical contexts and involving completion of units of real work tasks. We have referred to our testing of systems prior to system deployment at this level as "clinical simulations" (see Figure 2), where we collect video views from all computer screens (using screen recording software), as well as external video views of the room (using camcorders or ceiling mounted cameras). We have found such simulations are typically carried out in a laboratory-based software engineering environment, but can also be carried out in a hospital or healthcare setting itself, with all its accompanying complexity and realism (an example of this level of analysis will also be provided in a subsequent section). Finally, ensuring the safety and usability of a system such as an EHR at both Levels 1 and 2 may not ensure user adoption and system safety, as complex organizational issues may be at play (e.g. a change in work roles and responsibilities due to system deployment that may adversely affect uptake of the system). In the remainder of this paper we will provide examples of our methodological approach as we have applied it at Levels 1 and 2 of user interactions with EHRs and related technologies (see Figure 1).

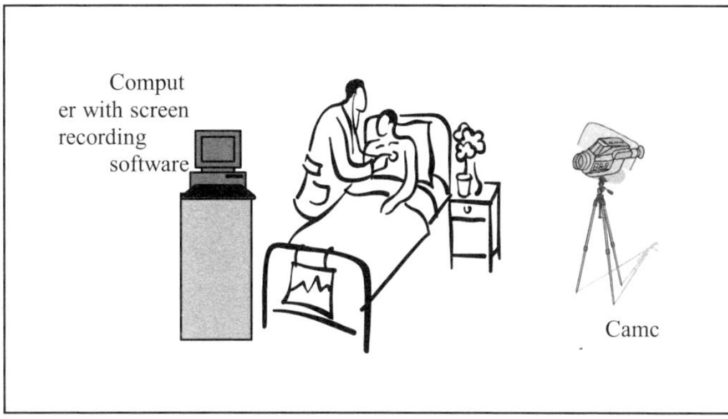

Figure 2. Set up for conducting clinical simulations in healthcare settings.

3. Example of Predicting Technology-Induced Error Identified from Level 1 User Interactions

In order to investigate the potential for specific user interface features to lead to technology-induced error, in a series of studies we employed methods arising from the usability literature, coupled with video analysis of both usability problems and technology-induced error. In this work we have focused on predicting errors that might result from the use of computerized physician order entry (CPOE) applications. In the study we developed a range of tasks, including asking subjects (i.e. physicians) to enter medications from a medication list into a prescription writing application. In doing the task we asked subjects to "think aloud", or verbalize their thoughts while doing the task. Using this methodology, we also video record the screens of the users' interactions with the system. This was accomplished using low-cost screen recording software [10]. Once the sessions were completed we then transcribed, time-stamped and coded the resulting movie files of user interactions. Over the past fifteen years we have developed coding schemes for analyzing such data for usability problems and technology-induced errors (see [2], [11-12] for more details about methods for coding, coding schemes and the categorization of codes arising from our work). Such schemes include categories for usability problems and technology-induced errors such as display visibility problems, navigation problems, problems with consistency of the user interface or layout, and issues related to content not being displayed in a clear manner (see [11-12] for more details). To apply our methods to predict potential sources of technology-induced error, we first coded the video data of physician interactions to identify usability problems (see below for an excerpt of a coded section of the video of a physician's interaction with the application). The excerpt shows the subject's "thinking aloud", as well as his actions using the application (e.g. entry of a medication and dosage) and note that numbers refer to the video counter (from a video analysis coding tool we used – Transana®). In addition, a medical expert independently coded the same interactions for either "slips" or "mistakes" in medication entry. Slips refer to mistakes that are caught by the physician before the prescription is processed, while mistakes refer to errors that are not caught by the physician (and which result in a recorded prescription error).

02:26 Subject: "Amoxillin, 250 capsule, po, two times a day, is that one of our options q8 darn, q8 hours times 7 days."

0:2:28 **SUBJECT ENTERS** 250 mg tid X 7 days (30 dispensed)

002:30 Subject: "Oh wait, I wanted to dispense 30 come back. Let me think about that, 7, 8, 24. He just got 6 extra tablets!"

USABILITY PROBLEM #1 – DISPLAY VISIBILITY – not clear that a drop down menu should be used in order to enter "q8h"

ERROR #1 MISTAKE – "tid" entered instead of "q8h"

USABILITY PROBLEM #2– DEFAULT INAPPROPRIATE

ERROR #2 SLIP - 30 dispensed instead of 21

This work has indicated that technology-induced error (as indicated by identified slips and mistakes) is highly related to specific user interface features. For example, for new users of the application described above, there was a high degree of association between coded usability problems (e.g. display visibility) and entry of medication errors. For example, 84% of the time a display visibility problem was identified. In conjunction with this there was identification of one or more variations in the medication entered by the physician (i.e. errors of some sort, e.g. errors in transcription) [9]. In subsequent work, we have used the rate of association of usability errors obtained from this Level 1 analysis as input into computer-based simulation programs to predict how the introduction of the system would lead to medication errors if introduced on a large scale [12-13]. We have also used this approach to make predications regarding the impact of fixing specific usability problems. It should be noted that this work was conducted at the level of individual application users interacting with a system individually and in isolation of complex health workflow. In the example provided in the next section, we describe a set of studies that involved not only analysis of Level 1 interactions with individual users, but also Level 2 interactions involving more complex work situations and involving more than one participant (see Figure 1 and 2).

4. Example of Predicting Technology-Induced Error Identified from Level 2 User Interactions

In a series of studies we have conducted with colleagues in hospital settings, we have been able to apply our approach to video analysis of user interactions with health information systems at multiple levels, starting at Level 1, involving individual users and moving to recording "clinical simulations" at Level 2, involving realistic scenarios of system use [2-3, 10-11, 13-14]. For example, in one study of the medication administration component of a hospital-wide EHR system, data collection involved asking 11 physicians and 6 nurses to interact with the system to carry out medication administration tasks. The data collected included two views: (a) a screen view obtained from installing a screen recording program (Hypercam®) on the computer where subjects accessed a medication administration system and (b) a view of the "hospital room" in which the clinical simulation took place [3, 10-11, 14-15].

In addition, using video analysis software we also linked transcripts of user interactions with fictitious patients and other providers (see excerpt of a coded transcript below). The excerpt gives an example of the video coded interaction of a subject (a nurse) interacting with the system. As can be seen, through review of the video we can time-stamp exact sequences of user interaction with the system (e.g. the nurse searches for a patient on the computer, reviews the orders and proceeds to execute the orders). In addition to having subjects carry out realistic simulation tasks, both individually and in groups, we also conduct post-task interviews with all participants, as illustrated in the below excerpt, where the subject is interviewed about problems they may have encountered. We have also graphically diagrammed out the impact of the system using workflow diagrams, before and after implementation of the system, identifying where and how the workflow has changed and developing ways of simplifying the workflow to make it safer (as overly complex work flows tend to increase opportunity to introduce errors) [16].

00:14 NURSE SEARCHES FOR PATIENT ON THE COMPUTER
00:45 NURSE VIEWS ORDER LIST ON THE SCREEN
00:51 NURSE SELECTS MEDICATION ORDER FROM LIST
00:55 VERIFICATION SCREEN APPEARS
NURSE WALKS OVER TO PATIENT TO CHECK IDENTIFICATION
00:59 NURSE TALKS TO PATIENT - "Nice to meet you. I will now give you an IV drip"
01:09 NURSE SCANS PATIENT IDENTIFICATION (FROM PATIENT'S WRIST BAND)
01:10 VERIFICATION SCREEN AUTOMATICALLY UPDATES
NURSE WALKS BACK TO COMPUTER
01:25 NURSE VIEWS EXECUTION INFORMATION ON THE COMPUTER
NURSE WALKS OVER TO PATIENT AND SETS MEDICATION BAG
NURSE WALKS BACK TO COMPUTER
03:15 NURSE CONFIRMS ADMINISTRATION OF MEDICATION ON THE COMPUTER

POST-TASK INTERVIEW:

Experimenter: Did you have any difficulty with the task?

Subject: I'm used to this operation, but sometimes it is hard to use the barcode reader when the barcode is not clearly printed.

Experimenter: Did you have any difficulties with the barcode reader?

Subject: In today's operation there were no problems. But in the real situation, sometimes the scanner doesn't respond to the barcode. Also, sometimes the cord of the scanner is too short to reach the patient.

Experimenter: Did you have any difficulty during the work process?

Subject: In general, I want a more simplified system for the verification process. The more patients there are, the more difficult the verification would become. Sometimes in the emergency we would have to skip this procedure due to its time-taking process and someone might need urgent help, but with this system I don't think I'd be able to do that.

Using the approach we have described above we have been able to conduct high fidelity clinical simulations (i.e. that have a high degree of realism in that they are conducted in-situ in hospital rooms, with health professionals of varying levels of expertise as participants) [14-16]. In addition, as we have outlined elsewhere, the cost for conducting such realistic clinical simulations is low, using portable recording techniques (i.e. installation of screen recording software and external cameras in settings and rooms that are actually used in the healthcare setting and therefore already existent) [11, 14-15]. In addition, such studies can be adjusted to include both Level 1 and Level 2 analyses. For example, in the above study, we initially conducted evaluations of individual users interacting with the medication administration study in isolation, moving to conducting studies involving multiple participants [3].

The results from such study have led to identification of a range of different types of technology-induced errors that emerge when workflow is considered. For example, in the study described above we found that the medication administration system worked well and increased patient safety by requiring that patients' bar codes (on their wrists) be scanned, and that there is a well defined verification process for administering medications (e.g. verification of the right medication etc.). However, under certain conditions, for example, emergency conditions where a physician or nurse using the system was called away from the computer, certain types of new safety issues arise. In this case, the clinical simulations were able to determine potential technology-induced errors prior to widespread system release (i.e. many of the technology-induced errors that were found during clinical simulations in our study (e.g. [14-15] have been found by others conducting research in the area after implementation (e.g. in [17]). For example, from the clinical simulations it was found that that nurses experienced bar code scanning failures, slow system response times and under emergency conditions there is a clear need for an emergency override function, as other physicians and nurses can become "locked out" from the patient information [14-15]. This type of error arises at Level 2, involving users interacting with the system in collaboration with the team (in terms of communication and workflow). It is an example of an unexpected impact of a system, which necessitated customization of a commercial product prior to release [3, 16].

5. Discussion and Conclusion

In this paper we have discussed a multi-level video-based approach to ensuring the safety of systems such as EHRs prior to their widespread release. The approach involves low-cost, high fidelity video analysis of user interactions at increasingly complex levels of interaction, starting with Level 1 interactions involving individual users and moving to Level 2 where team and group interactions come into play. The approach began by focusing on usability problems, but we have adapted it to identify specific classes of technology-induced errors that need to be identified to ensure systems will be safe once deployed. It should be noted that we are promoting increased levels of user-system testing: (a) in artificial laboratory-style testing conducted by vendors, and (b) simulation based testing of systems within the actual complex environments where EHRs will be deployed (and at multiple levels of user interaction). Along these lines we continue to work with a range of healthcare institutions as well as vendors in disseminating the methodological approach we have described in this paper.

References

[1] A. Jha, D. Doolan, D. Grandt, T. Scott, D. Bates, The use of health information technology in seven nations, *Int J Med Inf* **77** (2008), 848–54.
[2] E.M. Borycki, A.W. Kushniruk. Identifying and preventing technology-induced error using simulations: Application of usability engineering techniques, *Healthcare Quart* **8** (2005), 99–105.
[3] E. Borycki, A.W. Kushniruk. Towards an integrative cognitive-socio-technical approach in health informatics: Analyzing technology-induced error involving health information systems to improve safety, *The Open Medical Inform J* **4** (2010), 181–7.
[4] G.R. Baker et al., The Canadian adverse events study: The incidence of adverse events among hospital patients in Canada, *CMAJ,* **170**(11) (2004), 1678–86.
[5] D.W. Bates et al., Effect of computerized physician order entry and a team intervention on prevention of serious medication errors. *JAMIA,* **280** (1998), 1311–16.
[6] A.W. Kushniruk, M. Triola, B. Stein, E.M. Borycki, J. Kannry, The relationship of usability to medical error: An evaluation of errors associated with usability problems in use of a handheld application for prescribing medications, *Studies Health Techology Inform* (2004), 1073–76.
[7] R. Koppel et al., Role of computerized physician order entry systems in facilitating medication errors. *JAMA* **293** (2005), 1197–203.
[8] Y.Y. Han et al., Unexpected increased mortality after implementation of a commercially sold computerized physician order entry system, *Pediatrics* **116** (2005), 1506–12.
[9] K. Eason, Ergonomic perspectives on advances in human-computer interaction, *Ergonomics* **34** (1991), 721–41.
[10] A.W. Kushniruk, E.M. Borycki, Low-cost rapid usability engineering, *Healthcare Quart* **9** (2006), 98–100.
[11] A.W. Kushniruk, M. Triola, E. Borycki, B. Stein, J. Kannry, Technology induced error and usability: The relationship between usability problems and prescription errors when using a handheld application, *Int J Med Inf* **74** (2005), 519–26.
[12] A.W. Kushniruk, V.L. Patel, Cognitive and usability engineering methods for the evaluation of clinical information systems, *J Biomed Inform* **37** (2004), 56–76.
[13] E.M. Borycki, A.W. Kushniruk, J. Anderson, M. Anderson, *Designing and integrating clinical and computer-based simulations in health informatics: From real-world to virtual reality,* In C. Shekelzen (Ed.) Modeling, Simulation and Optimization, Vukovar, Croatia: In-Tech, 31–51, 2010.
[14] A.W. Kushniruk, E.M. Borycki, S. Kuwata, J. Kannry, Predicting changes in workflow resulting from healthcare information systems: ensuring the safety of healthcare, *Healthcare Quart* **9** (2004),114–8.
[15] A.W. Kushniruk, E.M. Borycki, S. Kuwata, H. Watanabe, Using a low-cost simulation approach for assessing the impact of a medication administration system on workflow, *Stud Health Technology Inform* **136** (2008), 567–72.
[16] E.M. Borycki, A.W. Kushniruk, S. Kuwata, H. Watanabe, *Simulations to assess medication administration systems*, In B. Staudinger, V. Hob, H. Ostermann (Ed.) Nursing and Clinical Informatics: Socio-technical Approaches, Hershey, New York: IGI Global, 144–59, 2009.
[17] R. Koppel, T. Wetterneck, J.L. Telles, B.T. Karsh, Workarounds to barcode medication administration systems: Their occurrence causes and threats to patient safety, *JAMIA* **15** (2008), 408–23.

Patient Safety Informatics
V. Koutkias et al. (Eds.)
IOS Press, 2011

doi:10.3233/978-1-60750-740-6-206

Mapping the ATC Classification to the UMLS Metathesaurus: Some Pragmatic Applications

Tayeb MERABTI [a,1], Hocine ABDOUNE [b], Catherine LETORD [a], Saoussen SAKJI [a], Michel JOUBERT [b] and Stefan J. DARMONI [a]

[a] *CISMeF, Rouen University Hospital, Rouen, France & GCSIS, TIBS, LITIS EA 4108, Biomedical Research Institute, Rouen, France*

[b] *LERTIM, EA 3283, Faculty of Medicine, Mediterranean University, Marseille, France*

Abstract. ATC classification is a WHO international classification used to classify drugs. The aim of this paper is to evaluate two lexical methods in English and in French to map ATC to UMLS. Several applications have been impemented to illustrate the use of the ATC mapping in English and French: (a) MeSH translation in Norwegian, (b) Drug Information Portal, and (c) ATC to PubMed tool. Two lexical methods were used to map ATC to UMLS. The first approach used a French natural language processing tool to map French terms of ATC to the French terminologies of UMLS. The second approach used the MetaMap tool to map English terms of ATC to UMLS. The English MetaMap provides slightly more mappings than the French NLP tool (3,170 vs. 2,992). On the other hand, the French NLP tool provides a slightly better precision than MetaMap (88% vs. 86%). Using a manual mapping between ATC and MeSH, the union of the validated mappings between ATC and MeSH provides 2,824 mappings (68.7% of ATC codes of the fifth level). Lexical methods are powerful methods to map health terminologies to the UMLS Metathesaurus. Manual mapping is still necessary to complete the mapping.

Keywords. Abstracting classification, drugs, multilingualism, semantics, terminology as topic, Unified Medical Language System, controlled vocabulary

Introduction

The ATC (Anatomical, Therapeutic and Chemical) classification is an international classification [1] used to classify drugs. The ATC classification is developed and maintained by the Collaborating Centre for Drug Statistics Methodology [2]. Since 1982, the Centre is situated in Oslo at the Norwegian Institute of Public Health. The Centre is funded by the Norwegian government. In 1981, the WHO Regional Office for Europe recommended the ATC system for international drug utilization studies. In 1996, WHO recognized the need to promote the use of the ATC system as an international standard for drug utilization studies. The Centre was therefore linked directly to the WHO Headquarters in Geneva instead of the WHO Regional Office for Europe in Copenhagen. The purpose of the ATC is to serve as a tool for drug utilization research in order to improve the quality of drug use. One component of this is the

[1] Corresponding Author: tayeb.merabti@chu-rouen.fr

presentation and comparison of drug consumption statistics at international and other levels. The ATC classification is available in the following languages: English, French, German, Norwegian and Spanish.

The EU-FP7 project Patient Safety through Intelligent Procedures (PSIP) [2], runs from 2008 till 2011 and develops - among others - a prototype that should provide contextualized information and alerts as part of an electronic prescribing process in a hospital. For that purpose, the ATC classification was chosen to classify the drugs as it is largely used in Europe.

The purpose of the Unified Medical Language System® (UMLS) [4] is to facilitate the development of computer systems that behave as if they "understand" the meaning of the language of biomedicine and health. The main component of UMLS is the Metathesaurus which contains in English around 130 medical terminologies and proposes mappings between terminologies. Currently, although ATC is a WHO classification, it is not (yet) included in the UMLS Metathesaurus.

The process of terminology mapping consists of identifying identical (or approximately identical) concepts or relationships between terminologies [5]-[6]. The objective of this work is to propose a mapping of the ATC classification to the UMLS Metathesaurus, using two tools in two languages: (1) using the MetaMap lexical tools [6] in the English Language for the ATC classification; (2) using French lexical tools in the French language [7] developed by the CISMeF team. The mapping that will be evaluated in this work will be the mapping between ATC and MeSH, which provides three pragmatic applications: (a) MeSH translation in Norwegian; (b) PSIP Drug Information Portal; (c) a software to access PubMed via an ATC code or a multi-lingual label.

1. Material and Methods

1.1. ATC Classification

The WHO Collaborating Centre for Drug Statistics Methodology publishes a new issue of the complete ATC index annually. In ATC classification system, the drugs are divided into different groups according to the organ or system on which they act and their chemical, pharmacological and therapeutic properties. The ATC Code has the general form LCCLLCC where (L represents a letter and C a number). In this system, the drugs are classified in groups at five different levels: the 1st level: anatomical group (1 alphabetical character): fourteen main groups. The 2nd level: principal pharmacological/therapeutic group (2 numerical characters). The 3rd level: therapeutic/pharmacological sub-group (1 alphabetical character). The 4th level: chemical/therapeutic/pharmacological sub-group (1 alphabetical character). The 5th level: sub-group for chemical substance: the individual active ingredient or the association of active ingredients (2 numerical characters). For example:

N The nervous system
N05 Psycholeptics
N05B Anxiolytics
N05BA Benzodiazepine derivatives
N05BA01 Diazepam

The 2nd, 3rd and 4th levels are often used to identify pharmacological subgroups when that is considered more appropriate than therapeutic or chemical subgroups. Each level of this classification corresponds to an ATC code and an ATC label. The label of the 5th level corresponds to the International Generic Name of the substance, when it exists. International non-proprietary names (INN) are preferred. If INN names are not assigned, USAN (United States Adopted Name) or BAN (British Approved Name) names are usually chosen. Each code is allocated according to its principal indication. However, the latter can vary from one country to another, which explains why there may be several ATC codes for the same drug according to the concerned country. The main focus of the Drug Utilization Research Group in Europe was initially to improve drug utilization through cross-national drug utilization studies based on the ATC methodology [10]. Approximately 10% of the drugs do not have the same ATC code between France and Denmark (according to an internal study carried out by the VIDAL company [11] for the PSIP project). It was thus necessary to adapt to the French context and the Danish context to overcome with the problem of the "variable" ATC. This adaptation was made possible thanks to the participation of the Vidal company which provided the appropriate files; one correspondence table INN-ATC by country.

During the mapping module, the correspondence between the ATC classification and the MeSH terms (descriptors and Supplementary Concepts (SC)), was realized in order to find the best matching. The precision was 90% and the recall was 87%. Concerning the three different methods to automatically index ATC (method by title, method by brand name and method by indexation), 3,634 out of 5,073 of MeSH manually indexed resources and 1,341 out of 5,177 of MeSH automatically indexed resources were ATC automatically indexed. Most of the DIP resources are ATC automatically indexed by the method by brand names (51.4% for manually indexed resources and 24.4% for automatically indexed resources), followed by the method by title and the method by indexation.

1.2. Mapping to the UMLS Metathesaurus in English

MMTX is an implementation in the Java programming language of the MetaMap software [6] used to map biomedical text to the UMLS Metathesaurus or, equivalently, to discover Metathesaurus concepts referred to in text. Mappings to UMLS are associated to a score describing the similarity between terms to be mapped and the equivalent concepts in UMLS. For example, the ATC code "L01CA02 - Vinblastine" is mapped to the MeSH and SNOMED international terms "Vinblastine".

1.3. Mapping to the UMLS Metathesaurus in French

French natural language processing tools and mapping algorithms were developed by the CISMeF team to map French health terminologies. These tools were used in previous works [8] and extended to link terms in multiple French health terminologies. This approach allows from a given term, to find a UMLS concept with French (or English) terms that are most lexically similar to it. Thus, to overcome some problems like inflections, stop-words, etc, basic natural language processing is necessary beforehand: (a) Removing stop words: frequent short words that don't affect the phrases such as "a", "Nos", "of", etc are removed from all terms; (b) Stemming: we use a French stemmer "Lucene" which proved to be the most efficient for the F-MTI automatic indexing tools using several health terminologies, as compared to the stemming tools developed by the CISMeF team and the stemming tools in [8]; (c) The mapping used by this approach may provide three types of correspondences between all terms in source terminologies and French terms of the UMLS Metathesaurus: exact correspondence, single to multiple correspondence, partial correspondence. In this work, only the exact correspondence was evaluated. This relation may also to be represented into SKOS (Simple Knowledge Organization System) language [12]. SKOS language is also used to represent French health terminologies into the French Health Multi-terminological Server [13] to integrate the main health terminologies available in French, including those not yet mapped to the UMLS (e.g. ATC, CCAM, which is a French classification for procedures, ORPHANET, which is a thesaurus for rare diseases).

1.3.1. Exact Correspondence

One ATC term and one French term in UMLS are in an "exact correspondence" if all words composing the two terms are exactly the same. Thus, according to this correspondence there is at most one UMLS concept corresponding to the ATC term. Formally, an "exact correspondence" between this ATC term and one French term in UMLS is defined if the two terms are lexically similar. For example, the ATC code "A11HA06 - pyridoxal phosphate" is mapped to the MeSH and SNOMED international terms "pyridoxal phosphate".

2. Evaluation

We use an existing manual mapping between ATC codes of the 5th level and MeSH terms to evaluate the two approaches. Out of 4,268 ATC codes of the 5th level, a number of 4,108 (96%) mappings were performed manually by a librarian & pharmacist (CL) between ATC and MeSH terms. For each approach, three sets of codes were created: (1) the validated mappings: all the mappings of this set are obtained by the manual and the automatic approach; (2) the second set corresponds to all the mappings obtained automatically and not manually; (3) the last corresponds to all valid mappings not obtained automatically. Nevertheless, for the 4,108 manual mappings only 2,971 correspond to 1 to 1 mapping (one ATC code to one MeSH term). For example, the ATC code "J01MB06 - cinoxacin" is manually mapped to the MeSH term "cinoxacin". Thus, in this evaluation we use only this number of mapping to evaluate the two approaches.

3. Results

3.1. Mapping to the UMLS Metathesaurus in English

Using this approach, there were 3,170 (74%) ATC codes out of the 4,268 ATC codes of the 5th level used in this study that are in an "exact matching" relation with at least one UMLS concept. Limiting this mapping to only the French terminologies included into UMLS, there are 3,062 (71%) ATC codes in an "exact matching" relations with at least one UMLS concept. These codes are in "exact matching" with 3,062 MeSH preferred terms and 1,631 SNOMED International preferred terms.

3.2. Mapping to the UMLS Metathesaurus in French

Using this approach, there were 2,992 (70%) ATC codes out of the 4,268 ATC codes of the 5th level used in this study that are in an "exact matching" relation with at least one UMLS concepts. These codes are in "exact matching" with 2,499 MeSH preferred terms and 1.728 SNOMED International preferred terms.

3.3. Evaluation Results

From the 3,170 mappings using English: (a) 2,740 (86%) mappings are in the set of manual mapping (validated mappings); (b) 430 (13%) mappings obtained automatically and not manually. Furthermore, 231 mappings were manually obtained and not automatically (Table 1).

From the 2,992 mappings using French: (a) 2,640 (88%) mappings are in the set of manual mapping (validated mappings); (b) 352 (11%) mappings obtained automatically and not manually. Furthermore, 331 mappings were manually obtained and not automatically (see Table 1).

Finally, the union of the validated mappings in French and in English provides 2,824 ATC to MeSH mappings (2,556 common in English and in French, 184 only in English, and 84 only in French) representing 68.7% of the 4,108 ATC codes of the fifth level. The use of the French lexical tool allows us to detect three misspellings in French ATC labels.

Table 1. Number of validated mappings and number of mappings obtained only automatically according to the English and French approaches.

Type of mappings	Number of validated mappings	Number of mappings obtained only automatically
English-based mapping	2,740 (86%)	430 (13%)
French-based mapping	2,640 (88%)	352 (11%)

4. Some Practical Applications

4.1. MeSH Translation in Norwegian

The Norwegian Knowledge Centre for the Health Service [14] gathers and disseminates evidence about the effect and quality of methods and interventions within all parts of the health services. The Centre has decided to translate the MeSH to their language. Instead of starting from scratch, they will: (a) first, use the Swedish translation performed by the Karolinska Institute [15], as these two Nordic languages are quite similar; (b) second, they will use the proposed mapping ATC to MeSH as the ATC exists in Norwegian.

4.2. PSIP Drug Information Portal

The PSIP Drug Information Portal (DIP) was developed to allow French health professionals and patients to access relevant French information about drugs from main institutional health sites (e.g. French Drug Agency or European Drug Agency) [16]. The main innovation of this PSIP DIP relies on its multi-terminology indexing, mainly

MeSH and ATC, but also using different codes, such as Chemical Abstracts Service (CAS) codes and its multi-terminology information retrieval based on the same terminologies and classifications.

4.3. ATC to PubMed

The third application is still under development. The objective is to create software to access PubMed via any ATC code (in any language). To do so, we have finalized the automatic mapping between ATC and UMLS by a manual mapping for the levels 1, 2, 3, 4 and 5 of the ATC. This manual mapping has been realized by a CISMeF medical librarian (CL) (N=5,359 (97%)). In most of the cases, this manual mapping was a 1 to N mapping (e.g. for the ATC code "D11AX18 - diclofenac", the MeSH mapping was "Diclofenac" and "Dermatologic agents"). For each ATC code, a predefined query was then created and could be launched on PubMed or on the PSIP DIP. For example, the PubMed query ""desensitization, immunologic"[MH] AND "allergens"[MH]" is associated to the ATC code "V01A".

5. Discussion and Conclusion

To the best of our knowledge, this is the first study to map ATC to UMLS using English (MetaMap) and French NLP tools. The English MetaMap provides slightly more mappings than the French NLP tool (3,170 vs. 2,992). The French NLP tool provides a slightly better precision than MetaMap (88% vs. 86%).

A number of algorithms and approaches have been proposed to create an automatic mapping between health terminologies. For example, Rocha et al. [17] and Cimino et al. [18] both proposed a frame-based approach to perform mappings between health terminologies. Other approaches were proposed using UMLS [19] as a knowledge resource to perform mappings between terminologies making use of synonymy, explicit mapping relations and hierarchical relationships [20]. However, approaches using UMLS are limited to the biomedical terminologies already incorporated into UMLS.

Besides the ATC classification heavily used in Europe, RxNorm [21] is a standardized nomenclature for clinical drugs and drug delivery devices. RxNorm is produced by the US National Library of Medicine. RxNorm provides normalized names for clinical drugs and links its names to many of the drug vocabularies commonly used in pharmacy management and drug interaction software. RxNorm's standard names for clinical drugs and drug delivery devices are connected to the varying names of drugs present in many different controlled vocabularies within the UMLS Metathesaurus, including those in commercially available drug information sources. These connections are intended to facilitate interoperability among the computerized systems that record or process data dealing with clinical drugs. A mapping between ATC and UMLS imply an indirect mapping between ATC and RxNorm that should have some interest in the future. A formal evaluation of this mapping is mandatory before clinical use. This lexical methods were recently applied to one other French terminology (CCAM) not yet included in the UMLS Metathesaurus [23].

The current method is appropriate for ATC labels at the fifth level, which corresponds to its deepest level. This lexical tool was not adapted to the ATC other levels (level 1 to 4) because the ATC label used in the drug context, it is very difficult to process by NLP tool: e.g. the ATC code "digestive system" means in fact "drug therapy of digestive system diseases". Furthermore, in some cases, an ATC label of level 2, 3, 4 or 5 should also take into account the ATC label of level N-1, N-2 or N-3: e.g. for A12BA01 - Potassium chloride, must be distinguished from B05XA01 - Potassium chloride. A12BA01 is indicated in case of hypokalemia (by oral administration), therefore the A axis is taken into account (alimentary tract and metabolism). The final MeSH query for the A12BA01 - Potassium chloride is then: Potassium chlorside[MeSH] and hypokalemia/therapy[MeSH] and administration, Oral[MeSH].

Therefore, the mappings between ATC and MeSH for the ATC labels of level 1 to 4 were performed manually by the CISMeF pharmacist expert (CL). The overall mapping was then sent to the Collaborating Centre for Drug Statistics Methodology in Norway for validation.

The mapping between ATC and other terminologies is not so easy because: (a) mainly, one substance could have various ATC codes depending on whether it is used alone or in association, the diseases to be treated, the route of administration, (b) chemical classification varies from one terminology to another (e.g. mecamylamine is considered as an amine in ATC and as a terpenes in the MeSH); (c) the ATC classification is not purely anatomical (e.g. H axis stands for systemic hormonal preparations, excl. sex hormones and insulins); (d) in some cases, the MeSH lacks precision (e.g. impossibility to differentiate from beta blocking agents non-selective and selective; (e) in some cases, the MeSH hierarchy has to be carefully checked: e.g. Neomycin has three narrower terms: Framycetin, Paromomycin, Ribostamycin but there is also ATC codes for Neomycin and Framycetin. Therefore, the MeSH query for neomycin has to be restricted to Non exploded; (f) in some cases, pharmaceutical actions in the MeSH are not complete (e.g. the MeSH Supplementary Concept benfluorex has the following pharmaceutical actions: appetite depressants and antilipemic agents. The ATC classification provide another pharmaceutical action: hypoglycemic agents. Finally, some ATC codes are not mapped to the MeSH because there is no equivalent in that thesaurus (e.g. D11AC09 xenysalate).

Mapping the ATC classification to the UMLS Metathesaurus was performed with good results with automatic NLP and mapping tools. The coordinated use of appropriate NLP and semantic tools, international standards and ontology driven tools increased the quality of the mapping.

Acknowledgments

The research leading to these results has received funding from the European Community's Seventh Framework Programme (FP7/2007-2013) under grant agreement n° 216130 – the PSIP project.

References

[1] A. Skrbo, B. Begović, S. Skrbo, Classification of drugs using the ATC system (Anatomic, Therapeutic, Chemical Classification) and the latest changes, *Med Arh* **58** (2005), 138–41.
[2] http://www.whocc.no/atcddd/, last access on February 2011.
[3] R. Beuscart, W. Hackl, C. Nøhr, Detection and Prevention of Adverse Drug Events - Information Technologies and Human Factors, IOS Press, Amsterdam, 2009.
[4] D.A.B. Lindberg, B.L. Humphreys, A.T. McCray, The unified medical language system, *Methods Inf Med* **32** (1993), 281–91.
[5] O. Bodenreider, The unified medical language system (UMLS): Integrating biomedical terminology, *Nucleic Acids Res* **32** (2004), 267–70.
[6] Y. Wang, J. Patrick, G. Miller, J. O'Hallaran, A computational linguistics motivated mapping of ICPC-2 PLUS to SNOMED CT, *BMC Med Inform Decis Mak* **8 Suppl 1** (2008), S5.
[7] A.R. Aronson, Effective mapping of biomedical text to the UMLS Metathesaurus: the MetaMap program, *Proc AMIA Symp* (2007), 17–21.
[8] S. Pereira, Multi-terminology indexing of concepts in health. (Indexation multiterminologique de concepts en santé). PhD Thesis, University of Rouen, France 2008.
[9] T. Merabti, Methods for mapping medical terminologies: contribution to semantic interoperability between terminologies (Méthodes pour la mise en relation des terminologies médicales : contribution à l'interopérabilité sémantique Inter et Intra terminologique). PhD Thesis, University of Rouen, France, 2010.
[10] U. Bergman, The history of the Drug Utilization Research Group in Europe. *Pharmacoepidemiol Drug Saf* **15** (2006), 95–8.
[11] http://www.vidal.fr/, last access on February 2011.
[12] http://www.w3.org/2004/02/skos/, last access on February 2011.
[13] M. Joubert, B. Dahamna, J. Delahousse, M. Fieschi, S.J. Darmoni, SMTS®: Un Serveur Multi-Terminologies de Santé. *Risques, technologies de l'information pour les pratiques médicales: Informatique et santé* **17** (2009), 47–56.
[14] http://www.kunnskapssenteret.no/, last access on February 2011.
[15] http://mesh.kib.ki.se/swemesh/swemesh_se.cfm, last access on February 2011.
[16] S. Sakji et al., Drug information portal in europe: information retrieval with multiple health terminologies, *Stud Health Technol Inform* **150** (2009), 497–501.
[17] R.A. Rocha, B.H. Rocha, S.M. Huff, Automated transaltion between medical vocabularies using a frame-based interlingua, *Proc Annu Symp Comput Appl Med Care* (1993), 690–4.
[18] J.J. Cimino, G.O. Barnett, Automated translation between medical terminologies using semantic definitions, *MD Comput* **7**(1990), 104–9.
[19] K.W. Fung, O. Bodenreider, Utilizing UMLS for semantic mapping between terminologies, *AMIA Annu Symp Proc* (2005), 266–70.
[20] O. Bodenreider, S.J. Nelson, W.T. Hole, H.F. Chang, Beyond synonymy: exploiting the UMLS semantics in mapping vocabularies, *AMIA Annu Symp Proc* (1998), 815–9.
[21] F. Parrish, N. Do, O. Bouhaddou, P. Warnekar, Implementation of RxNorm as a terminology mediation standard for exchanging pharmacy medication between federal agencies, *AMIA Annu Symp Proc* (2006):1057.
[22] http://www.nlm.nih.gov/research/umls/rxnorm/overview.html/, last access on February 2011.
[23] T. Merabti et al., An automated approach to map a French terminology to UMLS, *Stud Health Technol Inform* **160** (2010), 1040–4.

Part F

Validation and Impact Assessment of Patient Safety Informatics Approaches

Patient Safety Informatics
V. Koutkias et al. (Eds.)
IOS Press, 2011

doi:10.3233/978-1-60750-740-6-217

Lessons Learnt from Conducting a High Fidelity Simulation Test in Health IT

Kitta LAWTON [a,1], Kristine BINZER [b], Peter SKJOET [b] and Sanne JENSEN [a]

[a] *Capital Region of Denmark, Department of Health IT*
[b] *Capital Region of Denmark, Unit for Patient Safety*

Abstract. Testing IT-systems by use of simulation requires a thorough planning and preparation in order to create a realistic clinical environment. For a successful test through simulation a dedicated test team to control the environment is needed, as well as people to play the role of patients and staff. Relevant artifacts and elaborate scenarios ensure the narrative. This paper explores the preliminary work and execution of an extensive test of a Computerized Order Entry System prototype. Central to the setup of the test is a script which outlines the method by guiding the preparation and execution.

Keywords. Simulation, impact evaluation, usability, health IT, high fidelity test

Introduction

For many years the aviation industry has used simulation to test IT-systems. In health care simulation has mainly been used for training clinical skills [1-3], and only recently been adopted as a method for testing IT-systems before implementation [4-5]. Through simulation it is possible to test IT-systems in environments very close to reality; so called high fidelity test. In such, test clinicians are invited to use the IT-system in a realistic but controlled environment, resembling the clinical setting with respect to surroundings, patient cases, interaction with other staff members, IT-systems etc. Hence, the context feels and acts like reality, but is shielded from consequences to patients, whereby the simulation provides a psychological safe space for the participant in which to try out new systems.

Since 2007 the Capital Region of Denmark (CRD) has conducted simulations on a regular basis in order to qualify IT-systems to the clinic. These simulations range from simple set-ups during the development phase, to full scale simulations complimentary to a pilot project like the high fidelity test presented in this paper.

The simulations are held at IT-eXperimentarium (ITX) located at one of the regional hospitals [6]. The ITX is designed for simulation training and test, and consists of a full scale hospital ward including operating theatre, intensive wards, delivery room and medicine room; all equipped with cameras for capturing data. From adhering observation rooms it is possible to observe and direct the simulation.

[1] Corresponding Author: kitta.lawton@regionh.dk

In order to address the complexity of simulations, in particular high fidelity tests, a template script was developed by CRD Corporate IT department in 2008 [7]. This template script frames the method by outlining the considerations and activities to be carried out before, during and after the simulation.

The simulation test described in this paper was carried out in order to evaluate a prototype of a Computerized Physician Order Entry (CPOE) system developed for the European project Patient Safety through Intelligent Procedures (PSIP) [8]. The PSIP project seeks to provide clinicians with decision support based on identified risks and errors regarding medication. The alerts are designed to help the clinicians identify adverse events related to medication, and the decision support is integrated into the IT-systems used by clinicians in their daily routines. Furthermore, the CPOE prototype provides the clinician with information about diagnoses, allergies, biochemistry, medication and alerts from the decision support system in one single user interface.

The evaluation of the prototype is two-fold; to assess the impact of the PSIP prototype on the occurrence of medical errors related to prescription and to assess the usability of the prototype. The test was shared by four stakeholders within the PSIP project. These stakeholders were responsible for the functionality of the prototype, the data and test setup, and the two aspects of the evaluation, respectively.

The aim of this paper is to outline the lessons learnt in the preparation and execution of a large simulation test, in order to shed light on the possibilities of this kind of evaluation setup.

1. Method

The main preparatory tool to conducting a simulation test is a script that outlines the activities and delegation of tasks to be carried out before, during and after the simulation. The template script consists of two components; a template specific to each scenario and a general template including a list of multiple aspects to consider as part of the preparation for the test (Table 1).

The script works as a guiding standard to the execution of a high fidelity simulation test by thoroughly outlining items to be considered. Main aspects of this is the resources needed, minute time schedule, framework in which to construct the actual scenario, and artifacts to be included.

The execution of the test consisted of a six months preparation phase commenced in March 2010, two days of trial runs just prior to the test and three full days of testing from September 29th to October 1st 2010. Throughout the test days, two simulations were planned to be executed simultaneously twice a day.

Compilation of lessons learnt has been conducted by auditing the script in the light of the flow of the simulation test, as well as through discussions in the core team. By thematizing the experiences we have been able to extract the most important of experiences.

2. Results

The number of test cases and participants was determined based on the amount of data needed to assess the dual objectives of the test. The test was designed to involve twelve doctors, each seeing five patients during two simulations. The simulations were executed in two ward rooms simultaneously; first using the CRD system, and then rotating to the other room to use the PSIP prototype. The script was based on these requirements.

Table 1. Aspects of a simulation test to address in a script.

Consideration to be addressed in script		Containing a description of:
Test organization		The role and tasks of each member of the test team during and between simulations.
Settings for the test	Setting	The location including which rooms are available and when.
	Participants	Number and identity of simulation participants (in this case medical doctors) including required level of experience.
	Clinical scenarios	Design of clinical setup and the task of the participant during scenarios. The development of the scenarios with regards to level of information needed and the format of role-cards used for setting the scene for the simulation was described in a separate script.
	Technical setup	Required equipment during the simulation and the systems used, as well as the technical information such as connection of servers, re-stalling of data etc.
	List of artifacts	Artifacts needed to ensure the technical setup and evaluation, as well as the fidelity of the clinical situation.
	Test data	The data used for the test, the origin of these and the criteria on which they were selected.
Data collection		The methods used for collecting data.
Time Table and resources		Who is needed where and when, as well as the actual schedule for the test days (broken down to minutes when appropriate).
Evaluation	Method	Method of evaluation and schedule for this including allocation of tasks.
	Data analysis	Method of analysis, allocation of tasks and timeline.

2.1. Test Organization

The preparation phase was led by a core group of four people representing the stakeholder responsible for the test setup and data. The framework for the script was developed through an iterative process involving all stakeholders, whereas other more specific tasks including synthesis of case data, developing clinical scenarios, establishing test environments, and recruiting participants was led by the core group.

Throughout this phase the core group drew extensively on additional capacities within their own organization and from other stakeholders when needed. Assistance was mainly needed for data entry and creation of test environments in the different IT-systems. External assistance was mainly needed two to three months prior to the test and accumulated to three months worth of full time employment for one person. These competences and tasks were not included in the script.

During the actual execution of the simulations, the test organization grew to 16 people including five ‘patients’. For each of the two simulation ward rooms, we assigned an instructor, a co-instructor and a test coordinator/rounding nurse. Three patients were stationary in one ward room, and two in the other. The rest of the members of the test team assisted in both simulations when needed. The assigned responsibilities and means of communication for each team member are outlined in Table 2.

Table 2. Roles and responsibilities throughout the test days.

Role (Location)	Responsibilities	Communication
2 Instructors (observation room A and B)	Overall responsible for the simulation is running according to script and timeline.	Communicates through headset with the test coordinator.
2 Co-instructors (observation room A and B)	Assisting the instructor, and in control of the cameras including parts of data collection.	Communicates with instructor.
2 Test coordinators/rounding nurses (simulation ward room A and B)	Translation of instructions from the instructor to the doctor or patient without breaking the credibility in the narrative of the simulation. Assisting the participating doctor if necessary in order to ensure progress in the simulation (clinical or IT related help, but only if accepted by instructor).	Receive instructions from instructor via headset.
1 "Doctor on call"/ "Lab assistant" (moved between the two observation rooms when needed)	Medical specialist available for clarifying questions and medical advice from participating doctors.	Reached by a dedicated phone in observation room. Participating doctor call this via cell phone.
4 Technicians (present in room close to simulation ward rooms in order to ensure rapid assistance when needed)	Secure soft- and hardware for data collection, functionality and re-stalling of the RegH systems, and functionality of the PSIP prototype, respectively.	
5 Patients	Act as patients during simulation. Each patient plays the same role during all sessions.	

One of the instructors and the doctor in charge of the patient cases were responsible of introducing the participating doctors to ITX, the project and to the PSIP prototype. During this introduction the participating doctors had the opportunity to gain hand-on experience with the PSIP prototype in order to accustom her with the user interface and the functionalities. The aim of this introduction was to equate the doctor's routine and knowledge of the PSIP prototype to that of the usual CRD systems.

2.2. The Patients

The script template did not describe a profile of 'patients' to recruit, and how to recruit them. Neither did it describe how they should be introduced to the simulations, the expectations to their participation, payment etc. This, however, was defined as part of the invitation to the 'patients'. In this test we decided to recruit men at an age resembling the chosen clinical cases.

The core team distributed a document throughout the CRD Corporate IT, challenging colleagues to invite people in their network to participate. From the replies we were able to select five suitable men to play the patient roles.

The five 'patients' were invited into ITX in order to familiarize themselves with each other, the location and the test team. At this occasion we introduced the scenarios and the patients' role in the simulation. In order for them to visualize their level of participation, we performed one of the scenarios. They were each handed a manuscript containing the facts and symptoms of their individual patient case in detail. The manuscripts did not contain any specific lines to which they had to adhere. In order to respond naturally to questions, they were asked to make up the answers the best they could from their knowledge of condition and symptoms stated in the script, when examined during the simulations by the participating doctors.

2.3. Setting and Artifacts

The setting was described in details in the script. We used two complete ward rooms at ITX, each fully equipped for simulations (Figure 1). Additional rooms were used for office space, storage of spare equipment, as well as the briefing of participants before and interviews after simulations.

Each ward room was furnished with a complete set of clinical artifacts relevant for the scenarios. The 'patients' were placed in hospital beds or chairs. Participating doctors had access to laptop computers with relevant IT-system as well as a paper file for each patient. Other artifacts included doctor's coat, stethoscope, bed side flowers etc. Each team member was assigned the responsibility for specific artifacts being in place before each session.

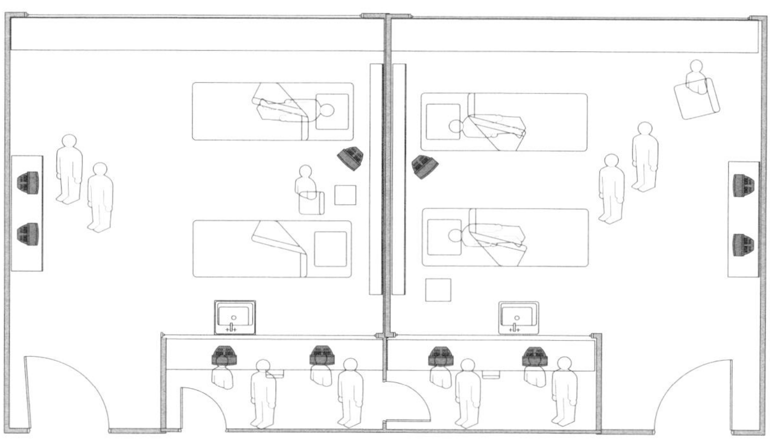

Figure 1. The two simulation ward rooms and observation room.

2.4. The Participants

The script template did not describe the clinical profile and competences needed for a specific simulation. The stakeholder of the impact evaluation requested us to recruit twelve participants with a wide range of clinical experience.

Participants were recruited through a written proposal send to the clinical administrators of six departments of internal medicine each employing approximately 20-30 doctors. The proposal contained information about the project, the purpose of the simulation, time, place and payment for participation. In general we met little interest, but one medical ward with prior experiences of projects regarding safe medication, referred seven participants at all levels of experience. In total we managed to recruit eleven doctors for the test, of which one did not turn up on the day of the test. We were not able to ensure emergency procedure in case of no show.

2.5. The Clinical Scenarios and Test Data

The five patient cases were chosen for their complexity in order to exemplify the functionalities of the PSIP prototype, as well as their potential to bring doctors to make errors concerning prescription of medication. Suitable test cases were selected from the PSIP database and refined through an iterative process by a medical doctor. They were all based on real patient cases and hospital files originating from male patients aged between 62 and 82.

The scenarios were described in separate sub-scripts and included a description of the patient's data including name, social security number and age. The medical history included all the information usually found in Danish medical records; previous and current diagnosis and plan for treatment, medication history and current prescriptions, allergies, social data such as marital status and information about physical capabilities.

The scenarios also included clinical observations at start of the simulation; e.g. temperature and blood pressure. Furthermore, each scenario involved a short narrative in order to set the scene for the participating doctor and nurse respectively. The expected actions of the participating doctor were added to the scenario for the purpose of directing the simulation.

2.6. The Technical Setup

It was necessary to have all the participating doctors to perform in both system set-ups, as the objective for the impact assessment demanded a comparison of the prescribed drugs for the 'patients' in the systems. In effect, the ward rooms were each fitted with two computers; one for the PSIP prototype and one for the CRD systems.

Due to the fragility of the PSIP prototype, this system was set up in closed circuit consisting of a laptop computer with the PSIP client connected to each a server.

The CRD set-up consisted of two systems: the medicine module (EPM3) for viewing the patients' drug regime and entering new prescriptions. The other system, Opus, is used for viewing diagnosis and patient notes. The participating doctors were familiar with the interface of the CRD systems, and the systems were pointed at the educational environments, containing the data of the test 'patients' only. The two lab-systems used in CRD were not included, as we were not able to access and set up data in those systems. Fortunately the recruited clinicians were used to work with lab data presented on paper as an alternative to computer access and we included these as part of the patient paper files. The data on specific test patients could be accessed in all the systems by use of name and personal ID number.

As we were not able to delete the prescription the doctors entered in the system, test data had to be restored in between sessions. This took approximately an hour, and had to be appointed by the server host.

2.7. The Emergency Procedures

A systematic way of describing emergency procedures was not a part of the script template. However, during the preparation phase it became clear that the PSIP prototype were prone to breakdowns. Although we secured the PSIP setup in closed circuits, we experienced several breakdowns during the simulations. The possibility of performing the test with stubbed alert data as an alternative to the actual CDSS was dismissed before the test. Such alternatives would be useful in less realistic evaluations, but was thought to lack the realism needed for comparing interaction and decision-making to that of the CRD systems.

Another disturbance affecting the test was a planned power cut to test emergency procedures at the hospital, which we were not informed about. This switched down the PSIP servers and could potentially have interfered seriously with session of testing.

2.8. Data Collection

When selecting means to record data, it is a trade off between immense amount of potentially redundant data, and the risk of failed data collection due to technical problems. The script listed four different ways of recording data for evaluation, as previous experiences have showed us that it is risky to rely on one or two recording systems.

The fixed equipment for data capturing in the ward rooms consists of two components; a camera fitted in the ceiling, which is controlled from the observation room in order to capture motion and sound, and a capturing setup at the workstation used by participants, enabling the test team to follow the clinician's interaction with the system real time. This equipment works on highly specialized software, which stores files not convertible outside the software. This poses a dependence on the technical staff at ITX. For the test we appointed a local technician to convert the files we needed. When converting the files, it is not possible to maintain the synchronization between motion in the room and the screen capture. Hence, the fixed equipment was complemented by freeware (CamStudio) used to record movement at the screen and a handheld camera to record all the simulations using the PSIP prototype. At some of the tests, the recording by using CamStudio failed. We therefore had to capture data about drug prescription by use of screen dumps. This last part was not described in the script.

2.9. Time Table and Resources

The script supported very well that every activity was scheduled minute-by-minute in order to ensure efficient use of time and the test participants were invited at different times according to the schedule. The sessions were planned with buffer time in order to accommodate any delays, breakdowns or other disturbances, which in effect allowed us some movement within schedule.

The days of testing consisted of two sessions of three hours each. Each session involved an introduction of the two participating doctors, the simulations and finally evaluation. Thus the script defined in detail which systems each participating doctor should use at a certain time during the session. Table 3 presents a breakdown of the schedule according to script for one session.

2.10. Evaluation

The evaluation consisted of observation and interviews. The script did not directly describe how the observations should be captured, the format of the interview guide for the semi structured interviews or a description of how data would be analyzed.

However, all relevant observers and stakeholders were present throughout the days of the test. The observers focusing on patient safety, usability, usefulness and impact evaluation respectively, moved freely between the observation rooms.

An observations form was handed out to the observers before the test, structuring observations and notes accordingly. The interviews were conducted by the same people in all sessions adding consistency to the format guided by an interview guide. The interviews were recorded by dictaphone.

Some participating doctors were interested in talking to a medical expert before the interview, in order to clarify clinical issues, which might have occurred during the simulation. This wish was addressed ad hoc during the test days.

Table 3. Part of Time Table for one session during the PSIP simulations. All doctors participated in a simulation using the CRD systems, and one simulation using the PSIP prototype, rotating the five patients.

Time	Activity	Room/Participant/Patient/system
9:00–9:15	Welcome and introduction to the project and to the simulations	Meeting room
9:15–9:50	Hands-on introduction to PSIP Presentation of the RegH systems	Meeting room
9:50–10:15	Set the scene and Simulation 1	Simulation room 1, doctor 1, patient a-c, PSIP Simulation room 2, doctor 2, patient d-e, PSIP
10:15–10:25	Change of rooms for the 2 participating doctors	Simulation room 1, doctor 2, patient a-c, CRD Simulation room 2, doctor 1, patient d-e, CRD
10:25–10:50	Set the scene and Simulation 2	Simulation room 1+2
10:50–11:50	Evaluation	Meeting room
11:50–12:00	Goodbyes and thank you	Meeting room
12:00–13:00	Restore of EPM3	Simulation room 1+2

3. Discussion

The script, including the sub-scripts for the five scenarios, functioned as a useful framework for the simulations. However, we found the preparation phase insufficiently addressed in the template and suggest adding a subscript describing the specific tasks, timeline and required resources needed as part of the preparation.

By the end of the preparation phase the script and the scenarios had reached extensive detail, which meant that team members and stakeholders would refrain from reading through the updated versions, limiting the value added to the iterative process. Hence, some input requiring changes to the set up was received only in the days prior to the test. However, the scenarios supported very well the simulation test. They made it possible for the participants as well as the persons acting patients to understand what to do during the simulation.

The use of 'real patients' of realistic age and gender as the patient in the scenarios proved to be a success. The 'patients' required a careful instruction as they had no experience with acting. Both test coordinators had nursing background, meaning they could support the 'patient' and cover for any lapses the patient may have. If real nurses are not available, instructions to the 'patient' could be communicated directly from the instructor to the 'patient' via discreet ear plug walkie-talkie in future simulations.

Appointing participants proved to be a challenge. As a result, we are establishing a panel of contacts within CRD. This should guarantee that each hospital provides relevant clinicians for future simulations and tests according to the kind of specialty and services the hospital is covering. Creating a realistic configuration in the CRD systems with the corresponding patient data for the simulation also proved to be a challenge thanks to limitations of the integrated logic of functionalities of production systems regarding patient safety. Those limitations especially posed restrictions in entering patient data preceding present time, e.g. time stamping lab-results and prescriptions. However, new technology offers different solutions, and we are presently scrutinizing the market. The PSIP prototype displayed numerous breakdowns. For future simulations of this type, we will require thorough pre-tests to ensure robustness of the system. The script template was supportive to an extent, in terms of setting up the technical framework for the simulation. However, it did not support the complexity of entering test data. Nor did it describe the challenges with interaction between the systems. The core group had extensive focus on this issue to make sure that all the systems would function during the period of test.

Dependency on the fixed equipment for data collection and delay in the conversion of captured data, delayed the data analysis. Furthermore, we were not informed of the planned power cut on the morning of third test day, which shot down the systems and the PSIP servers unexpectedly. Such unexpected dependencies can cause waste of time and effort, and evidently overturn the simulation. The handheld camera proved very useful, as playback is easy and ready without further converting. A drawback with this is that it takes a person handling the camera during simulation, which means an extra person in the wardroom. However, this did not seem to disturb the flow and participation in the simulations. We are currently scrutinizing the market for simpler ways in which to ensure data collection in the future.

To conclude we found the preparations and execution of this high fidelity test to be time and resource intensive. We therefore recommend carefully comparing the required level of fidelity to the objectives of the test and the available resources before commencing future simulation tests. However, resources invested in a simulation should be seen in comparison to resources wasted if an IT-system is implemented in the clinic with insufficient usability or unintended adverse impact on patient safety. Based on our experience we suggest simulation tests carried out according to a script, as a valuable and complimentary method for testing IT-systems.

Acknowledgments

The research leading to these results has received funding from the European Community's Seventh Framework Programme (FP7/2007-2013) under grant agreement n° 216130 – the PSIP project. Furthermore, we acknowledge the assistance from participants in the simulation test.

References

[1] W.M. Nehring, F.R. Lashley, Nursing Simulation: A review of the past 40 years, *Simulation & Gaming* **40** (2009), 528–52.

[2] K. Khan et al., Simulation in medical education, *Med Teach* **33** (2011), 1–3.

[3] W.C. McGaghie et al., A critical review of simulation-based medical education research: 2003-2009, *Med Educ* **44** (2010), 50–63.

[4] Society in Europe for Simulation Applied to Medicine, http://www.sesam-web.org/, last access on March 2011.

[5] H. van der Sijs et al., Understanding handling of drug safety alerts: a simulation study, *Int J Med Inform* **79** (2010), 361–9.

[6] Danish Institute of Medical Simulation, http://www.sesam-web.org/centers/herlev, last access on March 2011.

[7] S. Jensen, S. Koldby, Establishing IT Experimentarium (ITX) in The Capital Region of Denmark, 2008.

[8] http://www.psip-project.eu/, last access on March 2011.

Patient Safety Informatics
V. Koutkias et al. (Eds.)
IOS Press, 2011

doi:10.3233/978-1-60750-740-6-227

Impact Evaluation of Innovative Technology: Estimating the Impact of the PSIP Solutions

Elske AMMENWERTH [a,1], Werner O. HACKL [a], Sanne JENSEN [b], Kitta LAWTON [b], Daniel RIEDMANN [a] and Martin JUNG [a]
[a] *Institute for Health Information Systems, UMIT – University for Health Sciences, Medical Informatics and Technology, Hall in Tyrol, Austria*
[b] *Project Department, Corporate IT, Capital Region of Denmark, Denmark*

Abstract. Health informatics projects often develop innovative IT solutions for health care. Systematic evaluation of their impact and risks is an ethical imperative. However, field studies can often not be conducted because of immature solutions. On the other site, lab studies are not helpful when it comes to estimating the impact of an innovative IT solution. We faced this challenge within the PSIP projects where innovative tools for medication management are developed. In this paper, we present the approaches used within the PSIP project for estimating the impact of immature solutions, including surveys of future users, a Delphi study with experts, and a simulation study. The methodology and first results of those evaluations are presented, and lessons learnt for impact evaluation of immature solutions are discussed.

Keywords. Evaluation, Delphi study, user survey, impact evaluation, evaluation methodology

Introduction

Medication errors and resulting Adverse Drug Events (ADEs) are an important issue of global healthcare [1]. The EU-FP7 project PSIP (http://www.psip-project.eu), Patient Safety through Intelligent Procedures in Medication [2-3], runs from 2008 till 2011. PSIP develops, among others, innovative prototypes of clinical information system modules that can be used for medication management at the clinical work place to reduce errors and to increase medication safety. These modules offer different ways of presenting information and alerts on possible ADEs during drug prescription.

Both the clinical decision support system (CDSS) used in these tools [4], as well as the tools themselves, were new developments and thus need to be systematically evaluated with regard to potential impact and risks. Evaluation of innovative solutions is regarded as an ethical imperative for health informatics [5]. Evaluation can be done in lab studies, which provide a controlled environment, or in field studies which provide a more realistic environment. Lab studies typically show high internal validity, but less external validity, as the environment is not realistic. Field studies, in the contrary, show high external validity, but less internal validity as the situation cannot

[1] Corresponding Author: elske.ammenwerth@umit.at

be controlled as easily as in lab studies. Also, technology needs to be sufficiently advanced for field studies, to avoid disruption of clinical work and risks for patient safety.

Within the PSIP project, one overall objective was to learn more about the possible impact of the developed solutions. Impact evaluation especially of complex clinical tools is normally done in field studies. However, the prototypes developed in PSIP were not sufficiently mature to conduct field studies, as it was not the aim of the PSIP project to develop ready-to-deploy tools. We were therefore confronted with the problem that impact evaluation was needed, but related field studies not possible.

The objective of this paper is to describe the methodology and preliminary results while estimating the impact of the PSIP solutions on patient care and to discuss possibilities of evaluation immature IT solutions.

1. Materials and Methods

The PSIP solutions were designed to improve patient safety. Thus, impact on medication errors and ADEs was defined as major evaluation criteria.

As lab studies are not adequate to evaluate the impact of a new technology, but because field studies were found to be too risky, we decided to conduct a simulation study. The concept of "simulation studies" describes studies in settings that are as close to routine care as possible, but without endangering patients (and clinicians) [6]. For this, simulation studies often include simulation patients that are trained to behave like "real" patients. Simulation studies can be done at the daily workplace of the clinicians, or in specially designed simulation wards that resemble a real ward, but where only simulation patients are treated.

Besides the simulation study, we decided to exploit the knowledge of international experts and thus designed a Delphi study. This type of study allows for a systematic, iterative collection of expert opinions [7-8]. Compared to other methods, such as interviews, it enables the inclusion of a larger number of experts [9] and the derivation of quantitative assessments concerning the study questions.

Finally, to contrast the opinions of the experts to expectations of clinical users, we conducted a standardized questionnaire survey in several European hospitals.

We will now present more details of each of these three studies.

1.1. Simulation Study

The simulation test was performed over the three days in autumn 2010 in two simulation rooms in the IT eXperimentarium (ITX) in Copenhagen. The simulation was conducted by 10 clinicians that volunteered to participate. Five elderly simulation patients (62 – 82 years) were trained to reflect typical patient cases that were developed based on real cases. The cases comprised quite complex patient cases. Patients got detailed instructions describing their role, facts and symptoms of their cases. The doctors were then asked to perform a ward round on the five patients. They were asked to review the available clinical data, to talk to the patients, to decide on the next steps (e.g. new or modified prescription, lab orders), and to document this. For reviewing and documenting data, the physicians got access to a computer-based application system. This could be either the standard clinical information system of this hospital or a new protoype of the clinical information systems developed by the partner IBM and called “the PSIP system” in the following sections. The PSIP system provided a new user interface integrating diagnostic data, lab data, and prescriptions, and also offered the possibility to check prescriptions before their order.

The physician used the standard system for one half of the patients, the new PSIP system for the other half of the patients, with varying order of patients for each physician. Overall, half of the 50 simulation runs were done with the standard system, the other half with the new system. In addition, to reflect normal working processes, paper-based documentation was provided where needed.

Before the simulation, the physicians got an introduction into the setup and technology. During the simulations, a team member acted as nurse and helped in case there were questions with regard to the patient case. The physicians only got technical support if they experienced larger problems. After the simulation, the physicians were interviewed with regard to their experiences.

For data analysis, the prescriptions and other orders done by the physicians were documented (via camera and screen dumps) and compared to the expected outcome that has been defined beforehand by two physicians in consensus (gold standard). This gold standard comprised a list of 3 – 6 expected activities that should be performed for this patient (such as order an INR test, or order digoxin). The inclusion of both the standard system and the PSIP system allows to directly measuring the impact of PSIP on ordering patterns.

1.2. Expert Delphi Survey

Through a search of recent publications in PubMed, we identified 214 experts that had experience in electronic medication, and invited them to participate. During the Delphi study, the experts got a short description of both standard solutions as well as innovative solutions that were developed in PSIP, namely:

1. External drug information for clinicians: Allows reviewing detailed pharmaceutical information on a drug, and to check drug-drug interactions between selected drugs.
2. Passive alerting module: Displays, in an informative and non-interruptive way, all alerts that are relevant for a given patient. Can be part of a clinical information or EHR system. A prototype was developed within PSIP.
3. Active alerting module: Actively checks all new prescriptions and alerts the user if there are any interactions or other drug-related problems. Typically part of an electronic prescribing module in a clinical information system.
4. Proactive prescription simulation module: Allows simulating different prescriptions. It provides instant information on possible drug-related problems before the prescription is being finalized. Typically part of an electronic prescribing module in a clinical information system. A prototype was developed within PSIP.
5. Patient component: A personalized tool that provides the patient with information on recent prescriptions, possible drug-related problems, and access to patient-tailored drug information. A prototype was developed within PSIP.
6. ADE epidemiology information: A summarized overview on the number and types of ADEs that occurred in a given clinical unit. Can be provided in written or electronic form to a unit. Can help to increase awareness and reduce future errors. A prototype was developed within PSIP.

The experts were then asked to judge whether they feel that each tool can prevent ADEs, and how much they feel the impact could be. The aggregated results of the first round were then fed back to the experts, and each of them could revise his or her opinion in the light of the others opinions. The Delphi study was ended after this second round.

1.3. Future User Survey

Five hospitals or hospital groups from four countries were included in the study; results from three of them are available at the moment and will be reported. We invited 100 physicians from the University Hospitals of Rouen/France, 60 physicians from the hospital of Denain/France and 207 physicians from three hospitals in Copenhagen/ Denmark to complete the survey.

The questionnaire comprised of 15 questions on expectations and fears with regard to medication ordering systems and alerting functionalities. The questionnaire was developed based on items from [10-11] and [12]. A four-point Likert scale was offered for answers. The quesitonnaire was carefully translated into Frensh (in Denmark, the original English items were used). At the time of the study, Rouen did not have a CPOE system, while Denain and the Copenhagen hospitals had a CPOE system with some basic decision-support functionality such as drug-drug interaction checking.

2. Results

2.1. Simulation Study

Overall, 50 data sets are available for analysis (10 participants * 5 patients), half of them being documented by the standard system, the other half with the PSIP system. Each data set is just being analyzed and compared to the pre-defined gold standard that described the optimal clinical reaction (prescription, lab test ordering, and other activities) to the given patient case. Statistical analysis will reveal whether the PSIP group performed differently.

2.2. Expert Delphi Survey

From the 214 invited experts, 69 (32.2%) completed both rounds. The impact of the various solutions as estimated by the experts in the second round is indicated in Table 1. Active alerting, proactive prescription simulation and patient component are estimated to have the highest impact on ADE rates.

2.3. Future User Survey

Overall, we got 41 responses from Rouen (return rate: 41%), 26 responses from Denain (43.3%) and 94 responses from Copenhagen ("Region H") (45.4%). Figure 1 presents selected results.

Table 1. Estimated impact of various solutions on ADE rates (n=69 experts).

Type of solution	**"How many ADEs can be prevented by using the solution?" [%]** median	mean ± standard dev.
External drug information	10.0	11.3 ± 10.3
Passive alerting module	10.0	14.2 ± 9.8
Active alerting modules	25.0	31.2 ± 20.1
Proactive prescription simulation module	25.0	29.3 ± 18.6
Patient component	15.0	18.5 ± 12.4
ADE epidemiology information	10.0	13.1 ± 10.4

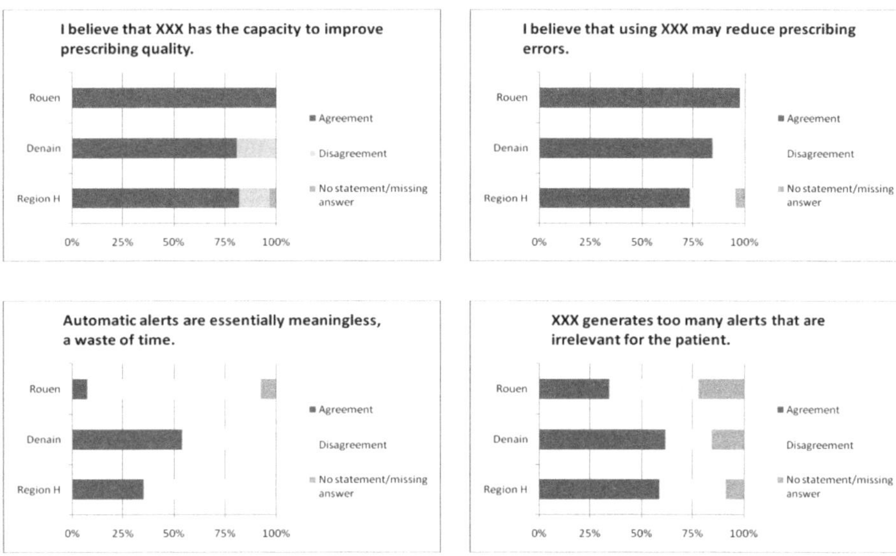

Figure 1. Aggregated answers to the question: "You are using the system XXX at the moment in your hospital to prescribe drugs. Imagine you will get automatic alerts on possible drug-drug-interactions or other drug-related problems in the future. What do you think about this?" (for Region H and Denain) and "Computer-based prescribing systems can offer some supporting functions, such as drug-drug interaction alerts. What do you think about this?" (for Rouen).

3. Discussion

We used a Delphi survey, future user surveys and a simulation study to estimate the impact of PSIP solutions on patient safety. For an international survey, a participation rate for two rounds of around 30% seems quite high. The experts found that maximum benefit can be obtained by an active alerting module and by a proactive prescription simulation module. Active alerting modules have been implemented already in many hospitals, and controlled studies showed their effectiveness to reduce errors and ADEs

[13]. Therefore it is not surprising that experts judge the impact here as rather high. Proactive prescription simulation is a concept developed within the PSIP project and not yet systematically investigated. Experts found this a concept with a potential high impact. Whether this is in fact true is being evaluated in the simulation studies that are just under way.

Third-ranked tool is a patient component that allows the patients to check themselves on possible drug-drug interactions and related problems. These patient components could be part of Personal Health Records (PHRs, see [14]), but will only be successful if these PHRs are integrated with the EHRs systems of the health care providers [15], so that the PHRs have access to up-to-date information on prescriptions, lab values, diagnosis and allergies. Within the PSIP project, a first prototype of a mobile patient component is just being developed and will be evaluated with regard to usability and potential impact in 2011.

In the user surveys, we found that future users are overall optimistic with regard to the impact of automatic alerting during electronic prescribing. Interestingly, users in the hospital with less support during prescribing at the moment, namely the hospital in Rouen, are more optimistic than users of the other hospitals that already have an electronic prescribing tool. In Denain and Region H, more than half of the users find that too many alerts are generated that are irrelevant for the patient. This points to a well-known problem with CPOE systems [16]. PSIP therefore tries to build contextualized decision-support, among others by including epidemiologic data of the given hospitals. Also other options of contextualization have been discussed, see [17] for details.

During the simulation study, we learned that the used PSIP solutions (a new clinical user interface with proactive prescription simulation) was not yet mature enough even for a simulation study. Several technical problems occurred that disturbed running of the simulation. Overall, it seems that there is a kind of logical flow of evaluations: Start with lab studies, focusing on technical issues and usability aspects. Only when the software is mature enough, go into simulation studies to get a feeling of workflow integration, usability and expected impact; only then go into field studies to measure the impact and unexpected consequences. This evaluation process corresponds in fact to the sequence of clinical trials (phase I – phase IV).

Delphi survey, future user surveys and simulation study addressed partly overlapping, partly different aspects; therefore a formal triangulation of results is not possible. However, we found that all three studies brought interesting insight into the expected impact of several of the developed PSIP solutions and PSIP concepts. Future controlled trials on specific interventions will allow verifying and quantifying the effects.

4. Conclusion

We discussed the problem of evaluating the impact of innovative solutions and presented some approaches to address this problem. Active and passive alerting as well as simulation of prescription and patient components all seem to have large potential, but many of these concepts still have to be developed further. We suggest an evaluation sequence consisting of lab studies, simulation studies and field studies, enriched by expert and future user surveys, to address the rising maturity of IT solutions and the corresponding shift in evaluation questions.

Acknowledgments

The research leading to these results has received funding from the European Community's Seventh Framework Programme (FP7/2007-2013) under grant agreement n° 216130 – the PSIP project.

References

[1] J. Schnurrer, J. Frölich, Zur Häufigkeit und Vermeidbarkeit von tödlichen unerwünschten Arzneimittelwirkungen, *Internist* **44** (2003), 889–95.
[2] Patient Safety through Intelligent Procedure in Medicine (PSIP). Available from: http://www.psip-project.eu/, last access on March 2011.
[3] R. Beuscart, W. Hackl, C. Nohr, *Detection and Prevention of Adverse Drug Events - Information Technologies and Human Factors*, IOS Press, Amsterdam, 2009.
[4] V. Koutkias, V. Kilintzis, G. Stalidis, K. Lazou, C. Collyda, E. Chazard, et al., Constructing Clinical Decision Support Systems for Adverse Drug Event Prevention: A Knowledge-based Approach, *AMIA Annu Symp Proc* (2010), 402–6.
[5] E. Ammenwerth, J. Brender, P. Nykänen, H.-U. Prokosch, M. Rigby, J. Talmon, Visions and strategies to improve evaluation of health information systems - reflections and lessons based on the HIS-EVAL workshop in Innsbruck, *Int J Med Inform* **73** (2004), 479–91.
[6] A. Roßnagel, E. Ammenwerth, A. Buchauer, H.-B. Bludau, Simulation Study for the Evaluation of Security Technology, In: G. Müller, K. Rannenberg, editors. Multilateral Security for Global Communication. Bonn: Addison-Wesley; 1999. p. 547–62.
[7] H.A. Linstone, M. Turoff, The Delphi Method: Techniques and Applications, 2002, Available from: http://is.njit.edu/pubs/delphibook/, last access on March 2011.
[8] N.C. Dalkey, The Delphi Method: An Experimental Study of Group Opinion. United States Air Force Project Rand, 1969, Available from: http://www.rand.org/pubs/research_memoranda/RM5888/, last access on March 2011
[9] K.C. Green, J.S. Armstrong, A. Graefe, Methods to Elicit Forecasts from Groups: Delphi and Prediction Markets Compared. Foresight: The International Journal of Applied Forecasting, (Issue 8 Fall 2007), 17–21.
[10] C.P. Hor, J.M. O'Donnell, A.W. Murphy, T. O'Brien, T.J. Kropmans, General practitioners' attitudes and preparedness towards Clinical Decision Support in e-Prescribing (CDS-eP) adoption in the West of Ireland: a cross sectional study, *BMC Med Inform Decis Mak* (2010), 10:2.
[11] D. Magnus, S. Rodgers, A.J. Avery, GPs' views on computerized drug interaction alerts: questionnaire survey, *J Clin Pharm Ther* **27** (2002), 377–82.
[12] Y. Ko et al., Practitioners' views on computerized drug-drug interaction alerts in the VA system, *J Am Med Inform Assoc* **14** (2007), 56–64.
[13] E. Ammenwerth, P. Schnell-Inderst, C. Machan, U. Siebert, The Effect of Electronic Prescribing on Medication Errors and Adverse Drug Events: A Systematic Review, *J Am Med Inform Assoc* **15** (2008), 585–600.
[14] D.C. Kaelber, A.K. Jha, D. Johnston, B. Middleton, D.W. Bates, A research agenda for personal health records (PHRs), *J Am Med Inform Assoc* **15** (2008), 729–36.
[15] D. Detmer, M. Bloomrosen, B. Raymond, P. Tang, Integrated personal health records: transformative tools for consumer-centric care, *BMC Med Inform Decis Mak* (2008), 8:45.
[16] H. van der Sijs, J. Aarts, A. Vulto, M. Berg, Overriding of drug safety alerts in computerized physician order entry, *J Am Med Inform Assoc* **13** (2006), 138–47.
[17] D. Riedmann, M. Jung, W.O. Hackl, W. Stühlinger, H. van der Sijs, E. Ammenwerth, A context model to prioritize drug safety alerts in CPOE systems: Development and validation of a context factor model, *BMC Med Inform Decis Mak* (2011), submitted..

Patient Safety Informatics
V. Koutkias et al. (Eds.)
IOS Press, 2011

doi:10.3233/978-1-60750-740-6-234

Scorecards: A New Method to Prevent Adverse Drug Events? Preliminary Results from a Clinical Field Study

Romaric MARCILLY [a,1], Werner O. HACKL [b], Michel LUYCKX [c,d] and Elske AMMENWERTH [b]

[a] *INSERM CIC-IT Evalab, CHU Lille, UDSL EA2694, Univ Lille Nord de France, F-59000 Lille, France*
[b] *Institute for Health Information Systems, UMIT – University for Health Sciences, Medical Informatics and Technology, Hall in Tyrol, Austria*
[c] *Faculté des Sciences Pharmaceutiques et Biologiques, UDSL2, Univ Lille Nord de France, F-59000 Lille, France*
[d] *Centre Hospitalier de Denain, France*

Abstract. In the field of the detection and prevention of preventable ADEs, several methods have been explored to decrease the rate of ADEs due to monitoring errors. This paper describes an innovative method that aims at improving patient safety by increasing ADEs' awareness of healthcare professionals. To this end, ADE-scorecards that provide healthcare professionals with retrospective data about ADEs' causes and rates have been developed. In order to evaluate the impact of this method on the ADE rate, in-field clinical tests have been set up. Data were collected by both qualitative (semi-structured interviews) and quantitative methods (log analysis and ADE rate calculation). Preliminary results reveal that ADE-scorecards are well-accepted by most of the healthcare professionals who intend to use them as discussion supports and/or learning tools. Thus, ADE-scorecards seem to be a relevant method to improve patient safety by increasing ADE-awareness of healthcare professionals.

Keywords. Scorecards, adverse drug events, monitoring errors, in-field clinical study

Introduction

Adverse Drug Events (ADEs) are a major public health issue: they endanger patients' safety (by causing or increasing risk for comorbidity or mortality) [1] and instigate significant extra hospital costs (by lengthening patients' stay and involving extra treatments) [2, 3]. Healthcare organizations worldwide are focusing upon their reduction.

[1] Corresponding Author: romaric.marcilly@univ-lille2.fr

Scientific Background

The European Union FP7 project entitled "PSIP - Patient Safety through Intelligent Procedures in medication" [4, 5] aims - amongst others - at reducing preventable ADEs characterized according to the NCCMERP taxonomy as "monitoring errors" [6]. The subset of ADEs targeted by the PSIP project includes Drug-Drug Interaction, Drug-Disease Interaction, and inadequate monitoring of clinical parameters or lab values (e.g. serum electrolytes, blood clotting parameters, blood pressure). The study in hand introduces the Human Factors' view of an intervention, so called ADE-scorecards, aiming at reducing preventable ADEs' rates and reports first results from a first field test with these ADE-scorecards.

In order to be able to prevent ADEs, the first necessary step is to detect them and especially to pitch on preventable events. Basically, there are two main detection methods, namely the voluntary safety reporting systems on one hand and the chart review on the other. The voluntary safety reporting systems consist in the form-based documentation of the potential ADE characteristics (including causes) by the physician, the nurse or the pharmacist who recognized the event (e.g. cf. [7]). This allows understanding how an event occurred (e.g. the patient got the wrong medication because he was not correctly identified). The information gathered with this method is mainly socio-technical and the registered ADE-causes are mainly organizational factors. Thus, the capable prevention methods following from voluntary safety reporting systems are mainly interventions aiming at consolidating and securing the medications' use process.

The second method used, the chart review, consists in a manual or a computerized reviewing of medical charts by healthcare professionals who are especially trained to ADE detection and prevention [8]. During the manual review process, the professionals look at a large amount of charts and search for events that could be potential ADEs caused by, for instance, drug-drug interactions, contradictions or overdoses. In the computerized review process, digitalized data are used to identify in patients' charts a signal that suggests the possible presence of an event; then, a professional goes to the chart to investigate this event further. Thus, the chart review method allows catching medical/pharmacological causes of ADEs. Consequently, the prevention measures carried out to counteract the ADEs detected with this method is to provide healthcare professionals with medical/pharmacological information about ADEs, for instance, through Clinical Decision Support Systems (CDSS).

Rationale for the Study

As well as catching only one type of causes of preventable ADEs (i.e. organizational ones for voluntary safety reporting systems and medical ones for chart review), both types of detection/prevention methods get use's limits. Voluntary safety reporting systems underestimate the actual number of ADEs (underreporting) [9]. Chart review methods are either performed manually and therefore are very time-consuming or require computerized data what could be cumbersome to get and use. Moreover, preventing ADEs by alerting healthcare professionals through CDSS is often problematic as alerts can be too intrusive, unspecific, or even disturbing and can cause "alert fatigue" which often results in alert overriding or deactivation of the alerting system [10, 11].

The PSIP project is interested in the medical causes of the ADEs; it falls in the second type of methods. It aims to:

- Innovatively produce knowledge on ADEs by performing automatic screening (by data- and semantic-mining methods) on patients' medical records. This method allows identifying within hospitals, their number, their type, their consequences and their causes.
- Investigate innovative possibilities for reducing ADEs' rates by developing systems using Human Factors engineering: the information gathered from the screening are not used only to provide healthcare professionals with ADEs' alerts. Other ways of prevention are explored.

One of the innovative ways explored to reduce ADEs' rates is a yet unexplored (at least, not reported in the literature) method. It consists in delivering to healthcare professionals monthly statistics about a particular set of ADEs in their own department, in the form of ADE-scorecards.

Scorecards are long-used in economics sciences and in various areas of industry and healthcare to support strategic management decisions [12]. In the context of ADE-prevention, scorecards could allow raising the awareness of the professionals about the ADEs' issue amongst their patients and acquainting them with their characteristics (causes, epidemiology etc.). As a result, scorecards could support identifying and undertaking strategies for reducing ADEs' occurrence.

Objectives of the Study

The objective of this paper is to investigate the impact of ADE-scorecards on healthcare teams' awareness of ADEs' issues in their own department and ultimately on the actual ADE rate. A clinical field study was set up to answer the following study questions:

- Q1: Do the clinicians, nurses and pharmacists use the scorecards (how often, why/why not, in which occasions and settings)?
- Q2: Do the users expect a benefit for patient safety due to ADE-scorecards? How? Do they intend to use them?
- Q3: Does the usage of ADE-scorecards in a clinical department lead to a change of ADE rates in this department?

1. Study Context

1.1. The ADE-scorecards

The ADE-scorecards' aim is to provide healthcare professionals (e.g. physicians, head nurses, nurses, pharmacists and may be quality management) with detailed information about the ADE cases (type and cause of ADEs, statistics) that occurred previously in their department in order to help them learn about how to avoid such ADEs in the future. Automatic Data Mining procedures [13] are applied to the hospital's Electronic Health Record (EHR) data gathered into a common data model [14] on a regular basis in order to determine the key figures on ADEs per hospital units (e.g. conditions leading the ADEs appearance). Thus, the ADE-scorecard website grants access to the scorecards with statistics on occurrences of 65 different classes of ADEs[2] (for a technical description [15]).

1.2. Interface Design and Development

The design of the scorecards results from a collaborative and iterative user-centered design process [16] involving healthcare professionals, epidemiologists, computer specialists, website developers and ergonomists. From the beginning of this work, an ergonomist was integrated in the designers-developers team to support cooperative design. Moreover, a sample of end users (4 physicians, 2 pharmacists, 3 head nurses, 6 nurses, 1 health care quality manager), were involved at different steps in the design by commenting on the mock-ups and the prototype, choosing features among parallel versions, and proposing new features and/or facilities. This design process aimed at ensuring that main users' needs were matched by the scorecards and that the developed interface was as usable as possible.

1.3. "Synthesis and Edition of detailed statistics" Page

By logging in, users are identified and thus, the interface's language is automatically adapted and only the user's department data are displayed. The first page the users meet is the "Synthesis and Edition of detailed statistics" page that contains (see Figure 1):

- A table/chart displaying the number of each detected ADEs' kind per month.
- A drop-down menu allowing to choose the displayed period of ADE statistics. A change in this menu immediately changes the data displayed in the previous table/chart.
- Next to every adverse effect's name, check boxes allow selecting the effects for which detailed ADE-scorecards pages will be generated.

1.4. "Detailed statistics" Page

For each selected ADE, an ADE-scorecard is generated which presents (see Figure 2):

- The characteristics of identified stays that describe the sample of stays presenting the adverse effect, including: number of patients concerned, average age, gender proportions, proportions of diseases that might have impact on ADEs (e.g. alcoholism, cancers, renal insufficiency) and the death rate (these deaths are not necessarily due to the adverse effect).
- The conditions (patients' conditions, administered drugs) potentially leading to an ADE with the confidence of association (percentage of stays for which the event occurs among the stays meeting the conditions), the median appearance delay (from the moment when all conditions of the rule are met, the period from which over 50% of events appeared) and the number of stays targeted.

[2] 65 ADE classes were defined, but up to now "only" 27 classes have been detected and, 21 classes have been detected during the time of this study in the test departments (cf. Table 2 for a list of those classes).

- A chart representing the distribution of the number of ADEs per month during the current year and a histogram displaying the median delay of appearance of the ADEs.
- Description of the conditions, which may contain a longer description of the rules, scientific explanations and references, and advice.
- Access to a synthetic view of the patients' record using an EHR visualization tool named "Expert Explorer" [17].This tool allows displaying closed stays' data in a visual, comprehensive and anonymized way through 8 tabs: stay (e.g. the age, the gender), steps (the medical units the patient went through), procedures, diagnoses, lab results (in tabular and charts forms), the administered drugs (in tabular and charts forms), a parallel view of lab results' and administered drugs' charts and the documents enclosed to the record.

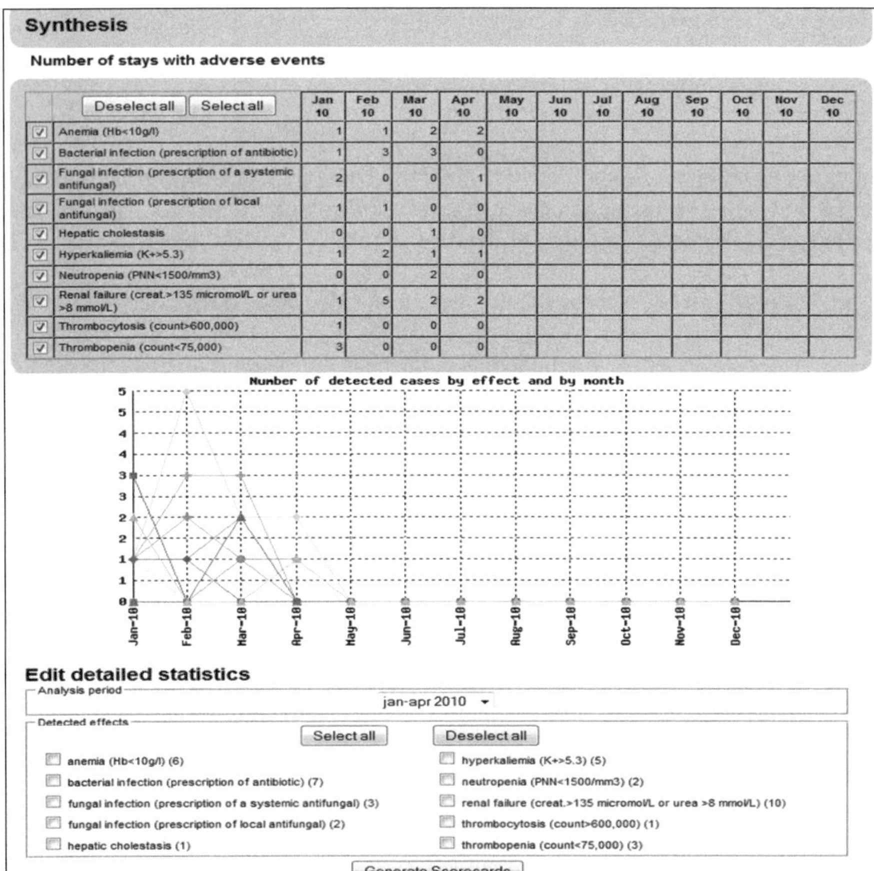

Deselect all / Select all	Jan 10	Feb 10	Mar 10	Apr 10	May 10	Jun 10	Jul 10	Aug 10	Sep 10	Oct 10	Nov 10	Dec 10
Anemia (Hb<10g/l)	1	1	2	2								
Bacterial infection (prescription of antibiotic)	1	3	3	0								
Fungal infection (prescription of a systemic antifungal)	2	0	0	1								
Fungal infection (prescription of local antifungal)	1	1	0	0								
Hepatic cholestasis	0	0	1	0								
Hyperkaliemia (K+>5.3)	1	2	1	1								
Neutropenia (PNN<1500/mm3)	0	0	2	0								
Renal failure (creat.>135 micromol/L or urea >8 mmol/L)	1	5	2	2								
Thrombocytosis (count>600,000)	1	0	0	0								
Thrombopenia (count<75,000)	3	0	0	0								

Figure 1. Screenshot of "Synthesis and Edition of detailed statistics" page.

2. Methodology

The in-field clinical test runs in a northern France 413-bed hospital and involves five wards (3 test wards and 2 control wards) and the hospital's central pharmacy.

2.1. Study Design

In order to answer the 3 study questions a combination of qualitative and quantitative study modules was designed. To study the impact of the ADE-scorecards on ADE rates (Q3) a quasi experimental field study with controlled intervention (=introduction of ADE-scorecards) on the variables monthly ADE rates (detected by the PSIP approach) investigated before and after the implementation of the ADE scorecards was chosen.

Log file analyses and qualitative, semi-structured interviews are conducted to answer study questions Q1, Q2.

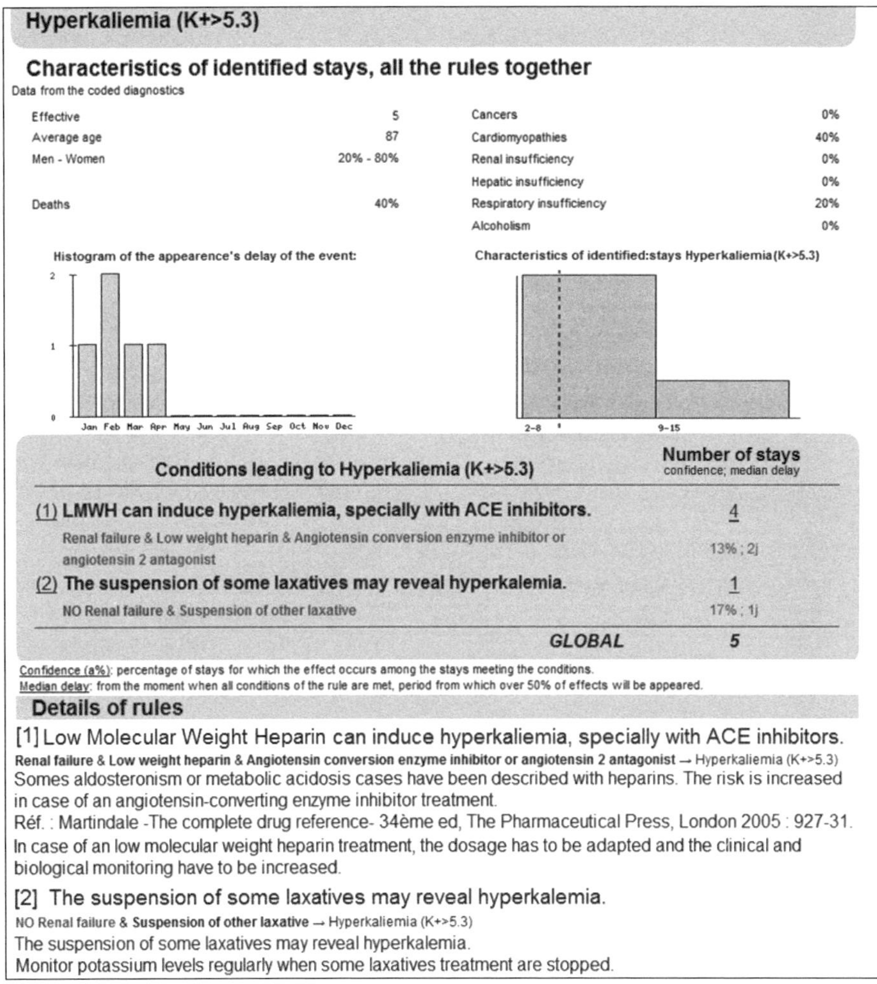

Figure 2. Screenshot excerpts of the "Detailed statistics" page.

2.2. Participants and Study Flow

In the test wards, scorecards were accessible to physicians but also (head) nurses and pharmacists as they are also fully involved in the drugs' management process. In each department, the same volunteers as in the design phase of the ADE-scorecards (except the quality manager) were involved (cf. Table 1). The scorecards give them access to the ADEs information concerning their own department; pharmacists get access to all three test departments' scorecards as they are involved in the drugs' management process of all medical wards.

Every user gets unlimited access to the ADE-scorecards. Additionally, the users are encouraged to consult at least a set of ADEs defined by the head physician of their department (cf. Table 1). At the beginning of the study in late June 2010, scorecards contained ADEs information for the four firsts months of 2010 and for all 2009, 2008 and 2007. Then, about every two months, users get informed of the upload of new ADEs' information in the scorecards.

Table 1. Description of the departments and practitioners participating.

Departments	**Involved healthcare professionals**	**Number of beds (approx. number of patients/year)**	**Effects of special interest (self defined)**
Department A	2 physicians, 1 head-nurse, 3 nurses	13 (out of 25) (1,340)	Hyperkaliemia Renal failure VKA overdose
Department B	1 physician, 1 head-nurse, 2 nurses	25 (800)	All
Department C	1 physician, 1 head-nurse, 1 nurse	10 (390)	All (especially interested in renal failure)
Control Department A	none	30 (880)	Ø
Control Department B	none	56 (1,500)	Ø
Pharmacy	2 pharmacists	n.a. (5,000)	All

Furthermore, to ensure that users will look at the new information at least once, two kinds of meetings of "scorecards' presentation" are organized at the beginning of the study and then after each upload:

- Physicians/pharmacists meetings animated by ergonomists and a physician (from another hospital) involved in the PSIP project.
- Head-nurses/nurses meetings animated by ergonomists.

These meetings have been negotiated three months before the beginning of the field test with physicians, pharmacists and (head) nurses. It was an occasion for them to look at examples of scorecards data and at PSIP information.

2.3. Data Collection and Analysis

Qualitative and quantitative data have been collected. During the meetings with the users semi-structured interviews were conducted and recorded using an audio recorder. The semi-structured interviews dealt with different topics: participants' current need of information about the ADEs occurring in the medical units, their consideration of the ADE-scorecards (how to use it), their feeling about the opportunity of using this tool to prevent/manage ADEs and their intention to use it.

Meetings with physicians and pharmacists permitted observing discussions between them and the "PSIP physician" about the information displayed and the details of the stays where patients encountered ADEs. From the second round of meetings information about the scorecards' use (Q1) were also documented.

Log files were recorded to know who was using the Web-based ADE-scorecards (e.g. physicians, nurses, pharmacists), when and more precisely which ADEs' page was accessed. Only the connections followed by an action on the ADE-scorecards website (e.g. change of page or of analysis period) were considered. Amongst them, we counted only logs separated by 60 minutes to avoid considering connections following technical disconnections.

Finally, to observe whether scorecards' implementation impacts on ADEs' rates, these rates were calculated as described in [13]. They allow two comparisons: (i) numbers of ADEs in the involved wards before against after the implementation of the ADE-scorecards and (ii) the evolution of the numbers of ADE in the involved wards against control ones.

3. Results

The introduction of the ADE-scorecards in three study wards started in late June 2010. The in-field clinical study being running since 5 months only, it is too soon to perform an interrupted time-series analysis on the evolution of the ADE rates and to get concrete answers to study question Q3 by now. Thus, only results related to the users' considerations about the ADE-scorecards and their use of this tool (study questions Q1, Q2) are presented hereinafter.

3.1. Usage of the Scorecards

From the start of the introduction of ADE-Scorecards on the 24th of June 2010 to the 8th of December 2010, a total of 69 connections shared out between the different medical units and groups of professionals. Nurses and head nurses in the study wards connected to the scorecards 31 times, physicians 8 times and the pharmacists consulted the scorecards in 30 cases. Pharmacists are looking at the ADE-scorecards more than the other professionals. Moreover, they looked at each and every ADE-scorecard available (23 out of the 23 that appeared in 2010) even if they looked more often at some effects (too high INR, renal failure, hyperkaliemia, bacterial infection and hyponatremia) than at others as depicted in Table 2.

No major differences were observed across the departments as for the nurses. Indeed, the differences of numbers of consultations are easily explained by the size of the units and the number of professionals involved (cf. Table 1). Moreover, even if they did not look at each and every ADEs' information available, they consulted a rather wide range of them. Finally, in the three departments, nurses expressed that ADE-scorecards could be useful to improve medications' management if it allows discussing with physicians.

On the contrary, as for the physicians, behaviors of use of the ADE-scorecards vary across the medical departments according to:

- **The actual consultation of the scorecards by the physicians**: outside any "scorecards presentation" meeting, while one physician consulted four times the ADE-scorecards (C), another one consulted them only once (B). The number of consultations is not related to the size of the department nor to the number of physicians involved. It seems rather that this difference comes from the physicians' interest in this tool: indeed, the physician who consulted the more the ADE-scorecards expressed a lot of interest in the scorecards (in terms of information about potential causes) while the one who consulted them once expressed that "retrospective data are not useful" to prevent ADEs.

Table 2. Prevalence of ADEs detected between January and June 2010 and number of consultations of the ADE-scorecards' pages related to the 21 classes of ADEs detected during the test time (as of 12-08/2010), according to the departments and the kind of healthcare professionals.

Effects	**Department A**			**Department B**			**Department C**			**Pharmacy**	
		nb of cons.			**nb of cons.**			**nb of cons.**			**nb of cons.**
	Prevalence	Nurses & Head Nurse	Physicians	Prevalence	Nurses & Head Nurse	Physicians	Prevalence	Nurses & Head Nurse	Physicians	Overall prevalence	Pharmacists
Anemia	4	3	4	3	5	0	1	3	7	8	12
Bacterial infection	8	1	1	14	0	0	1	0	4	23	16
Fungal infection (presc. of systemic antifungal)	2	0	0	4	0	0	3	0	1	9	5
Fungal infection (presc. of local antifungal)	0	0	0	1	0	0	2	0	3	3	4
Hemorrhage (presc. of hemostatic)	1	1	1	8	1	0	1	1	1	10	8
Heparin overdose	0	0	0	1	1	0	0	2	0	1	1
Hepatic cholestasis	0	0	2	9	1	0	2	2	4	11	5
Hepatic cytolysis	2	0	0	4	0	0	0	0	0	6	5
High a CPK rate	2	3	3	2	1	0	0	0	0	4	1
Hypereosinophilia	0	0	0	2	1	0	0	0	0	2	4
Hyperkalemia	22	8	11	11	8	0	9	4	13	42	21
Hypocalcemia	1	1	2	2	1	0	0	0	0	3	1
Hypokalemia	1	1	3	0	0	0	1	1	3	2	1
Hyponatremia	3	0	0	0	0	0	1	2	3	4	29
Increase of pancreatic enzymes	2	0	0	0	0	0	0	0	0	2	1
Neutropenia	0	0	0	1	4	0	0	0	0	1	1
Renal failure	26	1	1	18	4	1	9	1	5	53	25
Thrombocytosis	2	0	0	7	0	0	1	0	1	10	5
Thrombopenia	7	0	1	6	1	0	3	1	1	16	10
VKA overdose (presc. of vit K)	1	0	0	8	0	0	1	1	3	10	6
VKA overdose (INR>4.9)	11	5	6	10	1	0	1	0	2	22	27
Sum	95	24	35	111	29	1	36	18	51	242	188

- **The discussion about the information contained in the scorecards between nurses and physicians**: such discussions took place in only one department (C) even if nurses in other departments expressed their interest in discussing ADE information with physicians.

3.2. Users' Considerations about the Scorecards

Almost all (except one) physicians and pharmacists expressed that the display of information about the ADEs' statistics is useful for them to get a global and actual representation of the ADEs' prevalence in their respective units.

The detailed information was also appreciated by them and also by (head) nurses because some of the ADEs' causes were either known but not in mind ("it allows to have in mind some adverse effects of medications"), or unknown (e.g. nurses ignored that antibiotics increased the effect of vitamin K antagonists (VKA) on INR (international normalized ratio), and a physician ignored low-molecular-weight heparin could cause hyperkaliemia). In this way, professionals considered the scorecards as a learning-supporting/knowledge refreshment tool that could be also used to teach ADEs to medical and nursing trainees.

During the interviews, 11 participants out of the 13 answered to every topic tackled. All in all, 10 out of 11 participants said that ADE-scorecards could help them to prevent ADEs' appearance. The last participant would prefer to get alerts upon ADEs through a CDSS, which is compatible with the scorecards method. Nonetheless, every participant expressed his/her intention to use the ADE-scorecards in an ADEs' prevention approach.

4. Discussion

This paper aimed at describing an innovative intervention to reduce preventable ADEs related through an innovative way of ADEs' prevention consisting in delivering to healthcare professionals monthly statistics ADEs in the form of ADE-scorecards. The impact of such an intervention (in terms of patient safety improvement and healthcare teams' awareness of ADEs') as been studied the last five months in the clinical field. During this period, data that ADE-scorecards contain have been actualized twice and two rounds of "presentations meetings" have been performed.

4.1. Answers to Study Questions

ADE-scorecards have been used by almost all involved physicians and nurses in the three test departments and by pharmacists. Scorecards are used by healthcare professionals as a punctual source of information. Indeed, they consider the ADE-scorecards as a learning-supporting/knowledge refreshment tool for trainees as well as for themselves because it displayed innovative knowledge adapted to the medical unit clinical context. Moreover, healthcare professionals consider also ADE-scorecards as a tool supporting the dialogue between the different kinds of professionals involved in the medications' use process (pharmacist-physician and nurse-physician discussions).

Overall, ADE-scorecards allow healthcare professionals to be informed and aware of the ADEs' prevalence in their wards. This has been highlighted by most of the participants as a major benefit from the scorecards. The perceived utility of the ADE-scorecards is clearly expressed by most of the users. Consequently, all participants said that they would use the scorecards in an ADEs' prevention approach.

Due to the short duration of the study, the actual impact of ADE-scorecards' on ADEs' rate and on medical practices remains unknown for now. Indeed, changes in medical practices takes time to be implemented and cannot be observed after 5 months. In addition, the in-field clinical study method needs to take a step back to observe an actual impact over time. Thus, 5 months back is not a sufficient period to clearly assess of an impact of the scorecards neither on the medical practices, nor on the ADEs rates. More time is needed for such as study to check whether ADE-scorecards are an efficient tool to allow decreasing the rate of ADEs by improving healthcare professionals' ADEs-awareness.

4.2. Strengths and Weaknesses of the Study

One of the most important points of the study in hand is its innovative topic: it is the first time in the literature, at our knowledge, that the impact of the use of ADE-scorecards by healthcare professionals is evaluated and reported. Moreover, the study design, by combining qualitative and quantitative study modules, allows gathering different kinds of information about ADE-scorecards' use from complementary points of view (e.g. behavioral, considerations, ADEs rate). This mixed methodology allows getting a comprehensive view of the different issues related to ADE-scorecards' implementation.

However, one of these study modules (semi-structured interviews) implied to organize regular "scorecards presentation" meetings: thanks to them, we could gather feelings of the users and we ensured that they looked at the scorecards at least once. Now, these interventions surely influenced the participants as well as ADE-scorecards. They may have increased their ADEs-awareness. Thus, the respective impacts of the ADE-scorecards implementation and of the presentation meetings are closely intertwined. So, results' interpretation could not attribute potential changes in ADEs' rates and medical practices to the only ADE-scorecards. In order to observe pure impact of the ADE-scorecards another study without any intervention of PSIP physicians and ergonomists is under preparation in another hospital. Another potential bias is related to the fact that the participants were already involved in the design of the ADE-scorecards. Even if they did not see information about the ADEs' rates and causes for their own medical unit, their awareness of the ADEs issue could have been increased before the actual beginning of the study.

5. Conclusion

Even if the study in hand is still running, preliminary results show that ADE-scorecards could be a useful tool to increase the healthcare professionals' awareness of the ADEs' issue in their own department and thus to increase the safety of their own patients.

Acknowledgments

The research leading to these results has received funding from the European Community's Seventh Framework Programme (FP7/2007-2013) under grant agreement n° 216130 – the PSIP project.

The authors would like to acknowledge every healthcare professionals (physicians, nurses, head nurses and pharmacists) and technicians whose involvement made completion of this study possible.

References

[1] J.U. Schnurrer, J.C. Frölich, [Incidence and prevention of lethal undesirable drug effects], *Internist* **44** (1993), 889–95.
[2] D.W. Bates, N. Spell, D.J. Cullen, E. Burdick, N. Laird, L.A. Petersen, S.D. Small, B.J. Sweitzer, L.L. Leape, The costs of adverse drug events in hospitalized patients. Adverse Drug Events Prevention Study Group, *Journal of the American Medical Association* **277** (1997), 307–11.
[3] D.C. Classen, S.L. Pestotnik, R.S. Evans, J.F. Lloyd, J.P. Burke, Adverse drug events in hospitalized patients, Excess length of stay, extra costs, and attributable mortality, *JAMA* **277** (1997), 301–6.
[4] R. Beuscart, W. Hackl, C. Nøhr, *Detection and prevention of adverse drug events: information technologies and human factors*, IOS Press, Amsterdam, 2009.
[5] Patient Safety by Intelligent Procedures in medication, http://www.psip-project.eu/, last access on March 2011.
[6] National Coordinating Council for Medication Error Reporting and Prevention, NCC MERP: The First Ten Years "Defining the Problem and Developing Solutions". 2005. 23-5-2009.
[7] Association pour l'Assurance Qualité en Thérapeutique et l'Evaluation, http://www.adiph.asso.fr/aaqte/FormulaireREEM.pdf, last access on March 2011.
[8] A.K. Jha, G.J. Kuperman, J.M. Teich, L. Leape, B. Shea, E. Rittenberg, E. Burdick, D.L. Seger, M. Vander Vliet, D.W. Bates, Identifying adverse drug events: development of a computer-based monitor and comparison with chart review and stimulated voluntary report, *J Am Med Inform Assoc* **5** (1998), 305–14.
[9] S.A. Edlavitch, Adverse drug event reporting, Improving the low US reporting rates, *Arch Intern Med* **148** (1998), 1499–503.
[10] H. van der Sijs, J. Aarts, T. van Gelder, M. Berg, A. Vulto, Turning off frequently overridden drug alerts: limited opportunities for doing it safely, *J Am Med Inform Assoc* **15** (2008), 439–48.
[11] H. van der Sijs, A. Mulder, T. van Gelder, J. Aarts, M. Berg, A. Vulto, Drug safety alert generation and overriding in a large Dutch university medical centre, *Pharmacoepidemiol Drug Saf* **18** (2009), 941–7.
[12] R.S. Kaplan, D.P. Norton, The balanced scorecard--measures that drive performance, *Harv Bus Rev* **70** (1992), 71–9.
[13] E. Chazard, G. Ficheur, B. Merlin, M. Genin, C. Preda, R. Beuscart, Detection of Adverse Drug Events Detection : Data Agregation and Data Mining, *Stud Health Technol Inform* **148** (2009), 75–84.
[14] E. Chazard, B. Merlin, G. Ficheur, J.C. Sarfati, R. Beuscart, Detection of Adverse Drug Events: Proposal of a Data Model, *Stud Health Technol Inform* **148** (2009), 63–74.
[15] E. Chazard, A. Băceanu, G. Ficheur, R. Marcilly, R. Beuscart, Les «ADEs Scorecards», un outil de détection et de visualisation des effets indésirables liés aux médicaments, Proceedings Journées Francophones d'Informatique Médicale, Tunis, 2011.
[16] International Standards Organisation,. *Human centered design processes for interactive systems (Rep. No. ISO 13407)* (1999), International Standards Organisation, Geneva, 1999.
[17] A. Băceanu, I. Atasiei, E. Chazard, N. Leroy, The Expert Explorer: A Tool for Hospital Data Visualization and Adverse Drug Event Rules Validation, *Stud Health Technol Inform* **148** (2009), 85–94.

Patient Safety Informatics
V. Koutkias et al. (Eds.)
IOS Press, 2011

doi:10.3233/978-1-60750-740-6-246

Assessment of Three Systems to Empower the Patient and Decrease the Risk of Adverse Drug Events

Kitta LAWTON [a,1] and Peter SKJOET [b]
[a] *The Capital Region of Denmark, Department of Health IT*
[b] *Capital Region of Denmark, Unit for Patient Safety*

Abstract. One way to reduce adverse drug events (ADEs) is to empower the patient to participate in the control of medication. This empowerment can be supported in different ways by making knowledge and information available to the patient. This study examines the usefulness and safety of two different systems on the background of a paper-based medication list presenting prescribed medicine presently used in hospitals in Copenhagen. Each of the systems examined aims to reduce ADEs but presents information in different levels of detail, and anticipates different level of prior knowledge from the patient: a Web-based prototype presenting medication, lab-results and alerts, and a cell phone-based prototype presenting alerts. Six patients were introduced to each of the systems by performing small tasks and subsequently interviewed. The patients found the paper-based medication list useful and comprehensive for control of own prescribed medication. The Web-based prototype also proved to be useful, but drug and lab values were hard to correlate, and the alerts were hard to understand. The cell phone-based prototype proved less useful as the patients were challenged to vision the applicability of the system. Furthermore, it is a safety issue that the information the alert is based upon, stems from the patient alone. We conclude that, in order for the Web-based system as well as the cell phone system to empower patient and increase patient safety, further development of the systems is necessary.

Keywords. Patient empowerment, adverse drug event, patient safety, usability, usefulness

Introduction

Throughout the process from the doctor's prescription to the patient's intake of the drug there are several possibilities for Adverse Events. A report from the Danish National Board of Health states that approximately half the reported ADEs are due to events involving drugs [1]. In acknowledgement of challenges with ADEs due to drugs the European project Patient Safety through Intelligent Procedures (PSIP) [2] was launched in January 2008. Several prototypes have been developed in this project ranging from decision support modules for use by the doctor during prescription to a module on the patient's cell phone.

---

1 Corresponding Author: kitta.lawton@regionh.dk

The involvement of the patient in the process through mediated interaction with their own patient-specific information is one way in which to decrease ADEs while empowering the patient to play an active part in the management of their own health.

Health-IT aimed at informing and empowering the patient is not new; Netdoktor.dk is a Website that enables the patient to search for general information and place questions in the facilitated forum. Sundhed.dk is another Danish Website that also contains general information on health, but at which the patient can obtain access to her/her personal specific data about treatment, prescriptions, diagnosis etc. The two PSIP prototypes evaluated in this paper differentiate from those Websites by their dynamic and contextualized qualities that have the possibility to eliminate some ADEs. However, new ways of interacting with information could instigate new risks for ADEs.

This paper presents an assessment conducted at Hvidovre Hospital, Copenhagen Denmark, in order to extract information concerning the usefulness and issues of patient safety of the two PSIP patient modules. In the assessment we touch on usability, but have not conducted a full scale usability evaluation on the modules.

1. Method and Materials

1.1. Study Objectives and Setup

The overall objective of the study was to evaluate the usefulness and safety of the two patient modules. Through interviews we investigated the patient's response to three different systems aimed at providing information about drugs to the patient; the two PSIP patient modules, and a paper medicine list, which is presently used, and well known to patients in the Capital Region in Denmark. The data collection and analysis focused on three aspects of the systems:

- The meaningfulness: Does the patient understand how s/he can benefit of the system? And does the system provide the patient with information and knowledge that would inform her/his use of drugs?
- Patient safety: Does the information the patient receive from the systems have any potential impact on her/his behavior? Does the information in the system decrease or increase the risk or mistakes? [3].
- Usability: Were the functionality of the system clear and easy to understand? The usability evaluation focused on aspects like match between real world and system, consistency, standards and recognition [4].

The interviews were conducted in combination of a think-aloud-test and a presentation of the three different systems following each other. The interview was semi structured and focused on the objectives above and lasted for an hour. All interviews were taped.

Each patient would fill a short questionnaire regarding age and routine with IT and cell phones before the interview. At the end of each interview, we asked the patients to indicate the applicability of each of the three systems on a five-point scale. Immediately after the interview we performed an instant data analysis, in order to collect and document the participant's opinions regarding the three systems [5].

We included the paper-based medication list in order to provide a starting point for interviews about the usefulness of medicine information, as well as to obtain data about patient's present use of the paper-based medication list.

Relying on key literature on the number of test subjects for usability evaluation [6], we interviewed six outpatients in treatment with anticoagulants, represented by two men and four women, aged between 56 and 77. One must bear in mind, however, that while the limited number of test subjects would be satisfactory for a usability evaluation as well as for this preliminary assessment, a further investigation into development areas might require a higher number of test subjects.

One of the patient never used computers, and two did not use cell phones. The rest of the patients were experienced with the different uses of the Internet. Of the four cell phone users, three would use SMS as well as calls.

1.2. The Systems

The two PSIP modules (Web-module and cell phone-module) and the paper-based medication list represent three types of information about medicine to the patient, differentiating in proposed usage, level of personalization and expectation of patient's prior knowledge:

The paper-based medication list is printed from the medicine module at the hospitals in the Capital Region, and given to the patient at discharge from hospital or during hospitalization. It lists the different drugs that are prescribed to the patient, their dosage, frequency of intake, the route of administration and indication, as shown in Figure 1. It lists no side effects or possible ADEs, and it gives no indication of whether the medicine has been taken as prescribed. It is a plan for the patient to comply to.

Diovan 80 mg filmovertrukne tabl.		/ Stine Maria Rosenstrøm
Fast:		(Start: 20.10.10 18:06)
Kl.	**08:00**	
Dosis	1 stk.	
Indikation: **for blodtrykket**		
Administrationsvej: **Oral anvendelse**		
Simvastatin "Actavis" 40 mg filmovertrukne tabl.		/ Stine Maria Rosenstrøm
Fast:		(Start: 20.10.10 18:07)
Kl.	**22:00**	

Figure 1. Example of the paper-based medication list containing two drugs. For each drug is listed: Drug name and strength, and name of the health professional that approved the medication. Prescription date, administration time and dosage. Indication "concerning blood pressure". Route of administration "oral use". Often the paper-based medication list will proceed to numerous sheets of paper in order to encompass the amount of different drugs prescribed to the patient.

The Web-based patient module is designed for the hospitalized patients and outpatients, and gives the patient a day-to-day view of which drugs s/he has been taken, as well as her/his lab-results during hospitalization/consultation, as shown in Figures 2 and 3.

The cell phone patient module is accessible through the Internet at an Android cell phone [7]. The cell phone module does not access information about the patient, and identification is therefore not required. The patient enters her/his age, scans the barcode of the drug s/he is about to take, and provides input about drugs which s/he has been taken during the last 5 days, as well as her/his diagnosis and information about her/his lab-related conditions. This accumulates to general alerts specific to her/his age and condition, and presents a link to further information about the drug which might cause the event.

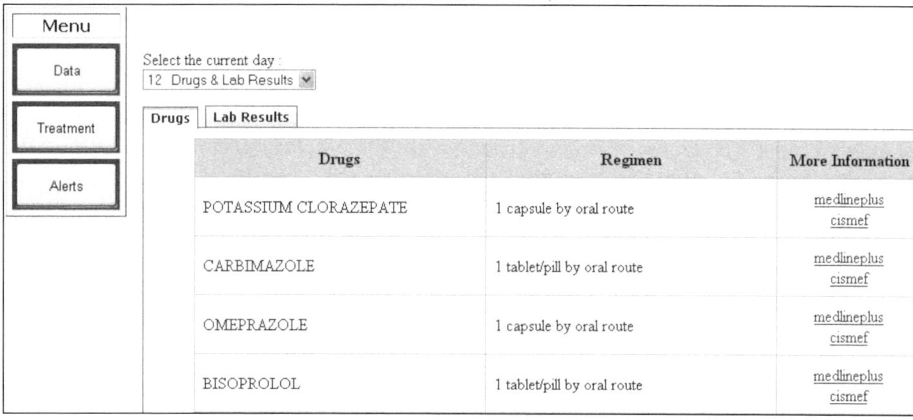

Figure 2. The medication list presents the drugs which the patient has taken at the specific day (day 12) and route of administration. "More information" gives access to a Website with generic information about medicinal products.

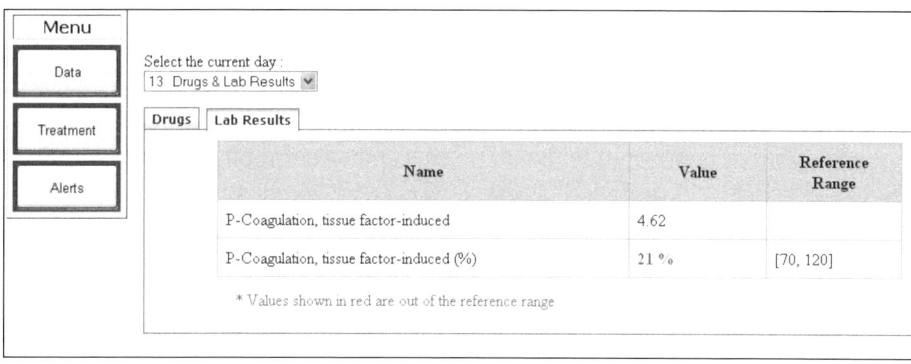

Figure 3. Lab-results presents the patients tests and their results at the specific day (day 79), as well as the frame of reference. Values are presented in red, where the patient's lab-results differentiate from the frame of reference.

The alerts presented on a specific day are the results of the previous five days of drug intake and lab-results, as shown in Figure 4. The patient module gives no information about prescribed drugs, and no text to inform about indication for intake. Also it gives no view of the individual day regime in terms of frequency of intake. It is a present and retrospective view of lab-results and intake of drugs.

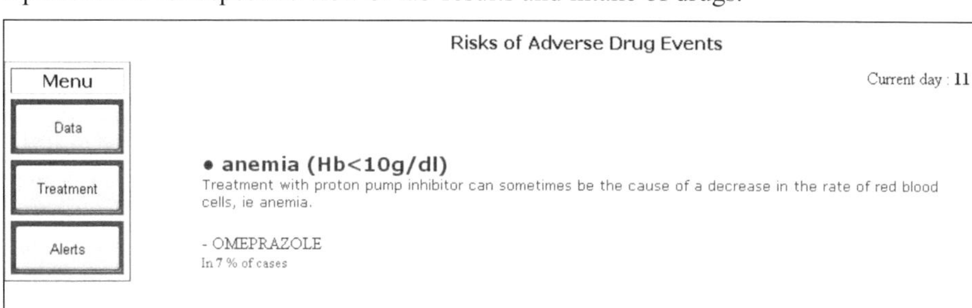

Figure 4. Alerts ("Advarsler") presents a list of possible ADEs and which drug that is associated to the alert. Example: Risk of haemorrhage ("Risiko for blødning"), a text that explains the risk in further details, the associated drug and how often the risk is present ("I 10% af tilfældene").

2. Results

2.1. The Paper-based Medicine List

Generally the patients use the lists to administer medicine at home, to consult the Internet for further information, and to take contact with their general practitioner, or other health professionals in order to discuss and inform about their prescriptions from hospital. Of the six patients, one had not seen the paper medicine list before.

In general the patients found the list very easy to understand and were able to explain what information the list encompassed.

One of the patients will always check the list for right doses. However full dose is not explained and the patient have to calculate from numbers of tablets. Two of the patients want the drugs to be listed in an aggregated chart to create an overview of the drug regime. Furthermore, there is a problem in the understanding of drugs taken week by week – when patient has to take the drug once a week the majority of the patients only thought they should take the one time. Also it is a safety issue if the patient has more than one days copy of the medicine list, especially if the list is not stabled.

One patient finds the overview problematic; s/he does not initially find the names of the drugs, s/he does not understand 'route of administration' and 'indication', but guesses right, though the route of administration 'subcutaneous' is not understood. The other patients know the lists and use them, yet find some of the terminology difficult e.g. 'indication', 'oral', and 'route of administration'. Despite these terminology challenges, the patients valued the paper-based medication list to be useful, as shown below in Table 1.

Table 1. The participants' assessment of the paper-based medication list.

	Very useful	Useful	Neutral	Less useful	Not useful
Paper list	1	5			

2.2. The Web-based Patient Module

The term 'Expected period of hospitalization' is confusing for the patients. Generally they think that this is the expected period of their stay, either from admission day, or from present day. One patient thinks that something must have gone wrong in the treatment to cause the stay to be extended by 35 days to the 79th day, which was the day at which we asked them look up information in the module.

All of the patients express uncertainty about the list of drugs; whether it is the prescribed or administered drugs. For the list to be meaningful, the patients request both to be available to them, and two of the patients request indication for each of the drugs and a link to the lab-result concerning the drug and vice versa. Generally they expected to find the indication for the ordination of the individual drug behind the link 'More Information', which however, leads them to the official Danish Formulary Handbook, with general information about the drug. At entering the Danish Formulary Handbook, only one of the patients understands that s/he has to enter further into the site to retrieve the core information about the drug. It troubles two of the patients that the time of drug intake is not visible, and one is aware, that some of the drugs should not be taken at the same time.

The lab-results are confusing for five of the six patients, as they do not understand most of the terms. One patient requests an explanation of which symptoms to be aware of, when some of the values in the lab-results are red. Generally, they find the red highlighted lab-values alarming, but are unsure how to react on the alerts. One patient requests that the prototype instruct her/his in what to do, i.e. to take another tablet, contact the doctor, etc. Concerning the red values in the lab-results one of the patients thinks that it is the intake of medicine that causes the value to be over or under the reference value. The way in which the values are given in the reference (i.e. 2.3 for INR) is misunderstood by all the patients.

Only one of the patients grasps the overall concept of the prototype, and understands the connection between the lab-results and drugs over time. However, the prototype does not enable her/his to understand whether s/he needs to take more or less Maravan. In order to understand the progress of her/his health, s/he asks for a better retrospective view of lab-results vs. the drug list.

The alerts are understood by the patients as general not patient-specific alerts, as the values are not directly interpreted to cohere to the values in the patient own lab-results. Furthermore, the risk of only 5% is generally overseen in a given alert, and one patient would immediately stop intake of the drug concerned and consult the doctor, if an alert is fired. The alerts are interpreted as results of excessive intake of the drug by two of the patients, and the symptoms of an ADE are not entirely clear to the patients; the text and explanations in the alert is hard to understand. Two of the patients understood bits of the message because they had previously been educated by the clinician to understand the term, e.g. anemia. The patient's positive assessment of the Web-based prototype (Table 2), despite the rather considerable challenges with understanding the information, could possibly refer to an overall positive attitude towards the possibility of access to patient's own data.

Table 2. The participants' assessment of the Web prototype.

	Very useful	Useful	Neutral	Less useful	Not useful
Web prototype	2	2	1		1

2.3. The Patient Cell Phone Module

None of the participant has any knowledge with the prototype or other similar systems.

To enter age, what drug they are scanning to take, and which drugs they have been taken is clear to the patients. One patient is asking if the application also alerts on interaction between drugs. However, the entering of diagnosis and lab related condition is difficult, as the patients does not necessarily distinguish the two from each other, and additionally often does not know her/his own lab related condition to enter.

Contrary to the two previous systems, the patient herself has to enter data in order to achieve information from the cell phone PSIP prototype. This poses patient safety issues, as it is crucial to the alert, that all information on diagnosis and lab related conditions is entered, and not just some.

Generally, the patient coheres to a regime prescribed by the doctor, and would therefore not consult a cell phone application for alerts. In situations of doubts about drugs, the patients would rather consult the doctor, and not the application.

The terms that determine the diagnosis and lab related conditions, as well as the alerts, are kept in medical terminology and like with the Web-based patient module, the patient is required some medical literacy to use the application. All the patients expressed uncertainty about what actions to take on the alerts. Patient's assessment of the cell phone prototype range from 'Not useful' to 'Very useful' (Table 3). As with the assessment of the Web-based prototype, we cannot exclude the possibility, that the positive assessment is based on the patient's attitude to the *concept* of accessing information via cell phone.

Table 3. The participants' assessment of the cell phone prototype.

	Very useful	Useful	Neutral	Less useful	Not useful
Cell phone prototype	1	1	1	1	2

3. Discussion

For all of the three systems, terminology and presentation are issues of concern. Terminology is clearly aimed at health personnel, and merely extracted from the systems to use in patient information. The medical terminology is not 'translated' into general language. Likewise, the presentation of the information especially in the Web-based module is not intuitive to the patients, and requires prior knowledge of how to read the information. This poses usability, as well as patient safety problems and concerns.

Common for the Web module and the cell phone module is that the patients are uncertain of how to react to the alerts; are the alerts more credible than the doctor who prescribed the medicine? How does the patient judge the likelihood of a risk, versus the consequence in stopping intake of the drug? In order to cope with questions of this kind, a thorough introduction to the modules is needed as well as education in interpreting the information.

The paper-based medication list is useful, provides reliable, static information on the patient's medication for the patient to take home, and importantly, to bring into dialog with other health personnel [8]. The paper-based list presents the patient with an overview of her/his medication, as well as with the information to administer her/his own medicine. This affords a feeling of being in control [6].

The Web-based patient module enables the patient to follow the progress of her/his health situation through access to lists of drug intakes and lab-results throughout the hospital contact. However, for the module to play a part in improving patient safety, it needs to provide a better context for the patient to understand the information: A retrospective comprehensive view of the progress in the lab-results and medicine intake. View of which drugs have impact on which lab-results and explanation of indication and view of prescribed drugs. However, the patients all show interest in access to their own data while hospitalized or attending hospital as an outpatient. The alerts could cause behavior that is unsafe because the patients do not find the alerts specific to their personal medical profile and therefore do not react upon them, or react in an inexpedient way. In this light, the patients need to be informed and instructed on how to understand the link between drugs, lab-results and alerts, as well as instructions in how to react on alerts.

The patients acknowledge that cell phone technology can play an active role in their control of their medication, although it is very unclear to all of the patients in which situations to use this module. In situations of doubts about drugs, the patients would rather consult the doctor, and not the application. To make sure the system provides the right response, the patients have to enter all information right which is an unsafe procedure which relies on memory.

There is no doubt that the respondents in this study – despite their age – are very positive towards more dynamic, contextualized information on their own health. However, further development is necessary if the systems should decrease the risk of adverse drug events and empower the patients to participate in the medication process. This development should be founded on studies within human factor in order to ensure unambiguous, intuitive and safe systems.

Acknowledgments

The research leading to these results has received funding from the European Community's Seventh Framework Programme (FP7/2007-2013) under grant agreement n° 216130 – the PSIP project.

Furthermore, we acknowledge the assistance from staff and patients at Hvidovre Hospital, Capital Region, Denmark.

References

[1] National Board of Health in Denmark, Temarapport 2005: Medicinhåndtering, http://www.dpsd.dk/, last access on March 2011.
[2] Patient Safety through Intelligent Procedure in Medicine (PSIP), http://www.psip-project.eu/, last access on March 2011.
[3] J. Reason, Understanding adverse events: human factors, *Qual Health Care* **4** (1995), 80–9.
[4] J. Nielsen, Ten usability heuristics, http://www.useit.com/papers/heuristic/heuristic_list.html, last access on February 2011.
[5] J. Kjeldskov et al., Instant Data Analysis: Conducting Usability Evaluations in a Day, NordiCHI '04, (2004), 23–7.
[6] J. Nielsen, Why you only need to test with 5 users, http://www.useit.com/alertbox/20000319.html, last access on February 2011.
[7] V. Koutkias, V. Kilintzis, C. Collyda, A. Triantafyllidis, Mobile Patient Component, *PSIP Internal Report,* Aristotle University of Thessaloniki (2010).
[8] T. Wibe, M. Ekstedt, R. Hellesø, L. Slaughter, Why do People Want a Paper Copy of Their Electronic Patient Record?, *Stud Health Technol Inform* **160**(Pt 1) (2010), 676–80.

Patient Safety Informatics
V. Koutkias et al. (Eds.)
IOS Press, 2011

doi:10.3233/978-1-60750-740-6-254

Validation of Completeness, Correctness, Relevance and Understandability of the PSIP CDSS for Medication Safety

Elske AMMENWERTH [a,1], Werner O. HACKL [a], Philippe MASSARI [b] and Stefan DARMONI [b]

[a] *Institute for Health Information Systems, UMIT – University for Health Sciences, Medical Informatics and Technology, Hall in Tyrol, Austria*

[b] *CISMeF, Rouen University Hospital & TIBS, LITIS EA 4108, Biomedical Research Institute, Rouen University*

Abstract. Medication errors and resulting Adverse Drug Events (ADEs) are an important issue of global healthcare. Within the European PSIP project that aims at developing solutions to improve medication safety, contextualized decision support modules aiming to prevent ADEs are being developed. The objective of this work was to thoroughly validate part of the CDSS (Clinical Decision Support System) and the underlying Knowledge Base, in order to detect incorrect or unclear alerts. We systematically developed a repository of test cases and used them for validation. The development of the test cases showed that there are differences among experts in interpreting the correctness of an alert, and that the clinical context is important when judging whether it is adequate. Overall, validation did not find major errors in the Knoweldge Base, but developed several recommendations for further improvement.

Keywords. Validation studies, medical order entry systems, medication error, adverse drug event, clinical decision support

Introduction

Medication safety is an issue that raises more and more concerns. In Germany, an estimated 28,000 deaths per year are associated with preventable medication errors [1]. Several groups recommend implementing electronic prescribing to reduce the number of medication errors [2-3]. In the U.S., only 5% of hospitals have fully implemented computerized physician order entry (CPOE) [4]. In Europe, this number is probably even lower.

The EU-FP7 project PSIP (http://www.psip-project.eu, Patient Safety through Intelligent Procedures in Medication) [5-6] aims at developing decision support modules to increase medication safety. The PSIP CDSS (Clinical Decision Support System) is based on a rule-based Knowledge Base [7].

The objective of this paper is to describe the methodology used for validation of the CDSS and the underlying Knowledge Base, to present results, and to discuss experiences and recommendations when developing test cases for CPOE validation.

[1] Corresponding Author: elske.ammenwerth@umit.at

1. Materials and Methods

While verification refers to internal static checks on a system, validation refers to checking the accuracy of results given by a system [8]. In our project, validation comprised of the following questions:

- How complete are the alerts provided by the PSIP CDSS?
- How correct are the alerts?
- How clinically relevant are the alerts?
- How understandable are the alerts to the users?

For validation, test cases can be used that cover the clinical setting that is addressed by the system. Within the PSIP project, the first clinical focus is anticoagulation and platelet aggregation inhibitors, as this presents an important source or errors in many countries, for example in the U.S. [9].

The validation comprised the following steps:

1. Development and management of test cases
2. Selection and application of test cases
3. Assessment of the outcome of the test cases

1.1. Step 1: Development and Management of Test Cases

In a literature review and by contacting experts, we tried to locate openly available CPOE test cases or test protocols. The Leapfrog group [10] uses test cases to validate CPOE systems, but those test cases were not openly available at that time. A Dutch group has developed and used test cases for CPOE systems [11] - however, those test cases do not involve anticoagulation prescriptions.

Therefore, we developed test cases, following the recommendations by Friedman and Wyatt ([12], p. 164): Test cases should be representative, of sufficient variety, from more than one site, and include simple and complex cases. The test cases were developed using national guidelines, drug information, scientific literature, patient safety incident reports, or real patient cases as possible sources. Each test case was checked and commented by at least one other expert from another country. Disagreements were solved by discussion. Test cases for which no agreement could be reached had to be excluded. Finally, each test case received ICD-10 codes (for diagnosis), IUPAC codes (for information on lab investigation) and ATC codes (for drug information).

To facilitate test case management, a Web-based platform was developed (Figure 1). This platform allows creation, modification, and commenting of test cases.

All test cases followed a pre-defined, semi-structured test case template that comprised background information, patient demographic data, patient history, information on the recent prescription, and description of the alert that is expected by the expert that developed the test case. This template was based on the overall data model developed in the PSIP project [13].

1.2. Step 2: Selection and Application of Test Cases

All test cases were transformed into the PSIP data model and then entered into the CDSS. The CDSS output was documented and then analyzed by two experts.

8. Gastric ulcer, recent surgery and NSAID

by Brian Bjoern — last modified Jul 16, 2010 07:07 AM

Test case data	
Date of creation	2008
Date of validation	25.3.2009
Developer of test case	B. Björn
Source of test case information (e.g. guidelines, ADE reports)	CIRS
Validator of test case	Prof. Pechlaner
Origin	RegionH, Unit for Patient Safety
Comments	
Date and Type of modification	
Status of test case	
Patient characteristics	
Age and sex	58, female
Weight and height	48 kg, 163 cm
Medical history	
Reason for hospital admission	Admitted from home after falling on the stairs. Is diagnosed with a hip fracture needing surgery.
Recent or prior diagnoses of the patient	Osteoporosis ** M81.9 Hypertension ** I10 Gastric ulcer, bleeding ** K25.0 Pertrochanteric fracture of the femur ** S72.1
Recent medications (that the patient is taking before current event)	Alendronate 70 mg once a week, anti-osteoporosis drug ** M05BA04 Paracetamol 500 mg x 3-4 as needed, analgesic ** N02BE01 Codeine 25 mg x 1-4 as needed, weak opiate ** R05DA04 (exceptional coding) Bendroflumethiazide 5 mg x 1, diuretic ** C03AA01 Zolpidem 7.5 mg at bedtime, hypnotic ** N05CF02 Omeprazole 20 mg when needed, antacid ** A02BC01
Recent relevant lab values (before current event)	
Known allergies	
Pregnancy (yes/no/unknown)	
Context (any further relevant information on patient context)	
Current event	
Department where patient is treated	Department of orthopaedic surgery; admitted from home
Clinical event (e.g. new findings, new problem, change of working diagnosis due to event)	Hip fracture needing surgery
New lab values	
New prescription	Standard analgesics plan, including an NSAID ** N02BA01
Qualification and role of prescriber (e.g. senior physician)	
Further information on process of care	
Expected outcome	
Text of alert	Avoid NSAID because auf history of bleeding gastric ulcer and recent surgery. There are good alternatives: preferred: opioids; if opioids undesirable: NSAID in combination with proton pump inhibitor. **NSAID are contraindicated in case of:** - **Active peptic ulcer (two or more episodes of proven ulceration or bleeding).** - **History of upper gastrointestinal bleeding or perforation, related to previous NSAID therapy.**
Priority (low, medium, high)	High
Explanation on expected outcome	Prescribing NSAID (which is ulcerogenic) to a patient with a history of bleeding gastric ulcer and recent surgery (which itself is a stressor that may cause a new ulcer). (In this case, the patient develops a bleeding gastric ulcer and undergoes gastroscopic treatment. The bleeding cannot be stopped and the patient dies.)

Figure 1. Example test case accessible via the Web-based platform.

1.3. Step 3: Assessment of the Outcome of the Test Cases

Two experts assessed the outcome. They used a structured assessment form to judge the completeness, correctness, relevance and understandability of each alert. During a 2-day workshop, the assessments of each clinician were compared and discussed to reach a consensus on the overall judgments. Kappa before consensus was calculated to quantify interrater reliability.

2. Results

Overall, 38 test cases were developed and reviewed. Nine clinicians and pharmacists were involved in creation of test cases, five in the review of test cases, and three in the validation itself. During test case development, two test cases have to excluded, as no consensus could be reached on the expected clinical outcome. Altogether, four validation runs were conducted between 2009 and 2010, reflecting the ongoing development of the PSIP CDSS. The largest validation run with 22 test cases was conducted in June 2010, together with two experts; we will report the results of this one. Overall, the 22 test cases generated 48 alerts.

2.1. Completeness of Alerts

When rating the completeness of each test cases, both experts agreed reasonably well (Kappa = 0.74). In six of the 22 test cases, the expected outcome was no present in the PSIP output. Reasons comprised test cases where time-relationships between two events were important (for example, pause a drug before surgery) and a contraindication to warfarin, both not yet being covered by PSIP.

2.2. Correctness of Alerts

Of all 48 alerts that PSIP generated, 19 (39.6%) were judged as correct, and 14 (29.2%) as incorrect; for the others, the two reviewers felt unable to decide. Detailed analysis of the alerts judged incorrect found that in most cases, an incorrect ATC-coding was used for Acetyl Salicyl Acid (here, ATC-code are different depending on the indication and dosage). This problem has been solved in the meantime. In the cases where the reviewers felt unable to judge, the PSIP alert presented information that the reviewers were not aware or not sure of.

2.3. Relevance of Alerts

From the 19 alerts that were judged as clinically correct, seven (36.9%) would have made a difference to patient care. The other alerts were judged as correct, but too unspecific for the given patient case (e.g. “NSAID can cause anemia by immuno-allergic mechanism”).

2.4. Understandability of Alerts

From 14 distinct alert texts, six (42.9%) were found as not easily understandable, for example: “Angiotensin-converting enzyme inhibitors and sartans may cause hyperkalemia due to a secondary hypoaldosteronism and this is facilitated by the presence of renal failure”. The reviewers felt that in those six cases, clarity of wording needs to be improved.

3. Discussion

3.1. Validation Outcome

Different versions of the PSIP CDSS were validated in four different validation rounds between 2009 and 2010. During the fourth validation run, PSIP already showed an increasing maturity and coverage. No major errors in the ruleset were found.

The validation detected some issues that should be revised to further improve the output; detailed recommendations, for example on the wording of some rules and on organization of output were made and have already been partly included in revisions of the PSIP CDSS. In this sense, validation was strongly oriented towards formative evaluation, and the recommendations helped to further improve the wording and presentation of alerts.

An important additional point that the reviewers made was that integration of clinical data into the decision-making process is crucial, to obtain maximum benefit of a CDSS. For example, depending on the diagnosis or treatment of a patient, anticoagulation therapy follow different aims, and thus not all cases can be treated by the same rules. Also, depending on the recent lab values of a patient, alerts may need to be modified. Thus, there is a need to adapt the presentation of alerts to the clinical context. As van der Sijs [14] showed for a Dutch medical centre, 91% of all drug safety alerts were overridden, often because they seem irrelevant for the individual patient. Adapting alerts to the clinical context may help the clinicians to focus on the most important alerts. Information usable for alert prioritization and alert filtering may comprise, among others, the clinical specialty of the user, the level of experience of the user, the ward, the hospital, the country, and the recent history of ADEs that occurred in a department.

Also, reviewers found that the explanations of rules is important for PSIP, as it partly presents alerts that describe very rare or often unknown relationships between certain drugs and their effects. Also, recommendations how to respond to the alert should be given to the clinical user.

Our two reviewers did not always agree on the expected outcome - the alerts that should be generated - of a given test case. Here, different cultures and working background may play a role. This experience stresses the need to have a structured multi-centre development and validation process for test cases.

Our test cases use international standardized terminology to be automatically processable, such as ICD-10 for diagnosis information, ATC for drug information and C-NPU/IUPAC for information on lab investigations. Hospital information systems must provide this information to allow decision-support within the prescription process.

3.2. Strengths and Weaknesses of the Validation Study

A large number of clinicians and pharmacists from three countries were involved in creating and reviewing the test cases, and in running and analysing the results. However, only two reviewers conducted the largest validation run, both of them being involved in development of some of the test cases. This can be seen as a weakness.

When analysing the validation output, we combined quantitative data with qualitative data from discussion and written comments; both were found helpful to analyse the data and to find recommendations.

4. Conclusion

We presented methodology and results of validation of the PSIP CDSS. Validation can contribute to formative evaluation and help to further improve the correctness, completeness, relevance and understandability of alerts. Validation results points to the need to optimize alert wording and alert explanation, and to the need to contextualize alerts to the clinical context.

Acknowledgments

The research leading to these results has received funding from the European Community's Seventh Framework Programme (FP7/2007-2013) under grant agreement n° 216130 – the PSIP project.

References

[1] J. Schnurrer, J. Frölich, Zur Häufigkeit und Vermeidbarkeit von tödlichen unerwünschten Arzneimittelwirkungen, *Internist* **44** (2003), 889–95.
[2] L. Kohn, J. Corrigan, M. Donaldson, *To err is Human: Building a Safer Health System*, National Academy Press, Washington DC, 2000.
[3] J. Smith, *Building a Safer National Health System for Patients: Improving Medication Safety*, Department of Health, London, 2004.
[4] D.M. Cutler, N.E. Feldman, J.R. Horwitz, U.S. adoption of computerized physician order entry systems, *Health Aff (Millwood)* **24** (2005), 1654–63.
[5] Patient Safety through Intelligent Procedure in Medicine (PSIP). Available from: http://www.psip-project.eu/, last access on March 2011.
[6] R. Beuscart, W. Hackl, C. Nohr, *Detection and Prevention of Adverse Drug Events - Information Technologies and Human Factors*, IOS Press, Amsterdam, 2009.
[7] V. Koutkias, V. Kilintzis, G. Stalidis, K. Lazou, C. Collyda, E. Chazard, et al., Constructing Clinical Decision Support Systems for Adverse Drug Event Prevention: A Knowledge-based Approach, *AMIA Annu Symp Proc* (2010), 402–6.
[8] R. Engelbrecht, A. Rector, W. Moser, Verification and Validation, *Stud Health Technol Inform* **17** (1995), 51–66.
[9] AHQR. Adverse Drug Events in U.S. Hospitals, 2004. Statistical Brief #29, http://www.hcup-us.ahrq.gov/reports/statbriefs/sb29.pdf, last access on March 2011.
[10] J.M. Grimshaw, I.T. Russell, Effect of clinical guidelines on medical practice: a systematic review of rigorous evaluations, *Lancet* **342** (1993), 1317–22.
[11] H. van der Sijs, Drug Safety Alerting in Computerized Physician Order Entry (Ph.D. thesis). Chapter 2.4: Functionality of drug safety alerting in computerized physician order entry systems. Amsterdam. 2009.
[12] C. Friedman, J.C. Wyatt, *Evaluation Methods in Medical Informatics, 2nd edition*, Springer, New York, 2006.
[13] E. Chazard, B. Merlin, G. Ficheur, J.C. Sarfati, R. Beuscart, Detection of adverse drug events: proposal of a data model, *Stud Health Technol Inform* **148** (2009), 63–74.
[14] H. van der Sijs, A. Mulder, T. van Gelder, J. Aarts, M. Berg, A. Vulto, Drug safety alert generation and overriding in a large Dutch university medical centre, *Pharmacoepidemiol Drug Saf* 18 (2009), 941–7.

Patient Safety Informatics
V. Koutkias et al. (Eds.)
IOS Press, 2011

doi:10.3233/978-1-60750-740-6-260

Completion of Structured Patient Descriptions by Semantic Mining

Dimitar TCHRAKTCHIEV [a,1], Galia ANGELOVA [b], Svetla BOYTCHEVA [b], Zhivko ANGELOV [b] and Sabina ZACHARIEVA [a]

[a] *University Specialized Hospital for Active Treatment of Endocrinology (USHATE), Medical University - Sofia*

[b] *Institute of Information and Communication Technologies, Bulgarian Academy of Sciences*

Abstract. This paper presents experiments in automatic Information Extraction of medication events, diagnoses, and laboratory tests form hospital patient records, in order to increase the completeness of the description of the episode of care. Each patient record in our hospital information system contains structured data and text descriptions, including full discharge letters. From these letters, we extract automatically information about the medication just before and in the time of hospitalization, especially for the drugs prescribed to the patient, but not delivered by the hospital pharmacy; we also extract values of lab tests not performed and not registered in our laboratory as well as all non-encoded diagnoses described only in the free text of discharge letters. Thus we increase the availability of suitable and accurate information about the hospital stay and the outpatient segment of care before the hospitalization. Information Extraction also helps to understand the clinical and organizational decisions concerning the patient without increasing the complexity of the structured health record.

Keywords. Information extraction, patient records processing, electronic health record (EHR), long-term impact on quality of care

Introduction

The key source of information about the process of care and its immediate outcome is, no doubt, the medical record [1]. Much data is structured in the Hospital Records by the Hospital Information Systems (HIS) – for instance, most numeric values of lab tests are automatically entered in predefined fields, and the drugs prescribed to the patient are maintained via the so-called Computerized Physician Order Entry (CPOE). However, essential findings are traditionally stored as free text descriptions. Thus the automatic text analysis is viewed as an information technology of vital importance, because it enables automatic generation of databases with structured patient data that can be explored for improving the diagnostics, care decisions, the personalized treatment of diseases, maintenance of adverse drug events, healthcare management and so on. The technology is language-dependent as it uses lexicons, terms and formalized grammatical knowledge. Despite of all shortcomings, biomedical text processing is a

[1] Corresponding Author:dimitardt@gmail.com

hot research area worldwide and attracts the attention of both academic and industrial communities.

This paper presents recent results which enable the production of an experimental repository for validating the approach of PSIP project (Patient Safety through Intelligent Procedures in medication). The validation takes part in USHATE, Medical University – Sofia. Essential information about patient treatment is automatically extracted from anonymized hospital Patient Records (PR) in Bulgarian language and delivered to the PSIP repository, as a complimentary data pool augmenting the HIS sources. More specifically, Semantic Mining (SM) and Information Extraction (IE) are applied for identification of medication events, diagnoses, and lab test values in the free text of discharge letters. The paper also discusses the possible long-term impact of SM and IE on quality of care. These advanced technologies can ameliorate the episode's description and facilitate the understanding of clinical and organizational decisions concerning the patient.

1. Background

The Hospital Information System of the University Specialized Hospital for Active Treatment of Endocrinology stores structured data about patient admission, transfer and discharge, diagnoses, procedures, clinical pathways, Diagnosis-Related Groups (DRGs), laboratory tests, drug prescriptions, structured vital signs and clinical findings, CPOE, pharmacy data and other medico-administrative data [2]. The discharge summaries are also recorded in the HIS.

More precise structured information is contained in the specialized database for pituitary and adrenal endocrine tumors set up in USHATE. This database registers all necessary demographic, medico-administrative, clinical and laboratory (incl. genetic) data, as well as imaging and therapy data for patients with endocrine tumors. An important fact is that the number of variables justified together with the endocrinologists increased to 882 [3].

The application of the European standard for Electronic Health Record Communication EN/ISO 13606 [4] and the implementation of published archetypes, concerning some medical data (blood pressure, laboratory data etc.) in the process of the design and development of these two systems make possible to assess the clinical significance of some clinical findings in the context of their examination.

The specificity of the clinical settings in USHATE is due to the fact that the Specialized Hospitals in Medical University – Sofia treat the most complicated cases of patients with all endocrine diseases. In this way many drugs, which the patients take for some of their accompanying illnesses, are not provided by the corresponding Specialized Hospital (e.g. drugs dispensed in ambulatory care for chronic diseases, reimbursed by the National Health Insurance Fund). Thus for patients treated in USHATE, there are drugs which are not available as separate records in the CPOE and the Pharmacy System in the USHATE HIS. Information about these drugs, their dosage and their side-effects is available only in the unstructured patient record text – for example in the discharge letters. In this way the unstructured texts of the hospital records in USHATE contain descriptions of sophisticated medical facts. Statistical observations of USHATE's hospital patient records show that the average number of drugs, discussed in a patient discharge letter, is 5,4 drugs per hospital record. However, according to the CPOE, there are 1,6 medications given to the USHATE patients. This means that much information about Adverse Drug Events (ADEs) is presented in the unstructured text part of the hospital records, where the drugs are usually described together with their dosage and frequency. The free text paragraphs also contain the numeric values of clinical tests, lab data and other medical information.

The discharge letters consist of the following sections: *(i)* personal data; *(ii)* diagnoses; *(iii)* anamnesis; *(iv)* patient status; *(v)* lab data; *(vi)* medical examiners comments; *(vii)* discussion; *(viii)* treatment; and *(ix)* recommendations. This structure is mandatory for all Bulgarian hospitals since it is published in the Official State Gazette, as a part of a legal Agreement between the Bulgarian Medical Association and the National Health Insurance Fund. The described structure enables appropriate contextualization of the extracted information but in the reality it is not strictly followed. Figure 1 shows some statistics about availability of the above-listed sections in 1,300 USHATE PRs. Despite the fact that the structure is mandatory, many PRs lack some sections due to the following reasons:

- merging of sections, most often for *(vii) discussion*, *(viii) treatment*, and *(ix) recommendations*;
- inclusion of sections only if they are applicable, e.g. *(vi) Medical examiners comments*;
- skipping a section or subsection, e.g. *Allergies and risk factors* which can be also merged with the anamnesis;
- domain-dependent choice: *e.g. Family medical history* is mentioned only for patient, whose relatives are diagnozed with diabetes.

The Bulgarian medical language and its specific particularities have to be taken into consideration too. In the hospital PRs, medical terminology is recorded in both Bulgarian and/or Latin language. There is no preferred language for the terminology so the two forms are used like synonyms. Sometimes Latin terms are written by Cyrillic letters especially when the medical expert prefers to avoid keyboard switching. In general the mixture of Latin and Bulgarian terms is traditionally established and commonly accepted, including in official documents. For instance, the International Classification of Diseases version 10 (ICD-10) is translated to Bulgarian terms; the list

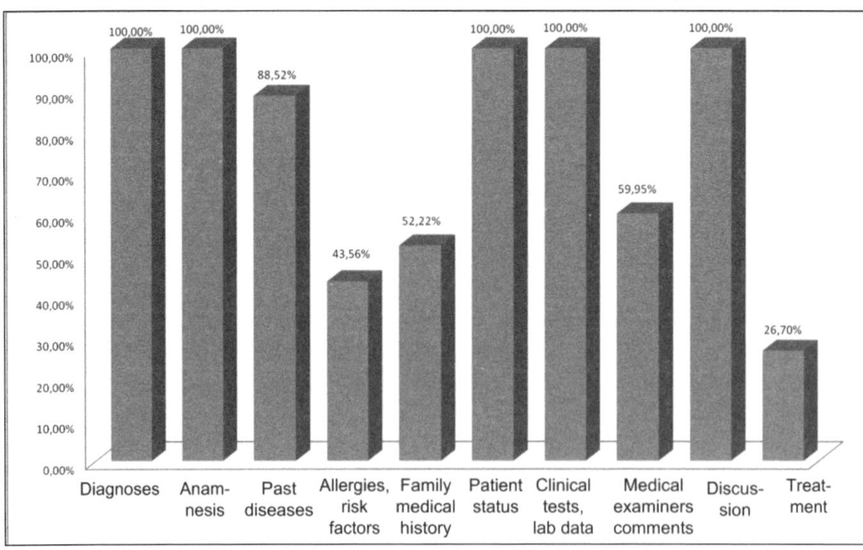

Figure 1. Percentage of PRs including standard sections.

of drugs in the USHATE's CPOE is supported with Bulgarian drug names even for drugs produced abroad (then the foreign words are transliterated by Cyrillic letters). However, the official list of registered drugs, published by the Bulgarian Drug Agency [5], contains the Anatomic Therapeutic Chemical (ATC) codes and the drug names in Latin alphabet even for drugs produced in Bulgaria. It is worth mentioning that all the *Application instructions* at [5] are written in Bulgarian and the drug names are given there by Cyrillic letters. In this way, the automatic identification of a term in the hospital patient record is a tricky task which requires more than a simple string match. Figure 2 shows some original excerpts of PR diagnoses: Latin names of diseases are transliterated by Cyrillic letters but alternatively might be given in Latin as well. The measurement units of clinical test are often entered with Latin symbols.

The automatic text processing needs background linguistic resources – lexicons and medical vocabularies, so one of the first issues is to prepare the necessary lists of multilingual terms. No computer dictionaries in the medical domain are available for Bulgarian language and we started to prepare lexicons from files containing specialized medical information. There are four primary electronic sources of medical vocabulary, which can be used as initial input for production of terminological lexicons:

- the nomenclatures ICD-10, which contains names of diseases in Bulgarian and ICD-9 CM used for codification of procedures;
- the CPOE and Hospital Pharmacy (parts of USHATE HIS) where drug names are supported together with the ATC codes – but only for 1,182 drugs used for treatment of patients with endocrinological diseases;
- various lists of medical terms available via the Internet for different purposes, among them the lists of drugs provided by the Bulgarian Drug Agency [5] and the site for medical information *www.medicine.bg* [6];
- the anonymized hospital PRs provided by USHATE HIS. Totally 6,881 anonymous hospital PRs (6,200 of them including discharge letters) were delivered from the USHATE HIS to the PSIP-compliant repository.

As the ATC classification [7] is not available in Bulgarian language, we have selected a part of it (covering the drugs occurring in the 6,200 discharge letters of our experimental corpus) and translated it to Bulgarian language. In addition to the 1,182 drugs prescribed via the USHATE HIS, some 355 drugs are taken by the USHATE patients. In this way our present drug vocabulary consists of 1,537 items.

Figure 3 presents the methodology for PSIP-repository preparation. The data available in the HIS, Hospital Pharmacy and CPOE are integrated with automatically extracted facts about diagnoses, medication events and values of clinical tests and lab data. The integration is done record by record. The extraction components mine independently the free PR texts and deliver information found in non-overlapping PR fragments. This approach relies on high-quality extraction components which analyse the text and extract patient-related facts with high accuracy.

> Диабетес мелитус – типус 1. Ретинопатиа диабетика пролиферанс. Статус пост ALC. Полиневропатиа диабетика. Хипертония артериалис гр. I. ….
> …Консултация с офталмолог: VOD= 0,8; VOS= 0,6-0,7; двуочно 0,9-1,0 със собствена корекция. Angiosclerosis vas. retinae hypertonica. Retinopathia diabetica simplex. макули без рефлекс.

Figure 2. Excerpts of hospital PRs in Bulgarian language.

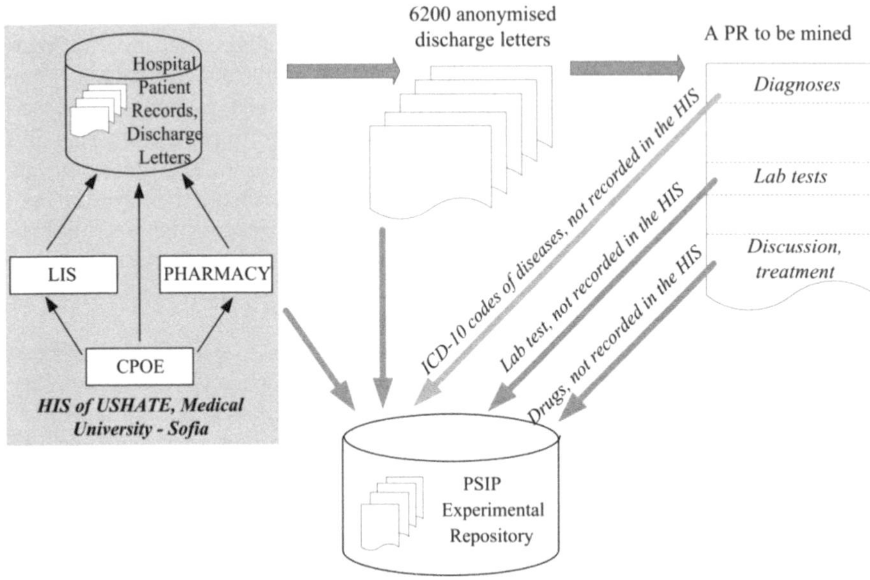

Figure 3. Integration of data from HIS and the three extractors into PSIP repository.

2. Methods: Semantic Mining and Information Extraction in USHATE

Three major extraction components have been developed and tested on the corpus of 6,200 discharge letters while preparing the PSIP-compliant repository in USHATE:

Component for automatic assignment of ICD-10 codes of diagnoses. As the Bulgarian hospitals are reimbursed by the National Insurance Fund via the "clinical pathways" scheme, it turned out that not all diseases are formally diagnozed by the USHATE medical experts. When a patient is hospitalized, they often select from the HIS menu one diagnosis which is sufficient for the association of the desired clinical pathway to the respective patient. The other diagnoses are entered in the PR section *(ii) Diagnoses* as free text. So while designing the repository to be delivered to PSIP, it became obvious that there is a significant percentage of PRs where patients take drugs for diseases which are not formally diagnozed in the respective HIS PRs. To tackle this issue, an already existing research prototype for automatic assignment of ICD-10 codes to diagnoses was extended and elaborated to cope with 6,200 PRs where thousands of ICD-10 diagnoses are mentioned. The initial prototype of this component processed about 50 ICD-10 diagnoses and was tested on less than 250 PRs [8]. Its PSIP-version is upgraded to tackle thousands of diagnoses. The component works in three steps: *(i)* shallow text analysis by regular expressions and patterns matching, *(ii)* searching disease names in the terminology resource bank (medical terminology dictionary, list of abbreviations rules and Latin – Cyrillic transliteration rules) and automatic assignment of ICD-10 code, and *(iii)* when *(ii)* fails, application of terminology binding rules that are manually added by experts. The regular expressions, applied at step *(i)* for shallow syntactic analysis, encode grammatical patterns of text phrases which describe diagnoses in the particular training corpus (of diabetic patients treated at Medical University Sofia). These patterns are extracted semi-automatically from the training texts by machine learning techniques.

Component for automatic extraction of medication events, based on ATC codes. This component is presented in more detail in [9]. The extraction works in several steps, starting by splitting the PRs into sections. The preprocessing task is very important since it provides the context for interpretation of the numerous drug names that might occur in a hospital PR. To ensure precise drug recognition, it is important to allocate the actual treatment within the PR pages discussing past, present and future medical facts. For instance the drugs, taken at the moment when the patient is hospitalized, should normally be described in section *(iii) anamnesis* under the title "accompanying treatment"; similarly, the drugs prescribed by the Hospital Pharmacy and taken in the hospital should be discussed in section *(viii) treatment*. Hence, the success in automatic PR splitting into sections turns to be an important prerequisite for further identification of various clinical events. For further discussion see [9].

Component for mining values of clinical tests and lab data. When a patient is examined in USHATE, the indicators of the clinical tests and lab data are entered to the hospital record via the USHATE HIS. However, the results of some lab tests can be brought as paper reports when the patient enters USHATE and then these results are usually typed in the hospital PR as free text description. Therefore, automatic mining of values is needed to discover all the results of important examinations.

As shown at Fig. 1, the results of clinical tests and lab data are listed in a specific PR section which is always included in the PR. The values are enumerated without predetermined order and without standardized names of the indicators. Most of them are alpha-numeric literals; about 16% of the tokens in our present corpus represent numerical values. The mining component has to recognize at first the indicator (i.e. the *name of the tested characteristic*), as well as the *value* related to the corresponding indicator. The *units* and *reference intervals* are desirable features, and the *time*, *condition* and *explanation* of further details are optional features.

The component has its own *vocabulary* (dictionary of 'keywords' constructed semi-automatically using a set of nomenclatures for clinical examination and lab data, their measuring units and reference intervals) and *rules* for recognition of the elements needed to form the values of interest. It analyses all the text in order to identify information about tests and examinations made outside USHATE. In this way the values, available in the USHATE HIS, were used as a gold standard for evaluation of the mining performance.

The mining algorithm is rule-based and copes with *(i)* the variety of name writings (abbreviations, omitted words in the name, joined words in the name, typos), *(ii)* various symbols used as separators, *(iii)* the varying format of the numeric values, *(iv)* arbitrary replacements of Cyrillic and Latin letters which look identical (e.g. the Cyrillic 'c' - pronounced 's' - is used for the Latin 'c') and *(v)* ambiguity in the recognition of the lab data section and the scoping of phrases related to certain indicator. As an illustration, we show a rule for packing tokens into a structural group:

<(><n><v><s><v><)> => <N> which means the following:

Find a sequence of tokens which:

starts with '('

followed by a phrase signaling referential values <n>,

followed by a number <v>,

followed by a separator <s>,

followed by a number <v>,

followed by a ')'.

If all tokens occur in the given order than this expression defines the group <N>.

This simple rule will be used to group the literals *'(norm – 8,7-42)'* in the text fragment *'testosterone -3.2 (norm – 8,7-42)'*. The rule has 18 variants reflecting the various separators and delimiters learnt from a training set of 1,000 PRs; we see empirically that it works successfully for the experimental corpus of 6,200 PRs.

3. Results

In general, we can accept that extraction accuracy higher than 95-97% is very good because human annotators would make some errors too. In IE there are two typical assessment indicators: *precision* (percentage of correctly extracted entities as a subset of all extracted entities, i.e. a measure of correct performance once an entity is found) and *recall* (percentage correctly extracted entities as a subset of all entities available in the corpus, i.e. a measure of the system's ability to find relevant entries in the text). Both measures are important since they explicate the system potential to cope with unknown texts. The so-called f-measure $F=2*Precision*Recall/(Precision+Recall)$ combines the precision and recall into one indicator. Overviews of relevant extraction competitions in biomedical text processing [10] show that the state-of-the-art accuracy is higher than 90%: the extraction of medication events achieves f-measure 93.2% for drug names, 94.5% for dosage, 93.9% for route, and 96% for frequency [11]; the automatic assignment of ICD codes to diagnoses achieves 89.08% accuracy [12]. The three top systems in the coding competition presented in [12] processed the negation, hypernyms and synonyms in some way and exploited the UMLS structure. These systems performed rule-based computations and two of them had in addition some machine-learning components.

Results achieved in PSIP mark the state-of-the-art for languages other than English. Paper [13] presents a detailed evaluation scenario where the extracted entities are compared to the suggestions by human experts or the information available in the EHR (which is already encoded). The extraction of ATC codes from free text in French is performed with f-measure 88% when compared to the manual extraction; compared to the CPOE content, the f-measure is 49%. The agreement between the automatic procedure for assignment of ICD-10 codes and the EHR content is 21%, which is partly due to the fact that the diagnoses encoded in HIS often reflect financial considerations.

The evaluation of our three extractors was performed on the collection of 6,200 anonymized PRs. The components delivered 160,892 drug records, 22,667 codes of ICD-10 diagnoses and 114,441 laboratory tests. The extractor of medication events recognized treatments with 355 drug names which are not reflected in the Hospital Pharmacy. All this information substantially deepened the description of patient cases in the PSIP repository. For example, in the Case 26137 the following information is delivered from the HIS and the extracting components:

- ***Diagnose***: the basic diagnose in the USHATE HIS is E668 *'Other obesity'*, and the extractor discovers in addition E898 *'Postprocedural adrenocortical (-medullary) hypofunction'* and E289 *'Other ovarian dysfunction'*;
- ***Medication***: there is only one entry found in the Hospital Pharmacy (Metamizole) and the medication extractor delivered eight records for taking Metfodiab for eight days;
- ***Clinical test and lab data***: there are 22 entries found in the USHATE HIS but the mining component adds seven more values mostly for hormones.

As for the automatic assignment of ICD-10 codes to diagnoses in the PR section *(ii) Diagnoses*, we present here some quantitative characteristics of the prototype and the input data. Most PRs in the PSIP corpus contain from one to seven diagnoses, and there are up to 30 diagnoses listed in the discharge letters (see Fig. 4). In total 6,650 phrases, separated by various delimiters, occur in section *(ii)* of our 6,200 PRs; these phrases formed the specific dictionary of the encoding component. An ICD-10 code was correctly assigned to 4,565 or them; no code is suggested for 2,085 phrases. The occurrences of diagnoses in section *(ii)* of all 6,200 PRs were 26,826; an ICD code was assigned to 22,667 of them (84.5%). Table 1 suggests an explanation about unsuccessful assignments of ICD-10 codes to phrases.

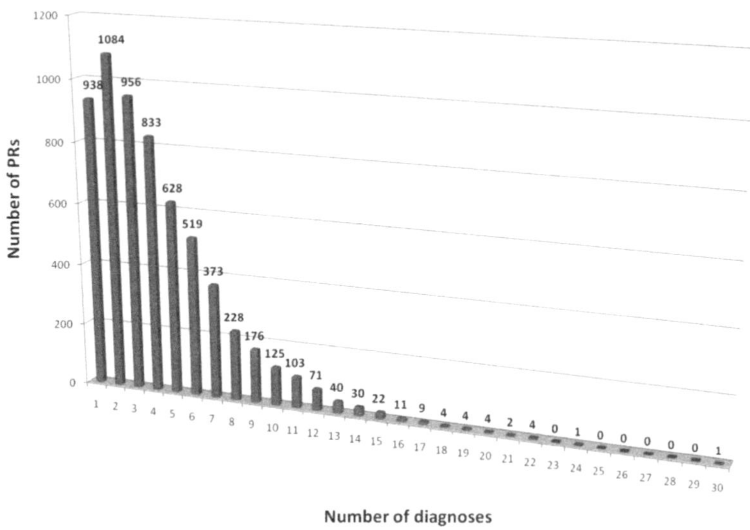

Figure 4. Number of diagnoses per PR in the PSIP corpus.

Table 1. Types of phrases in the PR section 'diagnoses' without associated ICD-10 codes.

Total	2085	Percentage
Latin	345	16%
Abbreviation	538	26%
Other	1202	58%

The component for extracting values of clinical tests and lab data was evaluated manually on 310 randomly-selected PRs (which is 0.5% of the corpus of 6,200 PRs). The precision is 98.2% (in the relatively closed world of laboratory examinations). As for the recognition of medication events and ATC codes extraction, drug names are found with f-measure 98.42% and the dosage – with 93.85% (more details are presented in [9]). At present we complete the evaluation of the extraction procedures which identify drug mode/route and frequency.

While recognizing drug names and diagnoses, the extracting components process negative phrases as single expressions according to an interpretation algorithm developed in a previous study [14]. Please note that in our grammatical patterns we try to address negative statements, elliptical constructions, and typical conjunctive phrases.

Experiments are done with simple inferences concerning temporal constraints. The preliminary correction of spell errors and other kinds of typos would also increase the IE accuracy if a spell-checker for Bulgarian medical text is developed.

4. Discussion

The Semantic mining modules are strictly oriented to Bulgarian language so the plans for their further development and application are connected primarily to Bulgarian local context. The exploitation potential is due to the high accuracy which might help for extracting data from large archives of patient record texts. However, the limitation is rooted in the linguistic rules that may require tuning and elaboration of the grammatical resources in case that the modules have to be applied to other PR archives (written by other medical experts) and in domains different from diabetes.

The components presented here are created as part of the research agenda of the PSIP project. They have also huge potential impact since they improve the clinical data, which concerns strategic medical issues like quality of care. For the assessment of quality of care it is important to have reliable data in six main dimensions of quality. These dimensions require that health care be [15]:

- *effective*, delivering health care that is adherent to an evidence base and results in improved health outcomes for individuals and communities, based on need;
- *efficient*, delivering health care in a manner which maximizes resource use and avoids waste;
- *accessible*, delivering health care that is timely, geographically reasonable, and provided in a setting where skills and resources are appropriate to medical need;
- *acceptable/patient-centred*, delivering health care which takes into account the preferences and aspirations of individual service users and the cultures of their communities;
- *equitable*, delivering health care which does not vary in quality because of personal characteristics such as gender, race, ethnicity, geographical location, or socioeconomic status;
- *safe*, delivering health care which minimizes risks and harm to service users.

Analyzing our results we observe the possibilities to increase directly the effectiveness of hospital care by improving the systematization and the understanding of patient needs in medication in the frame of the continuity of care process, belonging to the same episode.

Another important impact is to increase the hospital care safety, minimizing the medication risks, including the Decision Support Systems using all drug prescriptions – inpatient and outpatient - not registered in the hospital CPOE.

Further valuable axe is the increasing of the efficiency, by better extracting of all ICD codes related to patient status and the possibility to change the DRG group. This can help the future National case mix office in the determination of the relative indexes and the hospitals to associate the case to another better paid DRG. In Bulgaria the introduction of DRG system is planed for 2012.

In a long run the components, extracting diagnoses, medications, clinical tests and lab data, will be applied in various ways in Medical University – Sofia. They help to produce standardized vocabularies as a first step towards systematic archiving of various medical data (an issue that needs to be promoted in Bulgaria). These emerging extraction technologies can be used for automatic and semi-automatic filling of big specialized scientific databases extracting data from discharge summaries. The first example is the database for pituitary and adrenal endocrine tumors set up in USHATE which might be enlarged by automatic extraction of relevant information from the hospital patient records.

In this way the results obtained in PSIP will be exploited beyond the project, and will support the evolution of the Bulgarian national eHealth policy.

Acknowledgments

The research leading to these results has received funding from the European Community's Seventh Framework Programme (FP7/2007-2013) under grant agreement n° 216130 – the PSIP project.

The set up of the database of pituitary and adrenal tumors is funded by the project "Contemporary approach for diagnosis, frequency assessment, and geno-phenotype correlations of pituitary and adrenal tumors in Bulgaria", National Science Fund, contract No DO02-356/31.12.2008.

References

[1] A. Donabedian, The Quality of Care: How Can It Be Assessed?, *JAMA* **260** (1988), 1743-8.

[2] D. Tcharaktchiev, *Hospital Information Systems*, Kama, Sofia, 2003 (in Bulgarian).

[3] D. Tcharaktchiev et al., Database for patients with pituitary and adrenal tumors, *Social Medicine* **2** (2010) in press.

[4] Electronic Health Record Communication EN/ISO 13606-1, 2008.

[5] Bulgarian Drug Agency, http://www.bda.bg/index.php?lang=en, last access on March 2011.

[6] *Information for Medications in Bulgaria*, http://www.medicine.bg/lekarstva/, last access on March 2011.

[7] *ATC drugs classification,* http://atc.thedrugsinfo.com/, last access on March 2011.

[8] S. Boytcheva, Assignment of ICD-10 codes to diagnoses in hospital patient records in Bulgarian, In: Alfred, R., G. Angelova and H. Pfeiffer (Eds.). *Proc. of the Int. Workshop "Extraction of Structured Information from Texts in the Biomedical Domain" (ESIT-BioMed 2010*), ICCS-2010, Malaysia, Published by MIMOS BERHAD, ISBN 978-983-41371-3-7, July 2010, pp. 56–6.

[9] S. Boytcheva, Shallow medication extraction from hospital patient records, *Stud Health Technol Inform* **166** (2011), 119–128.

[10] *Third i2b2 Shared-Task and Workshop "Challenges in Natural Language Processing for Clinical Data: Medication Extraction Challenge"*, https://www.i2b2.org/NLP/Medication/, last access on March 2011.

[11] H. Xu et al., MedEx: a medication information extraction system for clinical narratives, *JAMIA* **17** (2010), 19–24.

[12] J. Pestian et al., A shared task involving multi-label classification of clinical free text. *ACL'07 workshop on biological, translational, and clinical language processing (BioNLP'07)*, Prague, 2007, pp. 36–40.

[13] B. Merlin, E. Chazard, S. Pereira, E. Serrot, S. Sakji, R. Beuscart, S. Darmoni, Can F-MTI semantic-mined drug codes be used for adverse drug events detection when no CPOE is available?, *Studies in Health Technology and Informatics* **160** (2010), 1025–29.

[14] S. Boytcheva, A. Strupchanska, E. Paskaleva, D. Tcharaktchiev, Some aspects of negation processing in electronic health records, In *Proc. of International Workshop Language and Speech Infrastructure for Information Access in the Balkan Countries*, 2005, Borovets, Bulgaria, pp. 1–8.

[15] Quality of care: a process for making strategic choices in health systems, *World Health Organization*, 2006.

Subject Index

Author Index